Elizabeth Ba~~~~

Physical Therapy Assessment
in Early Infancy

CLINICS IN PHYSICAL THERAPY

**TMJ Disorders: Management of the
Craniomandibular Complex**
Steven L. Kraus, P.T., guest editor

**Physical Therapy of the Geriatric Patient,
2nd Ed.**
Osa L. Jackson, Ph.D., R.P.T., guest editor

Physical Therapy for the Cancer Patient
Charles L. McGarvey III, M.S., P.T., guest editor

Gait in Rehabilitation
Gary L. Smidt, Ph.D., guest editor

Physical Therapy of the Hip
John L. Echternach, Ed.D., guest editor

Physical Therapy of the Shoulder, 2nd Ed.
Robert Donatelli, M.A., P.T., guest editor

Pediatric Neurologic Physical Therapy, 2nd Ed.
Suzann K. Campbell, Ph.D., P.T., F.A.P.T.A., guest editor

Physical Therapy Management of Parkinson's Disease
George I. Turnbull, M.A., P.T., guest editor

Pulmonary Management in Physical Therapy
Cynthia Coffin Zadai, M.S., P.T., guest editor

Forthcoming Volumes in the Series

Physical Therapy of the Low Back, 2nd Ed.
Lance T. Twomey, Ph.D., and James R. Taylor, M.D.,
Ph.D., guest editors

Physical Therapy for Closed Head Injury
Jacqueline Montgomery, P.T., guest editor

Physical Therapy of the Knee, 2nd Ed.
Robert E. Mangine, M.Ed., P.T., A.T.C., guest editor

Physical Therapy Assessment in Early Infancy

Edited by
Irma J. Wilhelm, M.S., P.T.

Formerly: Research Associate Professor
Division of Physical Therapy
Department of Medical Allied Health Professions
University of North Carolina at Chapel Hill
School of Medicine
Chapel Hill, North Carolina

CHURCHILL LIVINGSTONE
New York, Edinburgh, London, Melbourne, Tokyo

Library of Congress Cataloging-in-Publication Data

Physical therapy assessment in early infancy / edited by Irma J.
  Wilhelm.
      p. cm. — (Clinics in physical therapy)
    Includes bibliographical references and index.
    ISBN 0-443-08815-2
    1. Infants (Newborn)—Medical examinations. 2. Infants (Newborn)-
  -Development—Testing. 3. Physical therapy for children.
  I. Wilhelm, Irma J. II. Series.
    [DNLM: 1. Infant, Newborn—growth & development. 2. Motor Skills-
  -in infancy & childhood. 3. Physical Therapy—in infancy &
  childhood.   WS 420 P578]
  RJ255.5.P45 1993
  618.92'01—dc20
  DNLM/DLC
  for Library of Congress   92-49464
                                                        CIP

© **Churchill Livingstone Inc. 1993**

Distributed in the United Kingdom by Churchill Livingstone, Robert Stevenson
House, 1–3 Baxter's Place, Leith Walk, Edinburgh EH1 3AF, and by associated companies, branches, and representatives throughout the world.

The Publishers have made every effort to trace the copyright holders for
borrowed material. If they have inadvertently overlooked any, they will be
pleased to make the necessary arrangements at the first opportunity.

Acquisitions Editor: *Leslie Burgess*
Copy Editor: *Elizabeth Bowman-Schulman*
Production Designer: *Maryann King*
Production Supervisor: *Jeanine Furino*

Printed in the United States of America

First published in 1993   7 6 5 4 3 2 1

Contributors

Mary Jo Baryza, M.S., P.T.
Instructor, Department of Rehabilitation Medicine, Tufts University School of Medicine; Research Assistant, Research and Training Center in Rehabilitation and Childhood Trauma, New England Medical Center Hospitals, Boston, Massachusetts

Yvette Blanchard, M.S., P.T.
Doctoral Candidate, Boston University Sargent College of Allied Health Professions; Study Coordinator, Child Development Unit, Children's Hospital, Boston, Massachusetts

Suzann K. Campbell, Ph.D., P.T., F.A.P.T.A.
Professor, Department of Physical Therapy, University of Illinois at Chicago College of Associated Health Professions, Chicago, Illinois

Nancy Clopton, Ph.D., P.T.
Associate Professor, Department of Physical Therapy, Texas Tech University Health Sciences Center School of Allied Health, Lubbock, Texas

Stephen M. Haley, Ph.D., P.T.
Research Associate Professor, Department of Rehabilitation Medicine, Tufts University School of Medicine; Director of Research, Research and Training Center in Rehabilitation and Childhood Trauma, New England Medical Center Hospitals, Boston, Massachusetts

Carolyn B. Heriza, Ed.D., P.T.
Adjunct Associate Professor, Department of Physical Therapy, Saint Louis University Medical Center School of Allied Health Professions, St. Louis, Missouri

MaryBeth Mandich, Ph.D., P.T.
Associate Professor, Division of Physical Therapy, West Virginia University School of Medicine, Morgantown, West Virginia

Robert J. Palisano, Sc.D., P.T.
Associate Professor, Programs in Physical Therapy, Hahnemann University School of Allied Health Professions, Philadelphia, Pennsylvania

Martha C. Piper, Ph.D., P.T.
Professor and Dean, Faculty of Rehabilitation Medicine, University of Alberta Faculty of Medicine, Edmonton, Alberta, Canada

Anne Shumway-Cook, Ph.D., P.T.
Research Associate, University of Oregon Institute for Neuroscience, Eugene, Oregon; Research Coordinator, Department of Physical Therapy, Northwest Hospital, Seattle, Washington

Joyce W. Sparling, Ph.D., P.T., O.T.
Assistant Professor, Division of Physical Therapy, Department of Medical Allied Health Professions; Director, Maternal and Child Health Postgraduate Training Project, University of North Carolina at Chapel Hill School of Medicine, Chapel Hill, North Carolina

Jane K. Sweeney, Ph.D., P.T.
Chief, Army Medical Specialist Corps Research; Clinical Specialty Adviser in Pediatric Physical Therapy to the Surgeon General, Walter Reed Army Medical Center, Washington, D.C.

Jan Stephen Tecklin, M.S., P.T.
Chairman and Associate Professor, Department of Physical Therapy, Beaver College, Glenside, Pennsylvania

Irma J. Wilhelm, M.S., P.T.
Formerly: Research Associate Professor, Division of Physical Therapy, Department of Medical Allied Health Professions, University of North Carolina at Chapel Hill School of Medicine, Chapel Hill, North Carolina

Marjorie Woollacott, Ph.D.
Professor, University of Oregon Institute for Neuroscience, Eugene, Oregon

Preface

Infants at high risk for later developmental problems do not form a homogeneous group with similar medical histories, social or ethnic backgrounds, or developmental characteristics.[1] They may have been premature, full-term, or postmature at birth; appropriately or inappropriately grown; have genetic or congenital conditions; or have problems secondary to asphyxia, sepsis, intracranial hemorrhage or infarction, or prenatal drug exposure. They may come from families as diverse as street people or upwardly mobile professionals. They may be at risk for neuromotor disorders such as cerebral palsy, global developmental delay, behavioral problems, learning disabilities, or child neglect and abuse. Although physical therapists cannot hope to assess all of these potential problem areas, clearly the assessment methods we select must include more than just the neuromotor area.

The contributions to this volume reflect a number of changing concepts about the young infant and early development which, in turn, affect assessment. One concept is of the young infant as an interactive being with the capacity to influence and to be affected by his or her environment.[2] This dynamic concept necessitates assessing, in addition to neuromotor maturation and development, interactive behavior; coping skills; behavioral organization; and the contributions of the family, culture, and physical environment to the infant's functioning.

Another concept is of the young infant as having a developmental agenda of functional tasks to accomplish, necessitating the assessment of prerequisites and impediments to the development of function, in addition to the actual accomplishment of developmental milestones.[3] Finally, we must also consider the concept that high-risk infants may never follow the usual (or normal) developmental course,[4] thus necessitating less focus on attainment of normally performed activities, and more emphasis on assessing functional outcomes. At the same time as assessment must respond to these newer concepts of the infant, it must still provide basic information about the more conventional areas of sensorimotor performance, musculoskeletal development, and cardiopulmonary function.

The chapters of this volume provide theoretical and practical information in all these conceptual areas. In Chapter 1, Martha Piper explores and challenges some of the theoretical constructs underlying assessment in early infancy and suggests that we may need to focus more on identifying normality to avoid premature labelling of very young infants as abnormal. In Chapters 5, 6, and 7, Nancy Clopton, Jan Tecklin, and MaryBeth Mandich thoroughly discuss the basic clinical measurement approaches for assessing growth and development, the cardiopulmonary system, and oral-motor functioning in young infants. These approaches require a great deal of hands-on skill, clinical judgment, and knowledge of infant developmental processes and provide vital information on the interdependence of various subsystems in a dynamic model. In Chapters 8 and 9, Robert Palisano and Anne Shumway-Cook and Marjorie

Woollacott provide coverage of the vast areas of neuromotor, developmental, and postural control assessment from both practical and theoretical perspectives, while I have attempted, in Chapter 3, to describe neurobehavioral approaches specifically designed for the neonate, especially those that allow assessment of neonatal behavioral organization and competence. Jane Sweeney, Joyce Sparling, and Stephen Haley and colleagues (Chapters 2, 4, and 10) add the dimension of measuring function from a naturalistic perspective and in the context of the physical, family, and cultural environment. Carolyn Heriza, in Chapter 11, provides a comprehensive overview of the current status and future potential of assessment with "high-tech" methodology, and Suzann Campbell and Stephen Haley and colleagues (Chapters 10 and 12) describe some similarly "cutting edge" diagnostic techniques and assessment methods that are still under development. As a wrap-up, Suzann Campbell discusses some models of assessment and decision making to guide the work of the future.

In summary, this volume contains both breadth and depth of information concerning the theory, science, practice, and art of physical therapy assessment in early infancy. I sincerely hope it meets the needs of those physical therapists whose practices include assessing and treating neonates, young infants, and their families.

Irma J. Wilhelm, M.S., P.T.

References

1. Anderson J, Auster-Liebhaber J: Developmental therapy in the neonatal intensive care unit. Phys Occup Ther Pediatr 4(1):89, 1984

2. Brazelton TB: Saving the bathwater. Child Dev 61:1661, 1990

3. Haley SM, Baryza MJ: A hierarchy of motor outcome assessment: self-initiated movements through adaptive motor function. Inf Young Child 3:1, 1990

4. Bartlett D, Piper MC: Neuromotor development of preterm infants through the first year of life: implications for physical and occupational therapists. Phys Occup Ther Pediatr, 1992, in press

Acknowledgments

During the development of this volume, my work was supported in part by a training grant from the Bureau of Maternal and Child Health Care Delivery and Assistance, U.S. Department of Health and Human Services, and by the Department of Medical Allied Health Professions, Division of Physical Therapy, University of North Carolina at Chapel Hill. I am most grateful for this support.

In addition, I would like to thank all my family, friends, teachers, and professional colleagues who have supported this and other projects through the years and have helped me to grow personally and professionally. They are too numerous to name; they know who they are.

Contents

1 | Theoretical Foundations for Physical Therapy Assessment in Early Infancy

Martha C. Piper

Physical therapists are increasingly being asked to evaluate developing infants. This new role in infant assessment is largely the result of a change in the survival rates of infants at extreme risk for central nervous system (CNS) damage and a heightened appreciation for the potential impact of early intervention in minimizing the effects of a CNS insult. Because of their expertise in motor development, therapists are being called on to assess these young survivors and make recommendations about their care and management based on their findings.

Assessment is the complex and individually specific process of gathering information to identify areas of strengths and weaknesses and to interpret the findings for effective program planning. The actual testing of the infant is only one component of the assessment process. Other aspects include obtaining histories from parents and other professionals involved with the infant and observing the infant in his or her environment.[1] Infant assessments are usually performed to meet one of two objectives: (1) identification and classification or (2) programming for intervention and remediation.[2] At present, physical therapists are assessing infants in numerous milieus to meet one or both of these objectives.

The physical therapy assessment of young infants presents new challenges and issues for the clinician. While at first glance we may not want to question the merit of physical therapy assessments of infants, we still need to identify

1

the theoretical framework for the early assessment role. Lack of theoretical clarity can lead to inappropriate assessment strategies. What are the unique features of infancy that warrant early assessment? What do the results of infant assessments tell us? What distinguishes infant assessments from those conducted in childhood or adulthood? Are assessment results in early infancy valid? For any reasons should we not be assessing infants? Why do we believe that "earlier" is better than "later"? To answer these questions and others, we must examine the theories of early physical therapy assessment that form the rationale for the assessment techniques and practices.

In general, a *theory* summarizes and explains observations; it consists of a series of statements describing the laws, principles, and beliefs associated with the observations.[3] According to Shepard,[4] theory is an abstract idea or collection of ideas used to explain physical or social phenomena. A theory attempts to explain an observation and permits predictions to be made concerning the behavior studied. In physical therapy, assessment strategies should be grounded in a theoretical framework that provides a basis for the assessment approaches, the parameters to be assessed, and the interpretation of the results. Thus theories of physical therapy assessment in early infancy explain the rationale for early assessment, identify the features of early infancy to be measured, and predict how the measurements will be useful to the practice of physical therapy.

In this chapter, the theoretical framework for physical therapy assessment in early infancy is examined in terms of (1) the rationale for early assessment, (2) the essential components of early infant assessments, and (3) the usefulness of early assessment to practice. In addition to the theoretical foundations, information and evidence that either support or negate each theory will be presented. While theories per se are not directly testable, we can examine the validity of an individual theory by testing research hypotheses that have been derived from a theory. In this spirit of examination, we must recognize that theory is dynamic, evolving and changing as our experience and knowledge grow. Given the embryonic stage of physical therapy assessment in early infancy, we should not be surprised that our theoretical foundations are also fledgling in their development.

Clearly, some of the theories presented in this chapter may be discarded and replaced by others as we progress in our understanding of infancy and early assessment. More important than any one theory is the appreciation that theory is needed to guide daily practice and the making of clinical decisions. Without a theoretical foundation for clinical actions, we run the real risk of basing clinical assessments and their interpretations on our clinical biases and experience rather than on carefully formulated and documented ideas or sets of ideas, to be accepted or rejected through testable research hypotheses.

RATIONALE FOR EARLY ASSESSMENT

The earliest possible identification of infants and children who exhibit serious developmental disabilities, such as cerebral palsy and mental retardation, is an important goal of pediatric health care practitioners. This goal is based on a number of distinct clinical, educational, and social objectives, including the desire to identify the etiology of the diverse kinds of developmental disabilities, to institute early remedial measures for infants who manifest developmental delays, and to mobilize societal resources to prevent developmental disabilities.[5] Public Law (PL) 94-142, the Education for All Handicapped Children Act, exemplifies society's desire to identify as early as possible, through assessment, those children who are eligible for special education and related services. These laudable objectives are based on two underlying theories: (1) children who at some point in their childhood are diagnosed as having a developmental delay were also delayed as infants, and (2) those children who are deemed delayed in infancy will, without appropriate intervention, remain delayed as they age.

Good evidence exists to support the first theory, that is, that a large proportion of the children with developmental delays are indeed organically affected as infants. The majority of children with cerebral palsy and mental retardation have experienced either prenatal or neonatal insults; consequently, most of the children who are diagnosed as having cerebral palsy or certain forms of mental retardation have most likely been affected from the time of birth or before. While this is indisputable, the assumption that an infant who has organic deficits will always manifest the deficits through observable delays or dysfunction in infancy has not been proven. Although clinical investigations indicate that early infant assessments may reveal different patterns of observable behaviors in those infants who also demonstrate objective indicators of CNS dysfunction, such as intraventricular hemorrhage, not all affected children are accurately classified in infancy.[6–8] While this experience might be attributed to a lack of sensitive measures, it might also be explained by the fact that not all infants with CNS deficits demonstrate "abnormal" behaviors in infancy. Another possible explanation suggests that some forms of motor dysfunction may not be discernible until a certain level of motor development is achieved or emerging.

The validity of the second theory, that is, that children who are delayed in infancy will retain those delays as they age, is even less sound. This theory essentially assumes that development from infancy onward is solely the result of the maturation of the nervous system and reflects the neurologic integrity of the fetus or infant. It discounts the real possibility that the emergence of behavioral patterns throughout early childhood may reflect both brain maturation and environmental influences or some interaction of the two factors.

The potential effect of the environment on later development is gaining in importance and recognition with the recent interest in the systems theory of motor development. While this systems theory includes recognition of the maturational level of the CNS as an important component for the development of a specific motor behavior, it also includes the proposal that other variables influence the final motor behavior. These variables include the emotional state of the infant, the degree of motivation, cognitive awareness, the infant's posture while attempting a task, muscle strength, biomechanical leverages, and the task itself.[9] If indeed motor behaviors are the result of factors in addition to the maturation of the nervous system, assessment of early infant motor performance would only provide limited information about the eventual motor abilities in childhood.

Also impeding the validity of the second theory are the widely acknowl-edged transient effects of biologic insults on the brain. Even gross structural pathology associated with intracerebral hemorrhage or hydrocephalus can be consistent with apparently normal neurobehavioral development.[10] Although the factors that determine the varied neurobehavioral impact of apparently similar insults remain to be elucidated, clearly not all infants who exhibit "abnor-mal" neuromotor findings early in life will continue to manifest deficient devel-opment throughout childhood.

Despite technologic advances in imaging and assessing the structural com-ponents of the brain and the functioning of the CNS, the ability to predict outcomes accurately has not been substantially improved. Unfortunately, the use of neither neonatal cranial ultrasound nor evoked auditory and visual poten-tials has resulted in complete classification accuracy.[11-14] Thus we are increas-ingly being forced to question the assumption that early indicators of abnormalcy are accurate predictors of outcomes in later childhood. Clearly this is the case with many preterm infants, whose early development may differ from that of full-term infants but who may appear to be developing normally later in life.

The revisiting of these two theories may help to explain some of the diffi-culties experienced by persons intent on detecting, early in infancy, those children who will be delayed or who have cerebral palsy. Most infant or neonatal screening assessments, whether performed by physical therapists or other health professionals, have reasonable sensitivities but poor specificities and hence poor predictive values.[15-19] What do these rates actually mean? Essen-tially, early assessments have been successful in identifying those children who will exhibit cerebral palsy later in childhood but at the expense of classifying many infants as being abnormal who eventually are normal at later dates. These results lend support to the first theory, that children with cerebral palsy are affected as infants, and thus the sensitivities of the tests are high. These results do not, however, support the second theory that infants who are delayed are also delayed as children, hence the poor specificities of the test and resultant large numbers of false positives.

In the past, we have explained these disappointing findings on the basis of the poor predictive validity of the tests being used; that is, the test or assessment, per se, was at fault. The facts that our ability to classify children correctly has not improved remarkably as the psychometric properties of our assessment tools have improved and that the ability to visualize the CNS has been enhanced must lead us to question the appropriateness of the underlying theory of early detection.

In summary, two explanatory theories for early physical therapy assess-ment in infancy have been identified. A review of these theories questions the likelihood of accurately identifying in infancy all of those children who will have neuromotor deficits in later childhood. Because a variety of intervening variables and environmental factors may influence motor development and because many biologic insults on the brain may result only in transient symptom-atology, to assume that information gleaned from an infant assessment will accurately discriminate all of the children with motor problems from those children developing normally may be unrealistic.

ESSENTIAL COMPONENTS OF PHYSICAL THERAPY ASSESSMENT

The majority of well-known approaches to the motor and neurologic assessment of infants have been based on the neuromaturational theory of development. While most of these evaluative approaches, and subsequent measurement tools, were not developed by physical or occupational therapists, many have been adopted and used by therapists to assess the neuromotor status of infants. More recently, therapists have begun to construct their own tools with which to assess the motor performance of neonates, infants, and young children.

The neuromaturational theory of motor development, as enunciated by Gesell[20] and McGraw[21] has not only provided the conceptual framework for many of these assessments but also has determined the content of specific items. What then are the theoretical constructs that have provided the basis for the essential components of these infant assessments? Gesell[20] and McGraw[21] believed that maturation produces progressive, hierarchical changes in the structural components of the nervous system that in turn produce changes in motor output. Accordingly, the following assumptions have formed the basis of most of our assessments of early infancy.

First, at birth the cerebral cortex is not functioning, and movement, mediated by lower centers of the CNS, is reflexive in nature. Second, as the cerebral cortex develops, it exercises a controlling influence over neuromuscular functions and inhibits lower centers of the CNS. Third, development proceeds in a cephalocaudal direction. Finally, development must progress through a particular invariant sequence.[22]

These assumptions have spawned a variety of assessment tools. While many of the assessment approaches reflect aspects of one or more of the theories, clearly most of them are based on the overall neuromaturational framework. For example, several tools emphasize the evaluation of the reflexes that are present in early infancy and disappear with maturation with a view toward identifying those infants who either present "abnormal" reflex profiles early in life or who retain their early reflexes as they age.[23-27] These assessments are based on the first and second theories, that is, that initially motor development is under the control of the lower levels of the CNS and that only with maturation does the cerebral cortex assume a role in motor development. Other scales have been based on the theories that state that motor development progresses in a cephalocaudal direction and that the sequence of progression is predictable and invariant. These tools focus primarily on specific motor milestone acquisition.[28-30]

With increasing evidence that the neuromaturational theoretical constructs may be too narrow to explain all of the intricacies and various aspects of motor development, the appropriateness of not only the specific assessment tools but also the components of development that they emphasize are in question. The heightened interest in the dynamic systems theory that states that the CNS is only one subsystem of many that dynamically interact to produce movement suggests that a new or revised approach to infant assessment may be needed.

The dynamic systems perspective provides a different means of conceptualizing motor development and hence motor assessment. Rather than viewing motor behavior as the unfolding of predetermined patterns in the CNS, this perspective sees motor behavior as emerging from the dynamic cooperation of the many subsystems in a task-specific context. The dynamic systems theory offers a conceptual framework that is free of maturational determinism and implicates other elements such as the infant's biomechanical, psychological, and social environments.[22]

The adoption of the dynamic systems theory as the basis for early physical therapy assessments in infancy is attractive, as it would not only alter our approach to assessment but it would also permit us to retain certain aspects of our earlier orientation. Since the maturation of the CNS is acknowledged to be a contributor to motor development, infant assessments should most likely contain certain components of this theory. The challenge therefore is to identify those aspects of the neuromaturational theory that are valid and to expand the scope of our assessments to incorporate these identified components and the other important subsystems.

Heriza[22] identified three areas that should be addressed when assessing motor performance: the subsystems, the environment, and the task. Although in our current assessments we may evaluate many subsystems, we emphasize the importance of the CNS in directing motor outcomes. Heriza suggests that we need to evaluate many subsystems in addition to the CNS, such as the musculoskeletal system (joint mobility, muscle strength, and static postural alignment), movement patterns (motor milestones, reflexes and reactions, coordination, balance, endurance, and functional performance), sensation (visual, vestibular, proprioceptive, auditory, and tactile), and perception. Furthermore, she recommends the assessment of the various subsystems within a task context rather than testing in nonfunctional positions. Finally, she challenges therapists to change the environment during the testing to ascertain whether the infant can adapt to the changing context or whether the same movement pattern is used in all instances.

In summary, the adoption of a theoretical framework is critical to determining the thrust of infant physical therapy assessment. We are currently questioning our traditional neuromaturational theoretical orientation to infant motor development and hence to assessment. The application of the dynamic systems theory to infant assessment permits the inclusion of certain constructs and assumptions of the neuromaturational theory while at the same time expanding the scope of our assessment practices. The increasing awareness that we need to evaluate other subsystems in addition to the CNS in a task context in a variety of physical and social environments will help to shape our future assessment efforts.

USEFULNESS OF EARLY ASSESSMENT TO PRACTICE

The usefulness of any particular assessment approach or tool to clinical practice will vary according to the purpose of the assessment. Campbell[31] suggests that physical therapists use assessments to accomplish three things:

discriminate or identify normal as normal and abnormal as abnormal, predict later motor abilities from current performance, and evaluate or document change that has occurred. The theoretical foundations as well will vary according to the aim of the assessment. Nevertheless, with the exception of the predictive function, the theoretical assumptions for the discriminative and evaluative functions have some similarities.

First, we assume that by knowing the "normal" course of development we are able to discriminate those infants who are deviating in some fashion from the "normal" and identify them as "abnormal." In other words, we assume that deviations or differentiations from "normal" are "abnormal." Second, we measure change, either over time or as a result of intervention, in terms of an infant's progress in "normalizing" his behaviors. That is to say, positive gains are most often conceptualized as the infant's ability to approach or attain the "normal" behaviors for his age and sex.

These two theoretical constructs have dominated our assessment procedures in the past, whether they have been aimed at identifying normal as normal and abnormal as abnormal or at evaluating the change in an infant's performance over time or as a result of treatment. Have they served us well? What are the strengths and limitations of these two theoretical assumptions?

While numerous investigators have carefully described and documented the normal pattern of early motor development, in terms of sequence and rate of acquisition of specific skills, very few physical therapists have carefully studied, described, or defined the course of early motor development. With the exception of the substantial contribution by Lois Bly,[32] physical therapists have relied on other disciplines to define "normal." While this type of multidisciplinary collaboration should be encouraged, we should also recognize that the theoretical constructs and empirical descriptions arising from other disciplines may fall short of meeting our specific needs. For example, how does early motor development occur in the various postural planes? Must an infant develop postural control and hence motor skills simultaneously in prone and in supine? Is an infant who is delayed in prone necessarily delayed in all other postural planes? Current normative information provides very little information, other than acquisition of very gross motor milestones, to assist us in the sensitive assessment of acquisition of postural control, balance, or antigravity movements, to name only a few of the constructs essential to physical therapy.

In addition, current normative data have almost always been based on the full-term infant who has had uneventful prenatal and neonatal histories. These standards of "normalcy" have dominated our assessment efforts for identifying deviance and monitoring change and progress. With the increasing numbers of infants who are born prematurely or who have experienced prenatal and neonatal insults, such as substance abuse, respiratory distress, and intracranial hemorrhages, comes the growing recognition that the past criteria of "normalcy" may be inappropriate for these new groups of infants. For example, while we know that the early motor development of preterm infants varies from that experienced by full-term infants, we also accept that this variance does not necessarily always signify "abnormal" performance.[33]

This then is the heart of the question: should variability or differences in motor outcomes be interpreted as abnormal or deviant? Have our descriptions of normal development been too narrow? Do we need different "gold standards" for different groups of infants? What is an acceptable definition of "abnormal"? Is it always the absence of "normal" behaviors? Perhaps as important, what is an acceptable definition of "normal"? Does it vary according to the child, the child's family, the child's social and physical environments?

This leads us to the second assumption that positive progress of change is defined in relation to an infant becoming more "normal." Over the years, physical therapists have evaluated treatment progress in light of the child's ability to "normalize" movements in both quantitative and qualitative terms. While this orientation may be very appropriate for some infants, it may be unrealistic and inappropriate for others. Must infants only be evaluated in terms of their ability to acquire preambulation skills if they will never walk independently? Should infants who are capable of sitting with appropriate assistive devices be penalized because they are unable to sit independently? Clearly, we must continue to evaluate the effects of our treatment and monitor change over time. What is less clear, however, is what should be the focus of these assessments and what standards should be used to interpret these observations.

Finally, if we examine the predictive function of infant assessment, we must conclude that it is largely based on the theoretical construct that states that the overall developmental outcome of the child will be improved through the identification and treatment of delays early in infancy. This theory entails the underlying assumption that the eventual developmental outcome of the child will be enhanced as a result of prediction or early detection, that is, the earlier the better.

This theory has evolved from animal experiments that suggested "critical periods" and plasticity in the development of the CNS.[34-36] By identifying infants, early, who exhibit delays in their development and then intervening accordingly, therapists believe that they will be able to have an impact on the CNS and thus improve the long-term developmental outcome of the child. In this way, the importance of infant assessment and hence early detection has been inextricably linked to treatment and to the benefits derived from intervention.

To date, the validity of this theory is still uncertain. A variety of methodologic issues have prevented us from definitively testing hypotheses emanating from this theory. Specifically, the most severely affected infants are those who are normally identified first or earliest. Thus those infants who are identified earliest and receive treatment are often the least likely to benefit from intervention. Conversely, some children who exhibit suspicious development early in infancy will function normally in later childhood regardless of whether they receive treatment.[37]

More importantly perhaps is a growing appreciation for the potential negative consequences of "labeling" infants as "delayed" early in their lives. Parents have been shown to have lower expectations for and perceptions of children identified early in infancy as having a problem, regardless of the presence or absence of the problem later in childhood.[38] As a result of these facts, plus the results of studies that demonstrate that early neonatal assessments accurately identify those infants who are developing normally but also often falsely label normal infants as abnormal, the primary purpose of physical therapy assessments in infancy may need to be the identification of "normal" behavior rather than "abnormal" behavior.[39] The identification of "normal" infants and the subsequent reassurance of parents may prove to be more beneficial to the infants and their families than is the reverse approach: the early identification of deviance or abnormality. Regardless of the focus of infant assessments, the justification for and consequences of early detection need to be re-examined prior to advocating a proliferation of screening programs.

In summary, as our understanding of theories of motor development is enhanced, we should continue to review and revise the theoretical assumptions that form the framework for the infant assessments we use in our clinical practice and decision making. Previously, accepted theoretical standards of "normal" motor performance formed the basis of many of the assessment tools. These standards may no longer be applicable to all the infants physical therapists are now being asked to assess and treat. New theoretical frameworks are needed to reflect the new orientations to motor development and assessment and to ensure that the appropriate tenets are applied to subgroups of infants. The rationale for early detection is directly linked to the efficacy and effectiveness of early treatment and intervention. Until early detection and subsequent treatment can be shown to improve developmental outcomes, therapists should continue to assess carefully their clinical roles in early detection programs.

CONCLUSIONS

Physical therapists are becoming increasingly involved in the assessment of infants as a result of the growing numbers of disease survivors and a new awareness of the unique expertise the therapists can bring to the assessment procedures. Because the aims of infant assessment are numerous, the theoretical constructs vary according to the specific purposes of the assessment approach. The importance of understanding and examining these theoretical foundations is apparent. Without a substantiated theoretical framework, physical therapists are in danger of basing their clinical actions on false assumptions and untested biases.

Several explanatory theories for infant assessment have been presented and discussed in terms of their clinical relevance, appropriateness, and validity. Some of the theories are more attractive and acceptable than others; some exhibit more flaws and questionable assumptions than others. Despite the limitations of these theoretical constructs, they have all contributed to an overall understanding of infant development and assessment. The challenge we now face is to accept those tenets that have remained valid over time, reject those that have failed to explain what we observe on a daily basis, and create new explanations for the phenomena we experience. Only through building on our heritage and creating new, innovative theories will we expand the knowledge base that is critical for infant assessment.

ACKNOWLEDGMENTS

The author thanks Johanna Darrah for her critical reading of the manuscript and Annette Kujda for her assistance in its preparation.

REFERENCES

1. Huber CJ, King-Thomas L: The assessment process. p. 3. In King-Thomas L, Hacker B (eds): A Therapist's Guide to Pediatric Assessment. Little, Brown and Company, Boston, 1987
2. King-Thomas L: Responsibilities of the examiner. p. 11. In King-Thomas L, Hacker B (eds): A Therapist's Guide to Pediatric Assessment. Little, Brown and Company, Boston, 1987
3. LeFrancois GR: Psychological Theories and Human Learning. Brooks/Cole Publishing, Monterey, CA, 1982
4. Shepard K: Theory: criteria, importance, and impact. p. 5. In Proceedings of the II Step Conference: Contemporary Management of Motor Control Problems. Foundation for Physical Therapy, Alexandria, VA, 1991
5. Vaughan HG: Introduction: can developmental disabilities be predicted? p. 1. In Vietze P, Vaughan H (eds): Early Identification of Infants With Developmental Disabilities. Grune and Stratton, Orlando, 1988
6. Bozynski ME, DiPietro MA, Meisels SJ et al: Cranial sonography and neurological examination of extremely preterm infants. Dev Med Child Neurol 32:575, 1990
7. Dubowitz LM, Levene MI, Morante A et al: Neurologic signs in neonatal intraventricular hemorrhage: a correlation with real-time ultrasound. J Pediatr 99:127, 1981
8. Palmer P, Dubowitz L, Levene MI, Dubowitz V: Developmental and neurological progress of preterm infants with intraventricular haemorrhage and ventricular dilatation. Arch Dis Child 57:748, 1982
9. Thelen E: The role of motor development in developmental psychology: a view of the past and an agenda for the future. p. 3. In Eisenber N (ed): Contemporary Topics in Developmental Psychology. Wiley, New York, 1987
10. Vohr BR, Garcia-Coll C, Mayfield S et al: Neurologic and developmental status related to the evolution of visual–motor abnormalities from birth to 2 years of age in preterm infants with intraventricular hemorrhage. J Pediatr 115:296, 1989
11. Beverley DW, Smith IS, Beesley P et al: Relationship of cranial ultrasonography, visual and auditory evoked responses with neurodevelopmental outcome. Dev Med Child Neurol 32:210, 1990
12. DeVries LS, Dubowitz LMS, Dubowitz V et al: Predictive value of cranial ultrasound in the newborn baby: a reappraisal. Lancet 2:137, 1985
13. Fawer CL, Dubowitz LM, Levene MI, Dubowitz V: Auditory brainstem responses in neurologically abnormal infants. Neuropediatrics 14:88, 1983

14. Placzek M, Mushin J, Dubowitz LM: Maturation of the visual evoked response and its correlation with visual acuity in preterm infants. Dev Med Child Neurol 27:448, 1985

15. Allen MC, Capute AJ: Neonatal neurodevelopmental examination as a predictor of neuromotor outcome in premature infants. Pediatrics 83:498, 1989

16. Dubowitz LM, Dubowitz V, Palmer PG et al: Correlation of neurologic assessment in the preterm newborn infant with outcome at 1 year. J Pediatr 105:452, 1984

17. Harris SR: Early detection of cerebral palsy: sensitivity and specificity of two motor assessments. J Perinatol 7:11, 1987

18. Stewart A, Hope PL, Hamilton P et al: Prediction in very preterm infants of satisfactory neurodevelopmental progress at 12 months. Dev Med Child Neurol 30:53, 1988

19. Touwen BCL: Variability and stereotypy of spontaneous motility as a predictor of neurological development of preterm infants. Dev Med Child Neurol 32:501, 1990

20. Gesell A: The Embryology of Behavior: the Beginnings of the Human Mind. J.B. Lippincott, Philadelphia, 1945

21. McGraw MB: The Neuromuscular Maturation of the Human Infant. Hafner Press, New York, 1945

22. Heriza C: Motor development: traditional and contemporary theories. p. 99. In Proceedings of the II Step Conference: Contemporary Management of Motor Control Problems. Foundation for Physical Therapy, Alexandria, VA, 1991

23. Capute AJ, Accardo PJ, Vining EPG et al: Primitive Reflex Profile: Monographs in Developmental Pediatrics. Vol. 1. University Park Press, Baltimore, 1978

24. Chandler LS, Andrews MS, Swanson MW: Movement Assessment of Infants: a Manual. Rolling Bay, Washington, 1980

25. DeGangi GA, Berk RA, Valvano J: Test of motor and neurological functions in high-risk infants: preliminary findings. J Dev Behav Pediatr 4:182, 1983

26. Fiorentino MR: A Basis for Sensorimotor Development: Normal and Abnormal. Charles C. Thomas, Springfield, IL, 1981

27. Milani-Comparetti A, Gidoni EA: Routine developmental examination in normal and retarded children. Dev Med Child Neurol 9:631, 1967

28. Bayley N: Manual for the Bayley Scales of Infant Development. Psychological Corporation, New York, 1969

29. Griffiths R: The Abilities of Babies: a Study in Mental Measurement. University of London, London, 1954

30. Folio MR, Fewell RR: Peabody Developmental Motor Scales and Activity Cards: a Manual. DLM Teaching Resources, Allen, TX, 1983

31. Campbell SK: Framework for the measurement of neurologic impairment and disability. p. 143. In Proceedings of the II Step Conference: Contemporary Management of Motor Control Problems. Foundation for Physical Therapy, Alexandria, VA, 1991

32. Bly L: The components of normal movement during the first year of life. p. 85. In Development of Movement in Infancy. University of North Carolina at Chapel Hill, Division of Physical Therapy, 1980

33. Darrah J, Piper MC, Byrne PJ, Warren S: The utilization of the Movement Assessment of Infants risk profile with preterm infants. Phys Occup Ther Pediatr 11(2):1, 1991

34. Bishop B: Neural plasticity: part 2. Postnatal maturation and function-induced plasticity. Phys Ther 62:1132, 1982

35. Rosenzweig MR, Bennett EL, Diamond MC: Brain changes in response to experience. Sci Am 226:22, 1972

36. Schapiro S, Vukovich KR: Early experience effects upon cortical dendrites: a proposed model for development. Science 167:292, 1970

37. Piper MC, Mazer B, Silver KM, Ramsay M: Resolution of neurological symptoms in high-risk infants during the first two years of life. Dev Med Child Neurol 30:26, 1988
38. Cadman D, Chambers LW, Walter SD et al: Evaluation of public health preschool child developmental screening: the process and outcomes of a community program. Am J Public Health 77:45, 1987
39. Piper MC, Darrah J, Pinnell L et al: The consistency of sequential examinations in the early detection of neurological dysfunction. Phys Occup Ther Pediatr 11(3):27, 1991

2 | Assessment of the Special Care Nursery Environment: Effects on the High-Risk Infant*

Jane K. Sweeney

Preterm infants have been described as "physiologically displaced persons," ejected into the world to face a very unusual environment in the intensive care nursery.[1] Medically fragile infants in special care units experience an environmental paradox created by physiologic stabilization from specialized, often life-saving technology applied in an intermittently noxious, overstimulating caregiving environment. Iatrogenic physiologic risk is magnified by exposure to *both* the caregiving technology and the environment of neonatal intensive care. This chapter focuses on assessment of the ecology of this technologically complex extrauterine environment for newborn infants. The effects of the neonatal intensive care unit (NICU) environment on infants are examined and options for environmental modifications to reduce sensory stimuli are presented. A tool for assessing the effects of the environment on high-risk neonates is reviewed, and implications of environmental assessment and modification are described for neonatal physical therapy practice.

ECOLOGY OF NEONATAL INTENSIVE CARE

Anthropologic Orientation

In the spirit of Margaret Mead, the distinguished anthropologist who described primitive adolescent culture in *Coming of Age in Samoa*,[2] physical therapists must "come of age" in neonatal practice by balancing "physical"

---

* *Note:* The opinions and conclusions presented in this chapter are those of the author and do not necessarily represent the views of the Army Medical Department, the Department of the Army, or any other U.S. government agency.

movement science perspectives with reflective, observational behavior science approaches. The behavioral scientist role in physical therapy assumes new prominence in neonatal practice. Instead of behavioral modification and management familiar in general pediatrics, physical therapists engaging in neonatal practice take on the challenge of transitioning into the role of an anthropologist in general preparation for NICU service delivery, individual case management in the nursery, and environmentally appropriate and culturally sensitive family teaching.

As anthropologists in the nursery, neonatal physical therapists must observe, learn, and value the culture and ecology of the NICU before imposing physical therapy procedures or teaching into the environment. Recognizing and understanding the values, beliefs, attitudes, assumptions, and pressures of the newborn medicine subculture are critical components in professional socialization to the NICU.

Transition to a practice model of *observing* events, actions, and reactions instead of *doing* is often difficult for action-oriented, time-efficient physical therapists who derive high satisfaction and keen information from kinesthetic handling of patients. The observation-only role is frequently perceived as passive, nonproductive, and nonreimbursable. Observation of environmental effects on neonates may also be difficult for neonatologists and neonatal nurses focused primarily on medical crisis intervention and organ system stabilization. This crisis management approach may remain in the postcrisis period instead of transitioning into a developmentally supportive, holistic approach.

As custodian of the culture and ecology of the special care nursery, the head nurse or designated neonatal nurse clinical specialist is the optimum professional to orient and socialize the pediatric physical therapist to NICU practice. This process of orientation and integration into the culture sets the stage for collaborative service delivery between nursing and physical therapy that will include assessment and modification of the environment.

Light

Infants in intensive care frequently have continuous 24 hour exposure to fluorescent or cool-white light, which in some units may be augmented by light from windows, phototherapy equipment, or nonradiant heat lamps. Gottfried[3] found average illumination levels in one intensive care unit to be 530 lumen/m^2, peaking during the midafternoon. Glass et al.[4] reported a 5- to 10-fold increase in light intensity in hospital nurseries in the past 20 years. They identified a continuous median foot-candle level of 90 in two nurseries studied and postulated that high levels of continuous light exposure may contribute to retinopathy of prematurity, the alteration of normal retinal vascular development. They found a significant increase in retinopathy of prematurity in infants with birthweights below 1,000 g who were continuously exposed to high illumination (60 foot-candles) compared with weight-matched infants in protected lighting (25 foot-candles).

Adverse effects of continuous light on sleep patterns and weight gain in newborn infants have been identified.[5,6] Mann et al.[6] reported significantly increased weight gain (average of 0.5 kg), decreased feeding time, and increased sleeping periods for 20 infants in an experimental alternating day–night nursery in which light and noise were reduced from 7 PM to 7 AM.

In animal models, altered endocrine function, delayed gonad development, and chromosomal breakage were attributed to prolonged exposure to cool-white, fluorescent lighting.[7-9] Retinal and optic nerve damage in newborn animals from phototoxicity at light intensities similar to those in hospital nurseries have been described.[10,11]

Full visibility of the infant to monitor behavioral and physiologic changes and to allow ongoing immediate inspection of intravenous lines, endotracheal tubes, or nasal cannula are frequent justifications for continuous light in neonatal intensive care units. Architectural changes of indirect (Fig. 2-1) and individual infant lighting options and developmentally supportive caregiving models[12-15]

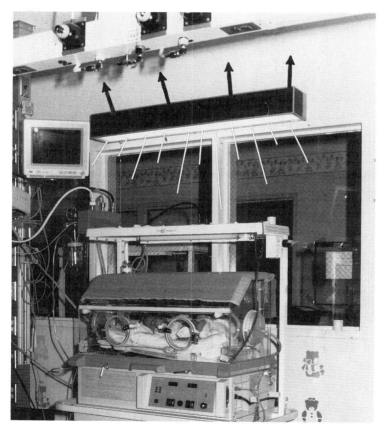

Fig. 2-1. Individually controlled lighting for direct (downward) or indirect (upward) illumination during care of a preterm infant in an isolette shaded with a towel.

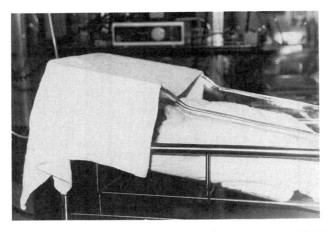

Fig. 2-2. Blanket draped over the bassinette to reduce continuous light on infants in the intermediate care nursery.

have contributed to recent decreases in levels of light stimulation in many neonatal care units. A survey of 155 hospitals with intensive care nurseries from 35 states revealed that the most common environmental modifications used for excessive light were blanket drapes over isolettes or bassinettes (Fig. 2-2) to shade infants' faces, low-intensity overhead lights, individual infant spotlights, and cycled day–night lighting procedures.[16]

Sound

Rather than being protected from environmental noise while placed inside a plexiglass box, infants in incubators are exposed to high, continuous mechanical noise, not unlike a busy street corner. The magnitude of sound in intensive care nurseries has been measured at an average of 85 dB, with inflections to 118 dB.[17] This noise level simulates light auto traffic with fluctuations to the level of large machinery.[3] Sound levels are known to increase during admissions, standard and emergency medical procedures, and daily rounds. Even nonjudicious manipulation of incubator porthole doors with a snap release of the knob may cause startle reactions in infants.

The acoustic environment of special care nurseries has been categorized as high intensity at low frequencies.[3,18] Because the low-frequency sounds are able to penetrate the incubator and muffle voice sounds from the environment, infants within incubators are predicted to have minimal association of voices with faces of caregivers.[19]

Abramowich et al.[20] found hearing loss in very low-birthweight infants to be negligible in the absence of other neonatal medical complications. In newborn animals, however, cochlear damage from environmental noise was apparent.[21] Future study is needed to determine the long-term effects of environmental noise on the integrity of the inner ear in infants with gestational ages of 24 to 28 weeks. Short periods of noise exposure of 80 dB, a level common in NICUs, have been associated with hearing loss in adults.[22] Experienced newborn-medicine staff exposed to a 1-hour tape recording of NICU sounds described symptoms of head and earaches and a disorganizing, "overwhelmed" feeling.[23]

Long et al.[24] identified physiologic consequences of NICU noise pollution in infants to include hypoxemia, disturbed sleep patterns, increased intracranial pressure, and tachycardia. The sources of noise causing inflections to 75 dB were the telephone, capillary tube centrifuge, cardiac monitor alarms, incubator drawers and ports, laughter, conversations directed over the length of the nursery, and nursery doors.

Noise reduction strategies in the nursery include padding doors; removing radios and centrifuges; eliminating loud conversations; conducting detailed case discussions away from the bedside during rounds; purchasing equipment with low noise levels; turning signals of alarms, loud speakers, and telephones to the lowest audible settings; wrapping music boxes with cloth; and placing carpeting and acoustic tile in the architectural structure of the nursery.[23,25] Other environmental noise-reducing procedures during caregiving include elimination of finger tapping on the top of incubators, placing items (e.g., clipboards or bottles) on the top of incubators, snapping porthole doors, and slamming or jarring incubator drawers.

Environmentally conscious neonatal nurses reduce high-pitched bubbling sounds by keeping ventilator tubing clear of water, by clearing suction catheter tubing outside of the incubator, and by turning off the suction machine when not directly in use. Caregivers can effectively decrease ambient noise levels by immediate silencing of monitor alarms (cardiorespiratory, oxygen saturation, temperature, infusion pump, ventilator) rather than waiting 20 to 30 seconds for infants to self-recover.

Caregiving Procedures

The frequency of physical handling of infants in neonatal intensive care during a typical 24-hour day has been documented at 130 times, with nonhandling periods lasting only 4.6 to 19.2 minutes.[19] In a similar study, the caregiving procedures for infants in intensive care were nearly twofold more frequent than handling in an intermediate care nursery.[3]

Hypoxemia, disrupted sleep patterns, apnea, and bradycardia are well documented physiologic costs of excessive handling of newborn infants in intensive care.[19,26–28] Speidel[29] found an average decrease in oxygen tension of 31 mmHg during 75 percent of the following activities: vital signs measurement, chest x-rays, blood sampling, pharyngeal suction, administration of intravenous infusion, and diaper changes. Dangman et al.[30] found a similar decrease (30 mmHg) in arterial oxygen tension after vital signs measurement and physical examination and a 40 mmHg decrease after endotracheal suctioning. Increases in heart rate, respiratory rate, or blood pressure were documented by other researchers after circumcision,[31] nasopharyngeal stimulation,[32] spinal tap,[33] and nasogastric feeding.[34]

The physiologic cost to infants of neonatal physical therapy intervention has been analyzed for only a few procedures. Chest physical therapy for neonates has been studied by several investigators with similar findings of decreased oxygenation, increased blood pressure, and increased heart rate during the procedure.[35-39] An 8 percent increase in heart rate and in mean arterial pressure occurred in medically stable, high-risk neonates during neonatal hydrotherapy sessions of 15 minutes duration.[40]

Neurologic assessment of 72 medically stable preterm and full-term neonates by an experienced neonatal physical therapist was found to be physiologically and behaviorally destabilizing to both gestational age groups of infants.[41] Preterm infants, however, had significantly higher heart rate, greater increase in blood pressure, and decreased peripheral oxygenation inferred from mottled skin color than full-term subjects. Preterm infants also demonstrated significantly more frequent behavioral signs of stress than did full-term peers: hiccoughs, yawns, arm salutes, and finger splay gestures. The neuromotor (tone and reflex) component of testing was the most stressful for both infant groups. The physiologic cost of neurologic assessment, even for healthy 3-day-old full-term infants, was an unexpected finding. The safety of neurologic assessment procedures for acutely ill or borderline stable neonates has not been established.

A neonatal physical therapy developmental intervention program for 14 preterm subjects at 34 to 38 weeks of gestation was analyzed physiologically by Kelly and colleagues.[42] While no significant changes in mean oxygen saturation occurred during intervention, a significant increase (7 percent) in heart rate from baseline values was evident. Analysis of the neuromotor intervention procedures was limited to six activities involving sidelying and supported sitting positions for eliciting head control, body righting, and midline upper extremity activities.

Because routine caregiving and common medical procedures for neonates in intensive care can no longer be assumed to be physiologically benign, protected caregiving guidelines have been developed. Minimal handling protocols,[43] clustering of procedures to allow rest periods,[44] and pacing of caregiving activities contingent with infants' cues[45] have been instituted to reduce the stress of intensive care on newborn infants.

ASSESSMENT OF ENVIRONMENTAL EFFECTS

Clinical Instrument

A major theoretical framework, the synactive model of infant behavioral organization,[46] was introduced by Als and colleagues in the late 1970s. This model of preterm infant behavioral organization provides a theoretical basis for understanding the behavioral interaction of physiologic, motor, behavioral state, interaction/attention, and self-regulation in infants attempting to cope with the stresses of the extrauterine environment and maintain homeostasis in the NICU.[46] To document the behavioral effects of the caregiving environment on infants in neonatal special care, Als et al.[47] developed the Assessment of Preterm Infant Behavior (APIB) and the Neonatal Individualized Developmental Care and Assessment Program (NIDCAP).[48] These instruments provide the examiner with a structure for developing a profile of an infant's responses to environmental demands and physical handling. Refer to Chapter 3 for detailed review of the APIB and synactive theory.

The NIDCAP includes a continuous, systematic observation at 2 minute intervals of an infant's autonomic, motor, behavioral state, and attention signals and a simultaneous documentation of vital signs and oxygen saturation responses from monitors. The observational protocol (Appendix 2-1) is conducted before, during, and after standard caregiving and handling procedures. A narrative description of the infant's behaviors in the NICU environment is then provided to establish an individualized care plan adapted for his unique response tolerance to environmental stimuli. This method of observing preterm infants too fragile to be examined developmentally provides the physical therapist with a naturalistic observation tool to assess an infant's baseline ability to handle the stresses of routine nursing and medical procedures to determine readiness for physical therapy evaluation.

Training

Examiner training[48] in the NIDCAP can be obtained at the National NIDCAP Training Center in Boston or at regional sites in North Carolina, Arizona, Colorado, California, and Oklahoma (Appendix 2-2). An alternative method is on-site training at individual institutions by a NIDCAP trainer for a minimum of three trainees. Arrangements for the training are coordinated through the National Training Center in Boston.

The NIDCAP training is conducted in four segments:

1. Preparatory reading
2. A 1- or 2-day introductory lecture/seminar and precepted NICU practicum by the trainer in the theoretical background and use of the NIDCAP instrument with infants.
3. Individual practice by the trainee to include
    a. observations of three preterm infants in intensive care, intermediate care, and at discharge to include each shift during the 24 hours of caregiving
    b. 20 infant observations before, during, and after caregiving procedures with preparation of individual developmental care plans: five healthy full-term infants and 15 preterm infant observations (five in intensive care, five in intermediate care, five at discharge) and
    c. observation and care plan documentation of three infants on the trainee's regular caseload with implementation of the individualized devel-

opmental care plan followed by re-evaluation of the effects of intervention using the NIDCAP instrument.

4. a 1-day reliability check with the trainer, either at the regional training center or at the trainee's NICU. Independent observations and developmental care plans are compared between the trainer and trainee on two infants. With reliability achieved, the NIDCAP training may be credited for 18 continuing education units.[48]

Research

A review of two outcome studies conducted by Als et al.[14,49] on the effects of developmentally supportive NICU care and the use of the NIDCAP and APIB clinical instruments shows an impressive pattern of shorter hospitalizations. This cost–benefit effect was due to earlier transitions from both ventilatory support and from gavage feeding and increased weight gain in the experimental group when compared with weight- and age-matched control infants born less than 32 weeks of gestation. In the first study of 16 infants, the experimental group of eight infants receiving NICU individualized developmental care from the tenth day of life until hospital discharge were found to have consistently increased cognitive and motor performance through three years of age.[14] This study has, however, been vulnerable to criticism due to the small sample size and phase-lag design rather than random assignment of subjects.[50]

An expanded second study[49] was a modified replication using random assignment of a larger sample (18 control; 20 experimental) of weight- and age-matched infants less than 32 weeks of gestation. Initiation of observation-based developmental care occurred from the first day of life until discharge from the nursery. The experimental infants receiving the developmentally oriented caregiving had significant reduction in the incidence of intraventricular hemorrhage and in the severity of chronic lung disease than control infants. The improved medical outcomes occurred in addition to the previously described benefits of earlier hospital discharge and increased weight gain.

A multicenter study, directed by Als,[48] is currently in progress at four sites. The methodology used in the modified replication study is incorporated at all sites. This collaborative investigation of individualized NICU developmental care is focused on comparing potential differences in infant developmental and medical outcomes on transported versus inborn infants and primary nursing care versus neonatal care without primary nurses.[48]

Becker et al.[51] used a phase-lag design to analyze the effects of developmentally supportive neonatal nursing care in 45 infants with birth weights less than 1,501 g and gestational ages less than 32 weeks. Infants receiving developmentally oriented nursing care from staff trained in NIDCAP procedures had shorter hospital stays, improved behavioral organization, fewer days on a ventilator, and earlier transition from gavage feeding than infants given routine care before NIDCAP training of the nursing staff. While data collectors were not blind to group assignment of subjects in the control and experimental phases, this clinical study demonstrated value in overall staff education in NIDCAP procedures, combined with ongoing assistance from developmental specialists, in changing infant outcomes. The use of general nursing staff education was in contrast to other studies,[14,49] in which reliance on developmentally trained primary care nurses occurred for behavioral observation-based care plans.

These studies[14,48-51] provide evidence of emerging positive effects of modifying the ecology of the nursery for preterm infants. In addition to an increasing pattern of improved medical, behavioral, and developmental outcomes for preterm infants receiving individualized developmental care in the NICU, the cost effectiveness of decreased hospital stay[48,50] at a minimum of approximately $1,100 per day, is striking.

IMPLICATIONS FOR NEONATAL PHYSICAL THERAPY PRACTICE

In preparation for environmental assessment, case management, interprofessional collaboration, and family teaching in the nursery, subspecialty training in neonatal physical therapy is required. This includes a precepted clinical practicum during which observation, physical handling, physiologic and behavioral monitoring, communication, and collaboration are modeled and supervised.

Neonatal Subspecialization

Because neonatal physical therapy practice demands expanded knowledge, competencies and practice models from general pediatric physical therapy,[52,53] subspecialty practice guidelines and advanced level competencies for physical therapy service in neonatal intensive care units were developed and disseminated by the American Physical Therapy Association (APTA) in 1989.[54] The advanced level competency areas in neonatal physical therapy are outlined in prevention, physical examination, treatment design and modification, treatment implementation, consultation and coordination, research, education, and administration.

The APTA directs that a precepted clinical practicum occur before independent assessment and intervention by physical therapists in the NICU.[54] Results from a survey of physical therapy directors in six large pediatric hospitals in a variety of geographic regions illustrated the APTA practice directive: 2.5 to 6 months of precepted training in the NICU were required after a minimum of 1.5 to 3 years of physical therapy experience in general pediatrics.[52] Subspecialty training promotes accountability in the care of high-risk neonates. Self-directed training in neonatal therapy is dangerous, because it is a trial and error experience at the infant's expense.

Case Management

A cornerstone in the *baseline* physical therapy assessment of high-risk neonates is evaluation of each infant's physical and caregiving environment and analysis of the effects of the environment on physiologic and behavioral stability before initiating neonatal therapy assessment or intervention procedures. A useful screening format for documenting ambient light, sound, activity levels, specialized equipment in use, and medical history is described in Appendix 2-3. This is an abbreviated version, from training materials developed by Als,[55] of a naturalistic observation of preterm and full-term infants. A comprehensive assessment of the nursery environment, including a manual, is work in progress by Als, with probable publication in approximately 2 years.

Prior to the evaluative handling of medically fragile neonates by the physical therapist, documentation of tolerance to routine nursing care helps to determine the readiness of infants for physical therapy assessment and begins a partnership with the nurse for assistance in monitoring the effects of physical therapy and for developing a collaborative caregiving relationship. The NIDCAP (Appendix 2-1) offers a clinically applicable structure for physical therapy evaluation of physiologic and behavioral changes at 2 minute intervals before, during, and after routine caregiving procedures. This format can then be modified or used intact as an observational risk management system for determining an infant's tolerance to neonatal physical therapy.

To exclude an observational baseline component may place an infant at unnecessary physiologic risk during neonatal physical therapy procedures. Now that the physiologic cost to high-risk neonates from assessment and intervention by physical therapists has been quantified for selected procedures,[35–38,40–42] medical–legal and ethical considerations drive the inclusion of prehandling physiologic and behavioral observation in neonatal therapy practice. The research of Gottfried[3] and Wolke[19] provides further support for this conservative handling approach, given that infants in the NICU can receive as many as 130 handling contacts from medical and nursing procedures within a 24 hour period.

Documentation and discussion of environmental and physical handling effects on infants during nursing care and physical therapy procedures leads to an initial environmental modification plan for developmentally supportive caregiving. This plan may then guide parent teaching on caregiving in the nursery; direct anticipatory guidance for the home environment; modify the pacing of medical, nursing, and therapy procedures; and establish the need for potential architectural changes for the entire nursery.

Neurologically impaired infants considered too fragile for handling by the physical therapist in a traditional practice model may now be included in the caseload when anthropology- and ecology-based approaches are used. This means a minimal handling approach in which infant assessment (NIDCAP format) by the physical therapist occurs during handling by the neonatal nurse in routine caregiving. The physical evaluator role is conducted through the hands of the neonatal nurse as both professionals observe and later document the effects of handling and the environment on the infant's physiologic and behavioral stability. Mutual decisions are then made for when the borderline stable infant may be ready for evaluative handling by the physical therapist. In the meantime, baseline reactions to the caregiving environment have been documented, and contact with parents may occur in preparation for later participation in developmentally supportive caregiving.

Change Process

Without the support and collaboration of nurses, physical therapists are not able to orchestrate environmental and caregiving changes in light, sound, positioning, feeding, or other individualized developmental strategies in the NICU. The power to change the physical, social, and 24 hour caregiving environment lies primarily with nursing rather than with the neonatal medical staff, many of whom may be in training (e.g., intern, resident, fellow) or on a rotating schedule as the attending neonatologist. The use of an environmental observation instrument by the physical therapist must be combined with nursing assessment and nursing concurrence on environmental issues for proposed environmental change to occur (Fig. 2-3).

Physical therapists may serve as effective catalysts for environmental change in the nursery. Using the specialty consultant format, most professionals

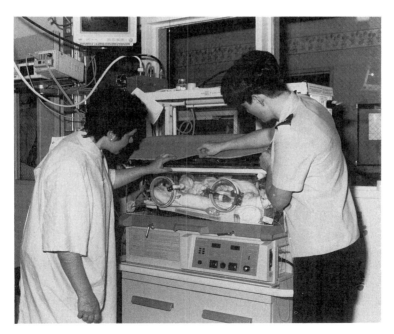

Fig. 2-3. Collaboration between physical therapist (left) and neonatal clinical nurse specialist (right) on environmental modifications for developmentally supportive caregiving.

have limited influence as agents of change in the nursery. Expansion of the developmental consultant role into a creative, interdependent, collaborative partnership with neonatal nursing staff can lead to innovative, widespread changes in caregiving and professionally rewarding, growth-enhancing interactions between the two disciplines.

Shepard,[56] described a process of building collaborative relationships among physical therapists and other health professionals using an organizational behavior model developed by Grinnell.[57,58] Modified for neonatal physical therapy, the partnership begins with a formal consultation stage, progresses through a "cold war"[58] stage of protective posturing and competition, to a harmonious sharing of work and successes before moving into a creative, collaborative partnership (Fig. 2-4).

During formal consultation in the nursery, the first stage in the adapted collaborative model of Shepard[56] and Grinnell,[57] minimal interaction occurs with staff on the newborn medicine service. The report is left in the medical record, and the formal assessment contains many abbreviations and pediatric therapy jargon. Participation in nursing or developmental rounds to discuss evaluative findings or coordinate care does not occur. This independent, consultative practice by physical therapists in the nursery may in fact be physiologically and behaviorally overstimulating to neonates when not carefully coordinated with and monitored by neonatal nurses.

During the second stage, the physical therapist is still considered a guest in the nursery but has expanded interaction with the nursery staff and an increased caseload. Although invited as a guest lecturer at inservice training, an undercurrent of competition and conflict may develop with attempted negotiation of role expectations and professional boundaries. Professionals from both disciplines are in an adjustment phase, coping with perceptions of intrusive and defensive behaviors from the other professional during neonatal developmental

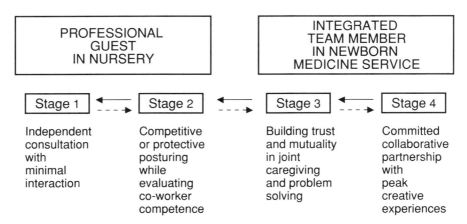

Fig. 2-4. Transitions in collaborative partnership development between physical therapists and neonatal nurses. (Data from Shepard.[56])

caregiving. It is a stage of protective posturing while evaluating the competencies and communication styles of coworkers. This is a strained, usually frustrating, exploratory stage that must be endured for collaborative characteristics to develop within the professional relationship. Resolution of the competition and testing issues allows the guest role to be abandoned.

Entry to the newborn medicine team occurs in the third stage, at which trust and mutuality are developed during sharing of work and successes in joint caregiving in the special care nursery. This is a stage of harmonious, collegial interactions marked by spontaneous clinical teaching at the bedside and regular participation in team conferences and rounds. The physical therapist is now a regular faculty member for inservice training and orientation of new staff to the nursery. Many highly effective nurse–physical therapist partners remain in this stage. Although specialty boundaries remain intact, excellent mutual problem solving and coordinated care processes occur with joint caregiving tasks.

In stage four a creative collaborative partnership has emerged from combining expertise, creative energy, and commitment to expand practice options and make innovative changes not possible while working independently. This stage is marked by peak experiences of unique productivity such as design of innovative clinical care protocols, creation of customized neonatal equipment, development of interdisciplinary neonatal specialization curricula, or unique consolidation of family teaching materials. Differences of opinion surface early in a climate of open communication; power is shared, flexible, and understated. Role overlap occurs on simple tasks as well as on projects developed jointly. With pooled knowledge and expertise, the collaborative partners may cross disciplinary boundaries to produce breakthroughs in complex or controversial projects.

Some physical therapists may travel through the early stages quickly; others may remain locked in the consultative or the exploratory, protective posturing stages as guests in the nursery instead of integrating into team membership. Caregiving crises followed by victories in the nursery may move therapists out of guest roles into expanded sharing of tasks and accomplishments (e.g., prevention of a scheduled gastrostomy placement by intensive, short-term oral–motor intervention and behavioral cue focused feeding trials by nurse–physical therapist partners). On the other hand, regression of the collaborative relationship can occur if the nonjudgmental, open feedback mechanism fails or the complexity of the task drives a more exploratory, protective, specialty-specific stance. If aware of developmental stages in creating professional partnerships, potential collaborators can focus on the end-stage desired and sustain the energy to work through the early stages of resolving competition or conflicts on joint tasks and modulating communication styles.[56,57]

"Good intentions and superb clinical skills will not alone support the realization" of neonatal therapy goals.[56] The quality of the professional or therapeutic relationship with neonatal nurses and parents is the critical ingredient to success in neonatal therapy intervention.

Interdisciplinary collaboration does not happen by chance; it is the outcome of focused professional development.[57] The NIDCAP clinical instrument for mutual assessment of the caregiving environment may be invaluable for initiating and bridging collaborative caregiving relationships in the nursery.

CONCLUSIONS

The special care nursery environment, including physical therapy procedures and interactions, can be physiologically and behaviorally destabilizing to newborn infants. Effects of the NICU physical and caregiving environment on infants can now be formally assessed through a naturalistic observation structure and the Neonatal Individualized Developmental Care and Assessment Program. An anthropologic orientation and a collaborative partnership model, rather than a consultative model, are recommended for holistic evaluation of infant response capabilities and mutual exploration by neonatal nurses and physical therapists of environmental change options. For safe and effective NICU practice, neonatal physical therapists must be willing to delay the "kinesthetics knowing" of physical handling of infants for assessing neuromotor, neurobehavioral, and physiologic stability. Instead, they must substitute naturalistic observation of nursing procedures for initial determination of baseline function and stability. In addition to coordinating developmental care for individual infants, mutual observation of the tolerance of infants to routine caregiving promotes transition to a collaborative partnership between the physical therapist and the neonatal nurse. The quality and growth of this professional collaboration will determine the depth of developmental care programs for infants and parents in neonatal special care units.

ACKNOWLEDGMENTS

Appreciation is expressed to LTC Deborah Leander RN, MSN, Katherine Shepard PhD, PT, FAPTA and COL Valerie Biskey RN, DSN, for support in concept exploration and in editorial review.

REFERENCES

1. Lucey JF: Foreward. p. xi. In Gottfried AW, Gaiter JL (eds): Infant Stress Under Intensive Care. University Park Press, Baltimore, 1985
2. Mead M: Coming of Age in Samoa. Dell, New York, 1928
3. Gottfried AW: Environment of newborn infants in special care units. p. 27. In Gottfried AW, JL Gaiter (eds): Infant Stress Under Intensive Care. University Park Press, Baltimore, 1985
4. Glass P, Avery GB, Subramanian KN et al: Effect of bright light in the hospital nursery on the incidence of retinopathy of prematurity. N Engl J Med 313:401, 1985
5. Shiroiwa Y, Kamiya Y, Uchyibori S et al: Activity, cardiac and respiratory responses of blindfolded preterm infants in a neonatal intensive care unit. Early Hum Dev 14:259, 1986

6. Mann NP, Haddow R, Stokes L et al: Effect of night and day on preterm infants in a newborn nursery: randomized trial. Br Med J 293:1265, 1986
7. Mayron L, Kaplan E: Bioeffects of fluorescent light. Acad Ther 12:75, 1976
8. Wurtman RJ, Weisel J: Environmental lighting and neuroendocrine function: relationship between spectrum of light source and gonadal growth. Endocrinology 85:1218, 1969
9. Gantt R: Fluorescent light-induced DNA cross linkage and chromatid breaks in mouse cells in culture. Proc Natl Acad Sci USA 75:3809, 1979
10. O'Steen WK: Retinal and optic nerve serotonin and retinal degeneration as influenced by photoperiod. Exp Neurol 27:194, 1970
11. Messner KH, Maisels J, Leure-duPree AE: Phototoxicity to the newborn primate retina. Invest Ophthalmol Vis Sci 17:178, 1978
12. Avery G, Glass P: The gentle nursery: developmental intervention in the NICU. J Perinatol 9(2):204, 1989
13. Cole JG, Begish-Duddy A, Judas MS et al: Changing the NICU environment: the Boston City Hospital model. Neonatal Network 9(2):15, 1990.
14. Als H, Lawhorn G, Brown E et al: Individualized behavioral and environmental care for the VLBW preterm infant at high risk for bronchopulmonary dysplasia: NICU and developmental outcome. Pediatrics 78:1123, 1986
15. Als H: A synactive model of neonatal behavioral organization: framework for the assessment of neurobehavioral development in the premature infant and for support of infants and parents in the neonatal intensive care environment. p. 3. In Sweeney JK (ed): The High Risk Neonate. Haworth Press, New York, 1986
16. Frank A, Maurer P, Shepherd J: Light and sound environment: a survey of neonatal intensive care units. Phys Occup Ther Pediatr 11(2):27, 1991
17. Gottfried AW, Wallace-Lande P, Sherman-Brown S et al: Physical and social environment of newborn infants in special care units. Science 214:673, 1981
18. Lawson K, Daum C, Turkewitz G: Environmental characteristics of a neonatal intensive care unit. Child Dev 48:1633, 1977
19. Wolke D: Environmental neonatology. Arch Dis Child 62:987, 1987
20. Abramowich SJ, Gregory S, Slemick M, Stewart A: Hearing loss in very low birthweight infants treated with neonatal intensive care. Arch Dis Child 54:421, 1979
21. Falk SA: Noise induced inner ear damage in newborn and adult guinea pigs. Laryngoscope 84:444, 1974
22. American Academy of Pediatrics Committee on Environmental Hazards: Noise pollution: neonatal aspects. Pediatrics 54:476, 1974
23. Catlett AT, Holditch-Davis D: Environmental stimulation of the acutely ill premature infant: physiological effects and nursing implications. Neonatal Network 8(6):19, 1990
24. Long GJ, Lucey JF, Philip AGS: Noise and hypoxemia in the intensive care nursery. Pediatrics 65:143, 1980
25. Kellman N: Noise in the intensive care nursery. Neonatal Network 1(8):8, 1982
26. Long JG, Philip MB, Lucey JF: Excessive handling as a cause of hypoxemia. Pediatrics 65:203, 1980
27. Murdoch DR, Darlow BA: Handling during neonatal intensive care. Arch Dis Child 59:957, 1984
28. Gorski PA, Hole WT, Leonard CH, Martin JA: Direct computer recording of premature infants and nursery care: distress following two interventions. Pediatrics 72:198, 1983
29. Speidel BP: Adverse effects of routine procedures on preterm infants. Lancet 1:864, 1978

30. Dangman BC, Hegyi M, Indyk L, James JS: The variability of PO_2 in newborn infants in response to routine care. Pediatr Res 10:422, 1976
31. Rawlings DJ, Miller PA, Engle RR: The effect of circumcision on transcutaneous PO_2 in preterm infants. Am J Dis Child 134:676, 1980
32. Cordero L, Hon EH: Neonatal bradycardia following nasopharyngeal stimulation. J Pediatr 78:441, 1971
33. Gleason CA, Martin RJ, Anderson JV et al: Optimal positioning for a spinal tap in preterm infants. Pediatrics 71:31, 1983
34. Mukhtar A, Strothers J: Cardiovascular effects of nasogastric tube feeding in the healthy preterm infant. Early Hum Dev 6:25, 1982
35. Fox WW, Schwartz BS, Schaffer TH: Pulmonary physiotherapy in neonates: physiologic changes and respiratory management. J Pediatr 92:997, 1978
36. Etches PC, Scott B: Chest physiotherapy in the newborn: effect on secretions removed. Pediatrics 62:713, 1978
37. Curran CL, Kachoyeanos MK: The effects on neonates of two methods of chest physical therapy. MCN 4:309, 1979
38. Gajodsik C: Transcutaneous monitoring of PO_2 during chest physical therapy in a premature infant. Phys Occup Ther Pediatr 5(4):69, 1985
39. Yeh TF, Lilien ST, Lew ST, Pildes RS: Increased O_2 consumption and energy loss in premature infants following medical care precedures. Biol Neonate 46:157, 1984
40. Sweeney JK: Neonatal hydrotherapy: an adjunct to developmental intervention in an intensive care nursery setting. Phys Occup Ther Pediatr 3(1):39, 1983
41. Sweeney JK: Physiological and behavioral effects of neurological assessment in preterm and full-term neonates, abstracted. Phys Occup Ther Pediatr 9(3):144, 1989
42. Kelly MK, Palisano RJ, Wolfson MR: Effects of a developmental physical therapy program on oxygen saturation and heart rate in preterm infants. Phys Ther 69:467, 1989
43. Langer VS: Minimal handling protocol for the intensive care nursery. Neonatal Network 9(3):23, 1990
44. D'Apolito K: What is an organized infant? Neonatal Network 10(1):23, 1991
45. Lott JW: Developmental care of the preterm infant. Neonatal Network 7(4):21, 1989
46. Als H, Lester B, Brazelton TB: Dynamics of the behavioral organization of the premature infant: a theoretical perspective. p. 173. In Field TM (ed): Infants Born At Risk. Spectrum Publications, New York, 1979
47. Als H, Lester B, Tronick EZ, Brazelton TB: Toward a research instrument for the assessment of preterm infants' behavior (APIB). p. 35. In Fitzgerald HE, Lester B, Yogman MW (eds): Theory and Research in Behavioral Pediatrics. Vol 1. Plenum Press, New York, 1982
48. Als H: Neonatal individualized developmental care and assessment program (NIDCAP): definition, training, and clinical application. p. 116. In Proceedings of the Seventh Annual Conference on Current Issues and Clinical Perspectives of Developmental Interventions in Neonatal Care, Anaheim, CA, November 6–8, 1991
49. Als H, Lawhon G, Gibes R et al: Individualized behavioral and environmental care for the VLBW preterm infant at high risk for bronchopulmonary dysplasia and intraventricular hemorrhage, study II: NICU outcome. In Proceedings of the Seventh Annual Conference on Current Issues and Clinical Perspectives of Developmental Interventions in Neonatal Care, Anaheim, CA, November 6–8, 1991
50. Zylke JW: Individualized care, as well as intensive care, may reduce morbidity among premature infants. JAMA 264:2611, 1990
51. Becker PT, Grunwald PC, Moorman J, Stuhr S: Outcomes of developmentally supportive nursing care for very low birth weights infants. Nurs Res 40:150, 1991

52. Sweeney JK, Chandler L: Neonatal physical therapy: medical risks and professional education. Inf Young Child 2(3):59, 1990

53. Sweeney JK, Swanson MW: At-risk neonates and infants: NICU management and follow-up. p. 183. In Umphred DA (ed): Neurological Rehabilitation. 2nd Ed. CV Mosby, St. Louis, 1990

54. Scull S, Deitz J: Competencies for the physical therapist in the neonatal intensive care unit (NICU). Pediatr Phys Ther 1:11,1989

55. Als H: Neonatal Individualized Developmental Care and Assessment Program (NIDCAP) Training Materials. Neurobehavioral Infant and Child Studies, Enders Pediatric Research Laboratories, Children's Hospital, Boston, 1981

56. Shepard KF: The effects of social environment on patient care. p. 73. In Payton OD (ed): Psychosocial Aspects of Clinical Practice. Churchill Livingstone, New York, 1986

57. Grinnell SK: Collaboration: a vital factor in group practice. Dent Clin North Am 16:357, 1972

58. Grinnell SK: Post conference reflections: autonomy and independence for health professionals? J Allied Health 18:115, 1989

APPENDIX 2-1

Observation Form for Neonatal Individualized Developmental Care and Assessment Program

OBSERVATION SHEET   Name _____   Date _____   Sheet Number _____

	Time:	52	54	56	58	9⁰⁰
	8	0-2	3-4	5-6	7-8	9-10
Resp:	Regular					
	Irregular	✓	✓	✓	✓	✓
	Slow	✓				✓
	Fast	✓			✓	✓
	Pause			✓		
Color:	Jaundice					
	Pink					
	Pale _(face)_	✓	✓✓	✓✓	✓	✓
	Webb					
	Red					
	Dusky	✓	✓	✓✓	✓	✓✓
	Blue					
	Tremor					
	Startle					
	Twitch Face		✓	✓	✓	✓
	Twitch Body	✓	✓	✓		
	Twitch Extremities					
Visceral/ Resp.	Spit up					
	Gag					
	Burp					
	Hiccough					
	BM Grunt					
	Sounds					
	Sigh	✓		✓	✓	
	Gasp					
Motor:	Flaccid Arm(s)					
	Flaccid leg(s)					
	Flexed/Tucked Arms Act/Post	✓	✓	✓	✓	✓
	Flexed/Tucked Legs Act/Post	✓	✓	✓	✓	✓
	Extend Arms Act/Post	✓	✓			
	Extend Legs Act/Post					
	Smooth Mvmt Arms					
	Smooth Mvmt Legs					
	Smooth Mvmt Trunk					
	Stretch/Drown					
	Diffuse Squirm	✓	✓✓		✓	
	Arch					
	Tuck Trunk	✓	A✓✓	✓P	✓P	P
	Leg Brace		✓	✓P	✓P	f
Face:	Tongue Extension					
	Hand on Face					
	Gape Face	✓	✓	✓	✓	✓
	Grimace				✓	
	Smile					

	Time:	0-2	3-4	5-6	7-8	9-10
State: 1A						
1B						
2A		✓	✓	✓	✓	✓
2B						
3A						
3B						
4A						
4B						
5A						
5B						
6A						
6B						
AA						
Face (cont.)	Mouthing	✓	✓			
	Suck Search					
	Sucking					
Extrem:	Finger Splay					
	Airplane					
	Salute					
	Sitting On Air					
	Hand Clasp					
	Foot Clasp	✓P	✓P	✓P	✓P	
	Hand to Mouth					
	Grasping		✓			
	Holding On	✓				
	Fisting					
Attention:	Fuss					
	Yawn					
	Sneeze					
	Face Open					✓?
	Eye Floating					
	Avert					
	Frown					
	Ooh Face					
	Locking					
	Cooing					
	Speech Mvmt					
Posture: (Prone, Supine, Side)		Side	→	→	→	→
Head: (Right, Left, Middle)		L	→	→	→	→
Location: (Crib, Isolette, Held)		Iso	→	→	→	→
Manipulation:		−	−	−	−	−
	Heart Rate	145	142	147	140	143
	Respiration Rate	34	42	54	46	54
	TcPO₂	97	47	97	97	47

(From Als, [55] with permission.)

30

APPENDIX 2-2

Training Sites for the Neonatal Individualized Developmental Care and Assessment Program (NIDCAP)

1. National NIDCAP Training Center, Boston, MA
   Brigham & Women's Hospital, Boston
   Children's Hospital, Boston
   Heidelise Als, PhD
   National Director, NIDCAP Training
   Associate Professor of Psychology
   Harvard Medical School
   Director of Neurobehavioral Infant and Child Studies
   Children's Hospital, Boston, MA
   Contact: Ted J. Gaiser, MTS
           Enders Pediatric Research Laboratories
           Room EN-029
           The Children's Hospital
           320 Longwood Ave
           Boston, MA 02115
           617/735-9249
2. CHO NIDCAP Training Center, Children's Hospital of Oklahoma
   Contact: Linda Lutes, MEd
           Oklahoma Infant Transition Program
           Room 3N-361
           University of Oklahoma
           940 North 13th St
           Oklahoma City, OK 73126
           405/271-6625
3. Oakland NIDCAP Training Center, Children's Hospital Medical Center
   Contact: Kathleen VandenBerg, MA
           Child Development Center
           Children's Hospital Medical Center
           52nd and Grove St
           Oakland, CA 94609
           415/428-3351

4. Saguaro NIDCAP Training Center, University Medical Center, Tucson
   Contact: Elsa Sell, MD
           University of Arizona Health Sciences Center, Room 3603
           501 North Campbell Ave
           Tucson, AZ 85724
           602/626-6627
5. Wake NIDCAP Training Center, Wake Medical Center
   Contact: James Helm, PhD
           Wake AHEC
           Wake Medical Center
           P.O. Box 14465
           Raleigh, NC 27620
           919/250-8276
6. Denver NIDCAP Training Center, Children's Hospital
   Contact: Joy V. Browne PhD, RN
           The Newborn Center
           Children's Hospital
           Box 535
           1056 East 19th Ave
           Denver, CO 80218
           303/861-3992

(From Als, [55] with permission.)

APPENDIX 2-3

Naturalistic Observation of Newborn Behavior (Preterm And Full Term Infants)

NATURALISTIC OBSERVATION OF NEWBORN BEHAVIOR
(PRETERM AND FULLTERM INFANTS)
Abbreviated Version

Name of Infant_____ Date_____
   Sex _♀_ Name of Observer _HA, LL, LL_
   Hospital & Record # _CH OK_ Parents' Names, Address, and Telephone #
_____

Maternal History:
   Pregnancy _4 prenatal visits, vag. bleeding_ Mother's Age _22_ G _7_ P _4_ Ab_2_ D_1_
   Labor & Delivery_____ Father's Age_____
   Other_____ Family Situation_____

Infant History:
   DOB _May 9.91_
   EDC _Aug '8 91_ (26?)
   Post Conc. Age at Birth _27_ wks____dys
   Mode of delivery _C-section_
   Birthweight _860_ g _25_ %
   Height at birth _30.5_ cm _<3_ %
   Head circ at birth _24_ cm _10_ %
   Apgars _5_ 1min _6_ 5min
   AGA_____ SGA_____ LGA_____
   Other_____

Current Status:
   Age Post Conception _37_ wks____dys
   Age Post Birth _10_ wks____dys
   Weight _1455_ g _<1_ %
   Height _385_ cm _<1_ %
   Head circumference _25_ cm _<1_ %

Respiratory Function
   Respirator _✓_ _for 49 days_
   Oxyhood _✓_
   Nasal Canula _✓_
   Highest inspired O2 _100%_
   No aid _—_
   Other_____ _—_

Respiratory Function
   Respirator _—_ rate_____
   CPAP _—_
   Oxyhood _✓ 70%_
   Nasal Canula _✓_ cc 31-63 FiO2____
   Inspired O2 required
   (prec, 24hrs) _1/32 - 1/16 ℓ_
   No aid _—_
   Respiration rate _38 - 80_
   Other _oxyg: 78 -100_

Medications
   Amp + Gent
   Indomethicin
   Lasix

Medications _Lasix_
   Dexamethasone

Mode of Feeding
   IV _✓_
   Gavage: nasal___ _✓_ oral_____
   Bottle_____
   Breast_____
   Type: breast milk___ formula _✓_ cal.____
   Caregiving Interval _Q2 - 3_
   Other_____

Mode of Feeding
   IV _✓ central line - hep lock_
   Gavage: nasal___ _✓_ oral_____
   Bottle_ —_
   Breast_ —_
   Type: breast milk___ formula _✓_ cal.___
   Caregiving Interval _q3_
   Feeding Interval _q 3° 27cc_

Complications _grade III ROP_
   Asphyxia_____
   RDS _✓_
   BPD _✓_
   Sepsis _—_
   IVH _—_ Grade_____
   Bili _✓_ Lights _✓_
   PDA _✓_ Repair _Endo_
   A. & B. _—_
   NEC _—_

Current Issues and Concerns
   O2 Dependency
   ROP
   Growth

Naturalistic Observation, p 2

Current Observation Circumstances   team II ✓

Location: Fullterm nursery_____ ICU_____ Intermediate____✓____ Isolation Room_____
             Parent's Room_____ NICU Parent Room_____ Home_____ Other_____

Environment: Table_____ Isolette __✓__ Mock Crib_____ Open Crib_____ Other_____

Bedding, Clothing, and Other Facilitation:
with soft cover   Mattress __✓__ Hammock_____ Waterbed_____ Sheepskin: natural_____ synthetic_____
       Bunting_____ Side rolls/Foot rolls __✓__ Clothing_____ Hat __✓__ Pacifier_____ Water gloves_____
big   Blanket: loose __✓__ secure_____ tight_____   in isolette
       Isolette/crib cover: partial_____ thin/light_____ thick/dark __✓__
       Personal items: pictures_____ photos_____ stuffed animals_____ decals_____
       Others: booties

Ambient Light, Sound, and Activity Levels:

Sound: 1 2 3 4 5 6 (7) 8 9
        1 is very quiet as if in a closed door parent room without interruption:
        9 is very noisy, for instance with radio on high volume, staff conversation, telephone ringing and
        monitors sounding
        Describe: ___alarms ongoing, staff talking about moonlighting, faucet___
        _____

Light: 1 2 3 4 5 6 7 8 (9)
        1 is a semi-dark room, shielded isolette, no overhead lights;
        9 is bright overhead and/or side lights, no covering on crib or isolette
        Describe: ___bright overhead light over isolette___
        _____

Activity: 1 2 3 4 5 6 7 (8) 9
        1 is very calm, quiet, soothing or no activity around the baby, e.g. no staff movement, or very soft
        unhurried walking, etc.;
        9 is hectic, continuously changing activity, with visitors, staff, x-ray machine, personnel hurrying
        about, water running, equipment being moved, etc.
        Describe: ___to + fro around beds + in room___
        _____

Caregiver(s) Observed: Physician_____ Nurse __✓__ Parent_____ OT/PT_____ Other_____

Manipulations Observed: (list in chronological sequence)___blood drawing, left alone (4)___
___feeding (6) repositioning (2)___
_____

Time and Duration of Observation: Pre-manipulation_____
                                           Peri-manipulation___16___
                                           Post-manipulation___14___
                                                    30 min.

_____

(From Als,[55] with permission.)

3

Neurobehavioral Assessment of the High-Risk Neonate

Irma J. Wilhelm

In the last several decades, as their role in the special care nursery setting has developed and expanded, physical therapists in pediatric practice have become increasingly involved with infants and, most recently, with neonates and their families.[1-5] As Sweeney[6] (see also Ch. 2) has described, neonatal physical therapy is a subspecialty within pediatric physical therapy practice that requires advanced training and competencies, including the ability to assess the neonatal environment. Advanced competencies also encompass the physical examination of high-risk neonates, including screening and in-depth assessment of neuromotor development and identification of movement disorders. The therapist is expected to conduct and interpret the results of standardized neonatal examinations in a reliable manner.[7]

Neonatal assessment methods can be used to examine individual differences in normal neonates or group differences in normal infants of differing cultural, ethnic, or racial backgrounds. They can also be directed at recognizing and describing departures from normal in compromised or high-risk neonates. Finally, we hope that neonatal assessment will be useful in describing change so that we can evaluate the effects of neonatal intervention and predict later developmental outcome, particularly for high-risk infants. The latter purpose has been the most problematic, as typically neonatal test results have not been very predictive of later outcome.[8] Several reasons are cited for this lack of predictiveness, including (1) the rapidly changing development of the neonate so that functions tested neonatally are very different from those tested at later ages; (2) the adaptability and plasticity of the neonate that allows a great deal of "recovery" from adverse perinatal events; (3) the influence of the environment on development, including the home, the caretakers, and society in general; and (4) the limited information that many of the currently available neonatal assessment instruments provide[8,9] (see also Chs. 1 and 12).

The focus of this chapter is on assessing infants at risk for developmental problems for the purposes of selecting those in need of therapeutic intervention, describing recovery from perinatal insults, predicting developmental outcome, and evaluating the effects of neonatal intervention. The aims of the chapter are to familiarize the reader with some of the types of neonatal assessment instruments that are available, to highlight and examine critically some selected tools that are appropriate for use by developmental therapists, and to suggest how those tools can be incorporated into physical therapy practice in the neonatal setting.

ASSESSMENT OF NEONATAL BEHAVIORAL STATE

Underlying any observation of neonatal behavior or functioning is the concept of behavioral state. Thoman[10] has written that "State is a contextual condition for all other behaviors of an organism. Thus, an understanding of state is fundamental for understanding behavior as well as neural and physiological functions." *Behavioral state* can be defined as a relatively stable, recognizable cluster of variables that occur and recur together and tend to be repeated.[11] In the neonate the variables most often used to distinguish behavioral states are eye movements, activity level, and respiratory pattern.

Full-Term Infant States

A number of systems for identifying and categorizing neonatal states have been developed since the initial works of Wolff,[12,13] who was the first to suggest an all-inclusive classification system. Classification systems vary somewhat, depending on the differences in the proponents' views of what *state* is, purposes for use of the systems, and professional backgrounds. Three systems are most commonly used in current neonatal research and clinical practice, those of Prechtl,[14] Brazelton,[15] and Thoman.[10] These systems have a number of similarities, but they also vary somewhat. The clinician must be aware of which system was used to describe states when reading the literature and interpreting reports of neonatal testing. The state categories included in each system are shown in Table 3-1, and examples of how some variables are described in each system appear in Table 3-2.

Prechtl,[14] a neurologist, believes that "States are distinct conditions, each having its specific properties and reflecting a particular mode of nervous function." He believes each state to be qualitatively different from the others and not levels on a continuum of nervous system arousal. He describes five mutually exclusive states using the dichotomized variables of respiration (irregular, regu-

Table 3-1. Neonatal Behavioral State Classification Systems

States	Prechtl	Brazelton	Thoman	
			Primary	Summary
Number	5	6	10	6
Sleep states	State 1	State 1, deep sleep	Quiet sleep	Quiet sleep
				Active-quiet transition sleep
	State 2	State 2, light sleep	Active sleep	Active sleep
	—	—	Active–quiet transition sleep	
Transition states	—	State 3, drowsy	Drowse	Drowse, daze
				Sleep–wake transition
			Daze	
			Sleep–wake, transition	
Awake states	State 3	State 4, alert	Alert	Alert
	State 4	State 5, eyes open, active	Nonalert waking	Nonalert waking
	—	—	Fuss	—
	State 5	State 6, crying	Cry	Fuss and cry

lar), eyes (open, closed), and movement (present, absent). The states are simply numbered from 1 to 5 (Tables 3-1 and 3-2).

Brazelton,[15] a developmental pediatrician, uses a behaviorally oriented state scale in which six states are named and described, some with dichotomous and some with more elaborate descriptions (Tables 3-1 and 3-2). This scale is an integral part of the Brazelton Neonatal Behavioral Assessment Scale (BNBAS).[15] The infant's ability to control state during the course of the examination is considered an important indicator of his or her current functioning.

Thoman,[10] an experimental psychologist, conceptualizes state organization within General Systems Theory and therefore believes that states are highly interrelated. She describes 10 Primary (sometimes collapsed into 6 Summary) States, and describes them with qualitative statements that definitely suggest continuity among the states (Tables 3-1 and 3-2). As does Brazelton, Thoman believes that the infant communicates with his or her environment and controls stimulus input by means of behavioral state.

Although the scales differ, some areas of agreement are evident. The scales all include two sleep states, described as differing in the parameters of body,

Table 3-2. Sample Descriptions of Neonatal Behavioral State Parameters

Description	Prechtl	Brazelton	Thoman
Respirations in quiet sleep state	Regular	Regular breathing	Relatively slow, regular, and abdominal in nature
Eyes in quiet awake state	Open	Open with bright look	Open, bright and shining, attentive, scanning
Motor activity in crying	Gross movements	High motor activity	—

eye, and respiratory activity, and two or three waking states, characterized by increasing levels of activity, one involving crying. The difference is primarily in the issue of transitions between and within state categories. Brazelton[15] and Thoman[10] describe one or more "drowsy" states that fall between sleep and wakefulness, while Prechtl[14] considers drowsiness to be a transition, but not a separate state. In addition, Thoman describes a transitional sleep state between quiet and active sleep. Much of the disagreement about transitions may relate to differences in the amount of time each proponent considers necessary for state parameters to be simultaneously present before the existence of a state can be declared. Prechtl considers anything less than 3 minutes to represent simply a transition between states, while Brazelton recognizes states that last at least 15 seconds, and Thoman records the prevailing state that occurs in a 10 second observational epoch.

Preterm Infant States

Thoman[10] and Prechtl[14] use their respective behavioral state classification systems for studying both full-term and premature infants. Thoman has stated that "We have found this classification of states, termed Primary States, to be appropriate for premature and full-term infants, and we have found them to be applicable throughout the first year of life, with no indication that they should not continue to apply at older ages." Prechtl et al.[16] do not recognize true states in the preterm infant because the state parameters do not occur or recur together for long enough periods until the infant approaches term-equivalent age (36 to 37 weeks).

Als et al.[17] have adapted the Brazelton state scale to assess premature infants. States are classified on one of two levels: *A* states are relatively undifferentiated and diffuse (premature infant) states, while *B* states are well-defined (full-term infant) states corresponding exactly to the states used by Brazelton.[18] A state is considered present when it has been recognized for about 3 seconds. This system also includes the notation of *AA*, which is used when the state becomes extremely disorganized and the infant manifests such danger signs as severe apnea and bradycardia, cyanosis, gastrointestinal upset or total flaccidity.[17]

Reliability of Neonatal State Assessment

Interobserver Reliability

State classification systems have been shown to have acceptable interobserver reliability. Prechtl[19] and Beintema[20] have reported 100 percent agreement among three observers in classifying the neonatal states of 80 infants during the course of administering the Prechtl and Beintema[21] neurologic examination. Colombo et al.[22] reported that over 95 percent agreement on a slightly modified version of the BNBAS state scale was achieved by the two experienced BNBAS examiners who collected data for their study of neonatal state profiles in 40 preterm and full-term infants. Thoman[10] has reported interobserver reliability of over 90 percent exact agreement for each state in a longitudinal study of 50 premature and full-term infants. Davis and Thoman[23] reported interrater reliabilities for a group of 9 premature and 28 full-term infants, ranging from 0.75 to 0.99 for seven of the states described by Thoman.[10]

Test–Retest Reliability

Test–retest reliability for neonatal assessment is not likely to be as high as one would expect if a relatively stable construct was being measured. Still, modest stability has been reported for measures of neonatal state. Colombo et al.[22] reported test–retest reliability with 37 premature and full-term infants retested at between 6 and 48 hour intervals, calculating both Pearson product moment correlation coefficients and intraclass correlations. Except for crying (0.56 and 0.76), all intraclass correlations were below 0.30 and all Pearson coefficients were below 0.56. These figures did not change appreciably when only the full-term infants were included in the calculations. The low correlations in this study could well have been partially the result of the fact that in 75 percent of the cases the two observations were made by different examiners and therefore true test–retest reliability was not being measured. Thoman[10] reported test–retest reliability for four weekly observations of 28 full-term infants. Reliability coefficients ranged from 0.46 to 0.76 for the Primary States and from 0.56 to 0.71 for the Summary States. The highest coefficients (0.70 or above) were for crying, active sleep, and alert states; the lowest was for sleep-wake transition (0.48).

Validity of Neonatal State Assessment

Discriminant Ability

Beintema[20] has reported age-related state differences using Prechtl's state categories in a longitudinal study. In the first 1 to 2 days of life, infants either had state instability or were predominantly in state 3 (eyes open, no gross movements). As the infants grew older, they were more likely to have predominant states of 4 (eyes open, gross movements) or 5 (crying). Theorell et al.[24] also reported age-related state differences in 20 healthy full-term infants observed for 6 hours within hours after birth and again on day 5 of life. On day 1, the infants spent from 33 to 50 percent of their time in awake states 3–5; this decreased to 7 to 13 percent on day 5. The percent of time in state 2 doubled between days 1 and 5, while state 1 percentage did not change. The durations of states 2 and 4/5 also varied, with state 2 duration increasing and states 4/5 decreasing between days 1 and 5. In general, day 1 was characterized by large and abrupt state changes and few epochs of stage 2. Prechtl et al.[25] examined behavioral state cycles in abnormal infants with either Down syndrome, hyperbilirubinemia, or high-risk pre- or perinatal histories who were observed for at least 6 hours between days 3 and 11 of life. Data were compared with the day 5 low-risk data from the previous study.[24] The state measures were distinctly different in the abnormal infants. Infants with Down syndrome had significantly increased percentages of time in awake states at the expense of decreased active sleep; infants with hyperbilirubinemia had decreased awake states with increased active sleep; and high-risk infants had increased quiet and decreased active sleep.

Davis and Thoman[23] compared behavioral states in 28 full-term and 9 low-risk preterm infants observed in their homes for seven hours at 2, 3, 4, and 5 weeks of age corrected for prematurity. Premature infants showed increased time in alert, nonalert waking and sleep–wake transition states and decreased time in drowse and in all sleep states. In addition, age-related changes were reported, namely, an increase in alert state and a decrease in active sleep over the 4 week period. Similar age-related changes were reported by Holditch-Davis[26] in a group of high-risk premature infants.

Colombo et al.[22] identified three neonatal state profiles from state observations of preterm and full-term infants. A "sleep" group had a high mean percentage of time in sleep states and high stability across observations made at two different times. This group included all the premature infants. An "alert-crying" group had equal mean percentages of time in active sleep, alert inactivity and crying, while an "unstable" group showed a predominance of active sleep and instability of profiles between the two observations. The groups also differed on some aspects of the BNBAS that was given at age 2 weeks. Infants in the sleep group had higher state regulation scores than the other two groups. Infants in the alert-crying group had higher modal orientation scores than did the sleep group.

Predictive Validity

Thoman[27] reported that categorization of infants as well organized or poorly organized, based on neonatal state observations, accurately predicted how their mothers described them during early infancy and at age 1 year. The mothers' descriptions were based on sleeping/waking habits, eating patterns, irritability, and mood changes. In another study, Thoman et al.[28] reported that low state stability scores derived from four weekly state profiles (weeks 2 to 5 of life) in a group of 22 healthy, full-term infants identified four infants who had significant later problems (one developed aplastic anemia at 30 months; one had seizures at 6 months; one suddenly died at 3.5 months; and one had severe hyperactivity at 30 months). Three other infants with low stability scores had low Bayley Mental Developmental Quotients at 21 or 30 months. No infants with stability scores above the median had any later developmental problems.

Moss et al.[29] in two studies with a total of 86 full-term, healthy neonates, reported that the range of states cluster of the BNBAS with Kansas supplements (NBAS-K)[30] correlated significantly with a visual discrimination task at age 3 months. They speculated that infants scoring high on this cluster are those with adaptive state organizational abilities who react with appropriate state changes to external stimulation and thus were able to respond with better visual discrimination of a novel stimulus at age 3 months.

Clinical Implications of Neonatal State Assessment

Korner[31] has suggested that state is often considered an obstacle to research that must be controlled, and less often as a precondition mediating the effectiveness of the infant's responses or as a variable to be studied in its own right. This statement applies equally to neonatal assessment. Behavioral state must be included in neonatal assessment systems because of its influence on infant responsiveness to testing and overall behavior.

Prechtl[19,32] states that behavioral state needs to be controlled during the course of a neonatal neurologic examination and also views state as a mediator of responsiveness. Instructions for administering and scoring each item in the neurologic examination include the optimal states in which the item can be administered as well as states that are contraindicated. In addition, the sequence of test items is designed to provide the maximum probability that each item can be administered in the optimal state. States are recorded at various points during the examination so that the pattern of state changes over the course of the examination is documented. Prechtl and associates[11,14] have demonstrated that state has a definite influence on some reflex testing. For example, monosynaptic reflexes (e.g., deep tendon reflexes, clonus, Moro) are very strong in state 1 (quiet sleep), intermediate in state 3 (quiet awake), but weak or absent in state 2 (active sleep). Conversely, polysynaptic reflexes (e.g., exteroceptive skin reflexes: root, grasp) are most active in state 2, weaker in state 3, and absent in state 1. Pressure responses (e.g., Babkin, palmomental) are strong in states 2 or 3 and absent in state 1. Nociceptive stimuli (e.g., Babinski) are strong in states 2 or 3 and slightly decreased in state 1. Auditory orienting is increased in state 3, and visual pursuit is only possible in state 3. Prechtl[14] concluded that these differences clearly demonstrate specific state dependency and support the concept of mutual exclusiveness and qualitative differences between states.

Brazelton[15] and Als et al.[17] include state in their behavioral assessments in a variety of ways. State is controlled in the sense that each item can only be administered if the infant is in certain state(s). State is also assessed in its own right through examination of alertness, state lability, consolability with or without intervention, level of arousal, rapidity of build-up to crying, and irritability. In assesssing premature infants, Als et al.[17] also examine the available range of states, the ability to move between states with flexibility and modulation, the ability to attain and maintain a quiet alert state with and without examiner assistance, and the degree and quality of responsiveness during the alert state.

In conclusion, the importance of assessing state during neonatal testing cannot be overemphasized. For that reason, the extent to which the assessment methods to be reviewed in this chapter include state control or measurement will be a major factor in how strongly they are recommended for use in pediatric physical therapy practice. In the discussion that follows, the assessment systems most highly recommended for use by therapists in neonatal settings will be reviewed in depth, although other tests will also be briefly described.

NEONATAL ASSESSMENT METHODS

Neurologic Assessment Systems

Neonatal neurologic assessments generally have as their major purposes evaluating the functional status of the nervous system, diagnosing peripheral and central nervous system abnormalities, identifying infants in need of further neurologic follow-up, and determining the effectiveness of medical treatment following a neurologic insult.[33] A number of systematic approaches have been developed that require neurologic training and expertise. These are briefly discussed so that therapists will understand their purposes, content, and interpretation. In addition, a short neurologic screening system that is appropriate for use by therapists is introduced and critically reviewed.

French Neurologists

A group of French neurologists, led by André-Thomas and Ste-Anne Dargassies, developed one of the first systematic neurologic examination systems specifically for assessing the newborn infant.[33-36] The system was adapted from the French adult neurologic assessment method, with its emphasis on the evaluation of muscle tone (see Ch. 9). Behavioral state is not measured, actively controlled, or manipulated during the examination. It is considered, however, in the sense that elicited responses are never deemed to be absent or diminished unless retested after an interval or under different conditions. This is because the influence of the infant's physiologic state (e.g., sleep, twilight state, wakefulness, hunger, contentment) on those reactions is recognized.[34]

According to the authors, "Neurological principles have determined the selection of signs [e.g., test items] and the relative importance that can be attributed to each of them."[34] Certain signs, however, were considered to have pathologic meaning, especially if they were asymmetric, persistent, or multiple. The system is applicable to neonates 1 to 10 days of age. It was developed to provide a neurologic diagnosis and to describe the neurologic mechanisms implicated.

Based on her work with André-Thomas, Ste-Anne Dargassies[37] developed an examination protocol for full-term infants that was used to establish a profile of the normal neonate. She has also developed sequential, stage-oriented neurologic examination techniques for assessing neuromaturation of premature infants between 28 and 41 weeks of gestation. The examination is designed to assess maturational level and characteristics of posture, activity, reactivity, mobility, muscle tone, reflexes and reactions, neurovegetative functions, and pathologic phenomena. The influence of behavioral state in the full-term examination is acknowledged in the sense that the examination is only performed when the infant is fully awake, and the infant is kept awake by the examiner. One interesting item, called *vigilance* is assessed. Vigilance is considered to be "a specific feature which has nothing to do with the state of consciousness."[37] It is "a quality of alertness such that the infant exhibits both receptivity and reactivity. He can accept or refuse to respond to a stimulus; . . . he can stay awake, calmly, without crying, as if in expectation."[37] In the premature infant, vigilance is not achieved until after 32 weeks of gestation. After that time, vigilance becomes more lasting and the infant is more often awake or more easily awakened. The preterm infant who has reached the age of a full-term newborn infant is described as more excitable and restless and having a short attention span compared with a full-term infant born at term. Ste-Anne Dargassies asked: "Is this a vestige or a prelude?"[37]

Although these pioneers in neonatal neurology have left a rich legacy for the neurologic study of the neonate, their assessment methods were, for the most part, based on a concept of the neonate as a "tonic animal with oropharyngeal and other automatisms and neuro-vegetative mechanisms."[34]

The Neurologic Examination of the Full-Term Newborn Infant

This neurologic examination system was originally developed by Prechtl and Beintema[21] and then revised and updated by Prechtl.[32] As has been discussed, Prechtl and Beintema[21] are recognized as the first to incorporate fully the concept of behavioral state into neonatal assessment. The purpose of this examination system is to document the condition of the nervous system in order to diagnose neurologic abnormalities and to identify infants in need of ongoing neurologic follow-up.[32,36] The instrument was designed as a measure of central nervous system (CNS) integrity, not as a measure of developmental maturation.[36] Underlying this examination is the concept of the CNS as a system that initiates, regulates, and adapts neuromotor behavior.[33,36] The examination therefore is not designed to detect local lesions, but to obtain information about complex neural functions.[32] The examination can be used with full-term infants (38 to 42 weeks of gestation) and with preterm infants who have reached that age, especially those at risk for CNS dysfunction on the basis of less than optimal pre- and postnatal conditions.[36] The items were selected to be age-specific and to represent functional subsystems of the CNS. The examination includes evaluation of physical features, tone, reflexes, automatic reactions, posture, and spontaneous movement.

Some reliability data based on the original version of the examination are reviewed by Harris and Brady.[36] Test–retest reliability ranged from 0.70 to 1.00, with behavioral state being most reliable and muscle tone least reliable. In another study,[20] significant test–retest reliability coefficients were obtained in examinations given on the first and second days of life for 26 of 30 items.

A number of research efforts that tend to support the discriminant validity of the system are reviewed by Francis et al.[38] The test discriminated infants born with prolonged vacuum extraction from normally delivered infants and full-term infants from preterm infants at term-equivalent age. The concurrent and predictive validity of the examination has also been examined. Beintema[20] has summarized some prognostic work performed by Prechtl and some concurrent findings of his own, based on the identification of three syndromes (apathy syndrome, hyperexcitability syndrome, and hemisyndrome) from the neurologic examination results. Overall, 73 percent of the children who had originally been classified by any one or more of the syndromes were still abnormal at 2 to 4 years of age. Those who had multiple syndromes had the worst prognoses.

Few investigators have used these syndromes for predictive purposes, but several other reports of predictive validity are available and were reviewed by Palisano and Short.[33] In two studies the neonatal neurologic results were compared with neurologic outcome at 2 to 4 years of age. In both studies the ability to predict abnormal outcome correctly (sensitivity) was over 80 percent, but the false-positive rate was also high (45 and 26 percent). In one other study, Bierman-van Eenderburg et al.[39] reported a false-positive rate of over 87 percent and the predictive value of a positive test of only 16 percent. In all fairness, Prechtl has repeatedly warned against using abnormal neurologic signs in neonates to predict future neurologic outcome, citing the transient nature of many of those signs and the rapid developmental changes in the infant nervous system. He recommends repeated examinations to monitor the resolution or permanency of neonatal signs.[19,32,33]

Neurologic Assessment During the First Year of Life

A somewhat more contemporary view of the newborn infant is taken by Amiel-Tison and Grenier.[40] In the preface to their book, they cite the effect on neonatal neurology of recent research on newborn infant competencies. The purposes of the system are to identify neuromotor differences or abnormalities and to monitor neuromotor development.[36] Although the examination is based on the works of the previously described French neurologists and relies heavily on reflex and muscle tone assessment, it also includes consideration of behavioral state. State is controlled in that the examination is only performed with the infant in an awake state (Prechtl states 3 or 4). The infant's caretaker is asked to describe the usual sleep and waking patterns, and the infant's predominant state of consciousness (normal, lethargic, hyperexcitable) and state changes are noted during the testing. The examination is designed to be given serially during the first year of life and can be used with preterm infants when they reach term gestation.

In one reliability study of the assessment of passive tone, two examiners had from 50 to 90 percent agreement within 10 degrees for hip adductors, heel-to-toe maneuver, popliteal angle, ankle dorsiflexion, and scarf sign ratings.[41] Wetzel and Wetzel[42] have reported percentage agreement of over 90 percent for repeated administrations of the examination, but provided little information on the numbers tested, the number of examiners involved, and the items examined for reliability. Very little validity information is available using the current form of the examination.[36]

In addition to the routine neurologic assessment, these authors also described a complementary neuromotor examination that is designed to affirm normality soon after birth[40] (see also Ch. 12). The examination is based on the concept that a newborn infant can perform activities usually acquired at a later age if head control can be artificially imposed to overcome the "physiological impotence of the neck," thus enabling the infant to perform "liberated motor activity".[40] The infant is examined in sitting or semireclining positions, with the examiner manually fixing the neck. The infant at first may fight the forces holding him, but within a few minutes calms down and begins to orient to the surroundings. Eventually, the infant begins to make spontaneous movements that resemble those of an older infant, and reflexes are much inhibited. The examiner can also then guide the infant in directed motor activities of various sorts, such as assisted movement from sidelying to sitting over the edge of the table, during which the infant may bear weight on the forearm and hand of the lower arm and may be able to reach for an object. The authors believe that the ability to perform liberated activities indicates sound CNS organization and is incompatible with brain damage. They see this method as essential for assessing high-risk infants who may have identifiable, but probably transient, abnormalities, as a means of reassuring their parents of the integrity of the infant's nervous system and the competence of their baby. The complementary examination anticipates future development, as it eliminates the effect of transient abnormalities. Used in combination with the classic examination, which serves to identify abnormalities, it is able to rule out permanent handicap. The classic examination, however, is more predictive of minor handicap at school age.[40]

These assessment systems are primarily designed for use by neurologists and neonatologists for identification of infants needing further neurologic evaluation and for aiding in diagnosing current neurologic problems. Developmental therapists may want to screen the neurologic functioning of high-risk neonates in the process of monitoring their developmental status. For that purpose, a relatively new neurologic screening instrument is appropriate for use by nonphysician personnel.

Infant Neurological International Battery

Brief Description

The Infant Neurological International Battery (INFANIB)[43,44] is a criterion-referenced battery of 20 items designed to assess the neurologic integrity of infants being monitored following treatment in neonatal intensive care units. It is appropriate for use with neonates and infants up to 9 months of age. Fourteen items can be assessed in the neonatal period; six others are added between 3 and 9 months of age. The items consist of measures of muscle range and resistance to passive movement (e.g., scarf sign, popliteal angle), reflexive responses (e.g., foot grasp, ATNR), equilibrium reactions (e.g., parachute responses), and quality of certain milestones (e.g., sitting position, weight bearing in standing).

Technical Evaluation

Test Development. A 32-item pool for the INFANIB was generated from four other methods of neurologic examination.[41,45–47] and assigned 5-point ordinal scales ranging from "severely abnormal" to "normal." The 32 test items were field tested by two physical therapists with a group of 308 infants aged 3 to 22 months who had been treated in the neonatal intensive care setting. The examiners also scored each infant on a 5-point degree of neurologic abnormality scale ranging from "severely abnormal" to "normal" and assigned each infant to a category of abnormality (e.g., spastic quadriplegia, hypotonia, transient abnormality). Correlations among the 32-item scores were subjected to factor analyses yielding five factors that described the data well. The four items that loaded most highly on each factor were selected to measure the factors, thus producing the 20-item final battery. The five factors are spasticity, vestibular function, head and trunk, French angles/resting tone, and legs. The internal consistency of each factor score ranged from 0.72 for legs to 0.89 for French angles and vestibular function. The total score internal consistency was 0.91 (0.88 for infants 7 months of age or younger; 0.93 for infants 8 months of age or older). The 20-item test was subjected to clinical testing by physical therapists and physicians. A number of clinicians had difficulty with the 5-point range; therefore the 5-point scale was collapsed to a 3-point scale. Cutting points for total scores were determined for three degrees of abnormality (abnormal, transient, normal) for each of three age groups (under 4 months, 4 to 8 months, over 8 months).

Evidence of Reliability. The source article includes no report of reliability measures. The authors acknowledge that interrater and test–retest reliabilities need to be examined and await further study.[43] The authors of an unpublished thesis research project done with 65 high-risk Colombian infants reported an intertester reliability for total scores of 0.97 (among seven physical therapy students trained for 5 days) and a test–retest reliability of 0.95 (Angel Castro V, De Sanchez IE, Landinez NS, unpublished data).

Evidence of Validity. The authors of the INFANIB[43] demonstrated the ability of the total INFANIB score to discriminate among the five degrees of abnormality/normality at two age levels (7 months or younger and 8 months or older). In addition, factor subscores were able to discriminate (over 80 percent correct) among categories of normality/abnormality except for the category of hypotonia (only 39 percent correct).

In a retrospective study using 243 premature infant hospital records, Stavrakas et al.[48] examined the ability of INFANIB factor and item scores obtained at corrected age of 6 months to predict the development of cerebral palsy in premature infants at corrected age of 12 months. Discriminant analysis with all factor scores showed the vestibular function factor to be most predictive of cerebral palsy (87.1 percent), followed by spasticity (86.8 percent). French angles were marginally predictive, while the head and trunk factor was not predictive. Items 1 (hands closed or open), 14 (tonic labryinthine-prone), 15 (sitting), and 16 (sideways parachute) were the most predictive (83.3 percent). The vestibular function and spasticity factors were also the most highly correlated with the Bayley Psychomotor Development Index.

Hansen and colleagues[49] used the INFANIB at discharge and at corrected ages of 6 to 8 months in a prospective study of outcome in 35 infants with cystic intracranial lesions. The predictive value of the INFANIB given at discharge was poor, as all but three of the infants were classified as abnormal or suspect at the time of discharge. The INFANIB given between 6 and 8 months of corrected age, however, correctly classified 86 percent of the infants as measured by the Baylay Scales at age 12 months or older. The sensitivity of the INFANIB was 96 percent, the false-positive rate was 13 percent, and the predictive value of a positive test was 97 percent. The specificity, however, was only 50 percent, and the false-negative rate was 20 percent. The predictive value of a negative test was 80 percent. Because this was a sample of extremely high-risk infants, the sensitivity and predictive values of a positive test may be higher than would be expected in a more typical sample of infants discharged from intensive care.

Qualitative Evaluation

The INFANIB can be completed and scored in a few minutes. The scoring sheet is used to record both the performance of the infant and the item, factor, and total scores. The examiner circles the correct item description as the child is examined and then uses the score sheet to match the description to that expected at the child's age in order to assign the score. Cut-off scores for the three age groups are given on the score sheet, as well as a space to record the category of abnormality. Detailed descriptions for administering the items are included in an appendix to the source article.[43] The source article does not include any examiner training requirements. The two physical therapists who participated in the test development were highly skilled in administering and scoring the quantified Milani-Comparetti and Gidoni method developed by El-lison et al.[50]

Summary Evaluation

This tool seems appropriate for follow-up of infants in special infant care clinics, in conjunction with developmental and behavioral testing. It does not, however, contain methods for either controlling or measuring behavioral state during the examination. A number of the items on the INFANIB would be repeated if the physical therapist were also using one of the neurobehavioral tests reviewed in the next section. Because of the paucity of information on the reliability of this tool, therapists planning to use it in their practices should establish their own test–retest reliability as well as interrater reliability rates if more than one person will be examining the same infants over time.

Neurobehavioral Assessment Systems

This category of examination includes both neurologic items and behavioral items. Most of these tests have their neural origins in the French neurologists' methods for assessing muscle tone[34,37] and in the methods of Prechtl[32] for assessing automatic reactions and postural responses. The behavioral items are usually adapted from the BNBAS.[15] The two most thoroughly developed of these scales are the BNBAS for use with full-term neonates and the Assessment of Premature Infant Behavior (APIB)[17] for assessing the competence of preterm and full-term neonates.

The Brazelton Neonatal Behavioral Assessment Scale

The BNBAS is based on a conceptual model of newborn organization that has several major premises: (1) that the healthy newborn infant is a competent social being who participates in shaping his or her own environment; (2) that the neonate is a complex being with a wide range of behaviors, including the capacity to demonstrate nonstereotyped graded responses, to inhibit responses, and to interact socially; and (3) that the neonate is a rapidly changing being who has developmental tasks to accomplish within a very short time after birth. The major tasks are to achieve control of behavioral states so that the quiet, alert state can be maintained, thus allowing the neonate to respond to his or her parents in an interactive, social manner.

The Brazelton Neonatal Behavioral Assessment Scale

Brief Description

The BNBAS[15] is made up of a number of ordinal scales. Eighteen elicited responses are measured on 4-point scales (ranging from 0, not able to be elicited; to 3, hyperactive response). These include a number of neonatal reflexive responses, as well as some vestibular responses and an assessment of passive muscle tone. The neurologic items are considered only a rough screen for neurologic integrity and are used primarily to assess the infant's ability to cope with the increasing amount of handling that occurs as they are administered. The meat of the examination is the 28 behavioral items that are scored on 9-point scales that include very detailed descriptions for each scoring point. The behavioral portion of the examination includes items for assessing response decrement to repetitive stimuli, motor abilities, visual and auditory orientation, and behavioral state expression and control.

The BNBAS is appropriate for use with newborn infants from 36 to 44 weeks gestational age, although the author suggests use of some supplementary items when examining infants born at 37 weeks gestation or earlier. These items are also scored on 9-point scales and are designed to assess the preterm infant's fragility and difficulty with self-regulation. The test is not appropriate for use with infants at less than 36 weeks gestational age or with any infant who is still on life support systems.

The infant's best performance is scored on the BNBAS, as the author believes that this is a way to control for the variability in performance, often out of the examiner's control, that might mask the infant's true capabilities. The NBAS-K[30] incorporates modal scoring of some of the items. Scores on the BNBAS are most commonly aggregated into clusters of behaviors for interpretation and data analysis. A number of clustering systems have been developed for this purpose.[51–54]

Originally developed for the purpose of studying individual differences in neonates that might contribute to the infant–parent relationship and for use in studying differences in groups of infants in cross-cultural studies, the uses to which the BNBAS has been put have expanded greatly since its first publication.[18] It has been used to study the effects of various prenatal and perinatal factors on neonatal performance (e.g., maternal malnutrition, intrauterine drug exposure, maternal diabetes, obstetric medication, cesarean section). Another use has been to predict parent–infant interaction and caretaking behaviors. Evaluation with the BNBAS at the time of discharge of preterm and high-risk infants as a basis for later special infant follow-up is another common use, as is its use as an intervention with parent participation to introduce parents to the behavioral capabilities and individual style of their infant.[38,55–57]

Technical Evaluation

Test Development. The manual provides little information on how BNBAS items were developed or selected, only that it "has been developed over a number of years with the help of a large number of direct and indirect collaborators."[15] The BNBAS has not been normed, but it is administered with reference to the behavior expected on the third day of life of a full-term neonate who weighed over 7 pounds at birth; whose Apgar scores were no lower than 7 at 1, 8 at 5, and 8 at 15 minutes after delivery; whose mother had 100 mg or less of barbiturates and 50 mg or less of other sedatives prior to delivery; who had an apparently normal intrauterine experience; and who required no special care after delivery.[15]

Evidence of Reliability. Training for clinical and research use of the BNBAS requires attaining interobserver reliability of 90 percent or better within one point on the 9-point scales and perfect agreement on the 4-point scales. This percentage can be maintained for several years with continued use of the scales.[38,58] Clopton and Martin[59] have noted that the reported reliability may be inflated because many of the scales contain some rarely used scores, resulting in a restricted functional range of scores. This in turn is exacerbated by allowing a 1-point discrepancy to count as an agreement. They recommend that exact agreement, which may be only around 50 percent, be reported. DiPietro and Larson[60] have suggested that differences in examiner style may introduce substantial variance into the BNBAS when the same infant is actually tested rather than just observed by a second examiner. In their study, however, this conclusion was reached on the basis of two observers testing the same infant, but on two consecutive days and using an invariant order of item presentation. Infants tested at such an interval would not be expected to have stable scores even if tested by the same individual. In addition, an invariant item presentation is not considered appropriate when administering the BNBAS, as it often precludes obtaining the infant's best performance.[15]

Test–retest reliability on the BNBAS is usually modest.[38,52] Although psychometricians may criticize this lack of stability in scores, most neonatal researchers believe that the lack of stability is reflective of the dynamically changing nature of neonatal behavior. Stability of test scores therefore may not be a valid criterion for judging the adequacy of any neonatal test.[38,52] On the other hand, Linn and Horowitz[61] have suggested that the individual infant's stability or variability (which ranged from 0.18 to 0.75 over 2 days in their study of 28 low socioeconomic status neonates) may be a variable worth studying in its own right as to its relationship with or effect on other variables, for example, maternal behavior.

The internal consistency of the various BNBAS item clusters has been the source of considerable study. When factor analysis is performed in an attempt to group items based on their statistical interrelationships, two dimensions of behavior are quite consistently demonstrated, one indicative of alertness and orientation, and the other of arousal and irritability. A motor dimension is sometimes found, but not as consistently.[52,62–64] The item groupings of the a priori clusters[51,62] sometimes are not corroborated in factor analytic studies, even though they have face validity. Jacobson et al.[54] have developed a revised set of seven clusters that demonstrate greater internal consistency and stronger test–retest reliability than the original clusters[52] on which they are based.

Evidence of Validity. The ability of the BNBAS to discriminate among groups of infants has been demonstrated many times.[38,55] Reliable differences have been noted among infants of different cultures and socioeconomic status, as well as infants differing in amount of maternal obstetric medication[65–67]; maternal diabetic status[68]; intrauterine drug exposure[69–72]; birth weight[73,74]; gestational age at birth[75]; perinatal and neonatal risk factors[73]; persistent pulmonary hypertension of the newborn[76]; and hyperbilirubinemia.[77] Gyurke et al.[64] compared three a priori cluster scoring methods for their ability to discriminate among healthy preterm, healthy full-term, sick full-term, and full-term infants with sick mothers. They concluded that to some extent all the methods distinguished healthy from medically at-risk infants on motor maturity and orientation dimensions but that no one system captures the richness of newborn behaviors. The BNBAS was sensitive to developmental changes in premature infants assessed longitudinally from 35 to 44 weeks postconceptional age.[78] Positive effects on various aspects of parent–infant interaction have been reported when the BNBAS is used as a parent education or intervention tool.[56,79]

Some ability of the BNBAS to predict later infant behavior or test performance has been reported. Lester[52,80] developed a method for measuring patterns of change (recovery curves) over three repeated examinations that predicted 63 percent of the variance in 18-month Bayley mental scale outcome in term and preterm infants.

Qualitative Evaluation

The BNBAS requires approximately 30 to 35 minutes to administer and 10 to 15 minutes to score, once an examiner has undergone the training process suggested. Examiner training involves a several stage program of consultation with trained examiners and self-training to achieve reliability.*

Once the observation is scored, the examiner will probably want to use one of the available systems for grouping the items into clusters in order to prepare a written or oral report of the examination and to pinpoint the dimensions that demonstrate the infant's strengths and weaknesses for future program planning.

Summary Evaluation

Learning to administer the BNBAS is an extremely valuable way to increase one's knowledge of normal newborn behavior and its possible effects on infant caregivers. This is because, as the examiner, one is not just administering and scoring items, one is also participating with the infant in an interactive situation so that one is in the position of being affected by, as well as eliciting, aspects of the infant's behavior. Competence in use of the BNBAS can also be a valuable first step in the process of becoming proficient in examining preterm and at-risk infants. It gives one the basic handling skills needed but without the worry of stressing a fragile infant while one is perfecting ones skills. It also instills in one the basic sequence for testing and scoring procedures upon which the APIB is

---

* Information about the training program can be obtained from Director of BNBAS Training, Child Development Unit, The Children's Hospital, 300 Longwood Ave, Boston, MA 02115.

based so that one has less to absorb should one wish to study that more detailed assessment system.

The Assessment of Preterm Infants' Behavior

The APIB is the most comprehensive neurobehavioral tool for assessing neonatal behavior.[17] It has a rich theoretical base derived from a number of developmental principles that are integrated into the principle of synaction[81–83]: (1) the principle of species adaptedness, an ethological principle that, at any stage of its development, an organism is to some extent "hard-wired" for species-specific behaviors that enable adaptation to its particular environment; (2) the principle of continuous organism–environment transaction, that an organism grows and differentiates in part through interaction with the environment; (3) the principle of orthogenesis and syncresis, that development proceeds from a state of relative diffuseness to one of increasing differentiation and organization; and (4) the principle of dual antagonist interaction, incorporating the notion of two basic types of responses, approach and avoidance, that must be in balance for the organism to function smoothly.

Based on these principles, the views of the full-term newborn infant and of the preterm infant differ within the synactive theory of infant development.[81–85] In the full-term infant the subsystems of autonomic, motor, and state organization are quickly restabilized after birth. The attention/interactive system is newly emerging and changes most rapidly, especially the stabilization of the quiet alert state, within the first several weeks of life. The preterm infant, on the other hand, while well equipped for existence within the intrauterine environment, is in a "mismatch" situation when forced to function in the extrauterine world. With preterm birth, medical technology is focussed on stabilizing the autonomic functions to sustain life, while the motor, sensory, and state systems are typically not given as much attention. As a result of premature birth, some of the infant's systems are triggered into functioning before they are mature, some are accelerated through medical intervention, motoric containment is lost, as is the constant cutaneous stimulation provided by the fluid environment, gravity is imposed on the motor system, sensory input is no longer muted, states are not yet fully differentiated, and maternal diurnal rhythms are lost. The agenda for the preterm infant therefore is to attain a well-defined sleep state and to stabilize autonomic functions. Movement and tactile and vestibular manipulations easily upset physiologic balance and sleep.

The APIB was developed as an instrument designed to identify and track the precursors of the typical subtle neuromotor, learning, and behavior problems seen so often in children who were prematurely born, even in the absence of any documented direct brain insult.[83] In this respect the parameters for assessment that are encompassed in the instrument are (1) the currently emerging developmental agenda of the infants and their state of development; (2) the current level of balance of the various subsytems; (3) the threshold of disorganization evident as the systems are tested; (4) the degree of modulation and regulation of the systems; (5) the degree of differentiation of the systems; (6) the degree of environmental structure, support, and facilitation needed for optimal functioning or returning to balance; and (7) the strategies used by the infant for self-regulation and the effectiveness of those strategies.[81-87]

The Assessment of Preterm Infants' Behavior

Brief Description

The APIB is an individually administered battery of ordinal scales proposed for use in documenting systematically the behavior repertoire of the premature infant; observing behavioral changes over time for charting development and measuring progress; and aiding parents in learning about their infant's strengths, areas of disorganization, and cues and to develop their skills in facilitating their infant's development. It is appropriate for use with preterm, at-risk, and full-term neonates, provided that the infant is medically stable in an open isolette or crib at room temperature and in room air.

The instrument is a refinement and extension of the BNBAS and uses the BNBAS maneuvers in graded packages of increasing stimulation. The packages include (1) sleep/distal stimulation (response decrement items); (2) sleep/uncover and turn to supine; (3) low-grade localized tactile input to extremities and face in supine (e.g., hand and foot grasp reflexes, root, suck); (4) medium tactile input combined with medium vestibular input (e.g., undressing, pull-to-sit, asymmetric tonic neck reflex); (5) massive tactile input combined with massive vestibular input (rotation in vertical suspension, Moro response); and (6) social interaction (with examiner) and orientation to inanimate auditory and visual stimuli. In addition to scoring the BNBAS scales, the APIB contains a number of additional scales designed to document premature infant behavior, including stress and regulatory behaviors. Before, during, and after administering each package the infant is also monitored along five subsystems of functioning (physiologic, motor, state, attention/interactive, and self-regulatory) and for the amount of examiner facilitation needed to attain optimal performance or to assist in returning to balance.

Technical Evaluation

Test Development. The APIB items are in part derived from the BNBAS. Additional items for documenting preterm infant behavior and subsystem functioning were created based on the developmental principles and parameters for assessment believed to be important for identifying precursors for later development and on the authors' extensive experience in observing the behavior of preterm and at-risk infants. No specific content validation or standardization procedures are described in the manual.

Evidence of Reliability. Interobserver agreement within one point on the 9-point scales and exact agreement on the 4-point scales for 90 percent of the items can be obtained with the extensive training required for APIB reliability.

Evidence of Validity. APIB systems, package, and examiner facilitation scores consistently discriminate preterm from full-term infant performance when infants are tested at equivalent postconceptional ages,[82,83,86,88,89] indicating that preterm infants are more sensitive and reactive to input, more easily stressed and overstimulated, and need more environmental structure and support than do full-term infants. In addition, system scores can be used to classify infants by behavioral organization and competence independent of maternal variables (e.g., age, parity, socioeconomic status, ethnicity) and gender, and not synonymous with (although influenced by) gestational age at birth.[86,90] This latter ability is seen as the first step in predicting later functioning if newborn competence and organization is an analog of later functional competence.

Classification into neonatal competency groups via the APIB systems scores has shown significant concordance with similar classification derived from scores obtained on a play paradigm, the Kangaroo Box (K-Box). The K-Box measures physiologic, gross and fine motor, cognitive, vocalization, affective, self-regulatory, object play, social interactive, facilitation needed, and pleasure and pride subdomains at 9 months and at 3 and 5 years of age.[83,86,89] Significant concordance has also been shown with a neuropsychological battery classification system.[89] Variables that especially discriminate the groups at the later ages are measures of spatial processing, freedom from distraction, sequential processing, gross and fine motor modulation, and affective social regulation. Als[89] has concluded that a profile of regulatory difficulties characteristic of preterm infants, especially those born very early, is consistent to 5 years of age and occurs in the absence of documented brain injury.

Like the BNBAS, the APIB has also been used in an intervention paradigm to educate parents about their premature infants. Culp et al.[91] reported that parents who observed an APIB examination and received feedback from the examiner reported less anxiety (fathers), more realistic perceptions of their infant (both parents), and more awareness of their infant's abilities (mothers) than did parents who did not observe the assessment.

Qualitative Evaluation

The APIB, although still considered primarily a research instrument, is gaining support as a clinical instrument as well. Although it is a long test to administer (30 to 45 minutes) and score (45 to 60 minutes) and requires an extensive committment for training, professionals in NICU practice are extremely pleased with the information it provides about individual infant functioning, especially for use in developmental consultation and discharge planning with professional colleagues and parents (Neonatal Developmental Team, Wake Medical Center, Raleigh, NC, personal communication).

Reliability training for research and clinical use of the APIB is the second level of the Neonatal Individualized Developmental Care and Assessment Program (NIDCAP) training, the first stage of which has been described by Sweeney (Ch. 2). NIDCAP naturalistic observational training is helpful but not required prior to APIB reliability training. APIB training consists of four stages. The first, preparatory stage is particularly necessary for nonmedical personnel and consists of establishing liaison with medical and nursing staff of the special care nursery, attending daily rounds, observing normal and high-risk deliveries, extensive reading, gaining competence in handling preterm and at-risk infants, observation at various times during a 24-hour period, learning the maneuvers of the APIB, and practice with at least one full-term and three to four NICU infants who are stable and nearly ready for discharge. The second stage is a demonstration day with an APIB trainer to clarify issues of administration and scoring. The trainer examines the baby, and trainees observe and then score and discuss the scoring and testing procedures. The third stage is the examination and scoring of at least 25 babies by the trainee in his or her own NICU. The final stage is the reliability session in which the trainee examines and scores two infants reliably with the trainer according to the 90 percent agreement criteria.**

Summary Evaluation

When the validity of the current lengthy instrument has been well established, and sufficient numbers of infants have been tested for reliable statistical methods to be applied, one would hope that the instrument itself will be examined for item internal consistency, item reliability, item redundancy, item definitional clarity, and the like so that the test can be simplified to the extent possible for clinical use. The APIB holds great promise as an instrument that can demonstrate continuity from the neonatal period to later developmental stages. The construct it measures—neonatal organizational competence—may be the area that has been so elusive in predicting from early to later developmental competence. If this is the case, the instrument will be invaluable for identifying infants at risk for neurobehavioral sequelae of perinatal complications and structuring of intervention programs to prevent or minimize those problems.

Other Neurobehavioral Assessment Methods

As valuable as these tools are, not everyone will be able to commit the time and resources necessary to achieve reliability for use of the BNBAS or APIB. Several other neurobehavioral examination systems are available, some of which are still under development, that have promise for assessing neonatal behavior in a number of domains. These include the Dubowitz' Neurological Assessment of the Preterm and Full-term Newborn Infant,[92] the Morgan Neonatal Neurobehavioral Examination,[93] the Neurobehavioral Assessment for Preterm Infants,[94] and the Neonatal Neurological Examination.[95]

** Two training centers provide APIB reliability training: [1] Boston Training Center, [Contact Heidelise Als, PhD] Enders Pediatric Research Laboratories, The Children's Hospital, 320 Longwood Avenue, Boston MA 02115, 617/735-8249; and [2] Saguaro Training Center [Contact Elsa Sell, MD] University Medical Center, 1501 North Campbell Avenue, Tucson AZ 85724, 602/626-6627.)

The Neurological Assessment of the Preterm and Full-Term Newborn Infant

Brief Description

The Neurological Assessment of the Preterm and Full-term Newborn Infant (Dubowitz)[92] is a criterion-referenced system that is applicable to all infants, including preterm and sick infants. Its purpose is to record the functional state of the nervous system and to document premature infant neurologic maturation and recovery from perinatal insult.

The test includes 2 habituation items to visual and auditory stimuli; 16 movement and tone items; 6 reflex items; and 9 neurobehavioral items (including orientation, defensive reactions, and several items assessing various state-related concepts). The Brazelton[15] state definitions are used, and the state of the infant is recorded as each item is administered. No particular states are required for testing of movement and tone items, but states are designated for testing habituation and the neurobehavioral items.

Technical Evaluation

Test Development.   The test was developed based on the authors' concern that no instrument was available as a day-to-day neonatal neurologic assessment tool. They set some basic requirements for such a tool, including reliability for use immediately after birth and for preterm and full-term neonates, sick or well; suitability for sequential examination, especially of the maturing preterm infant; and short, reliable, and simple to administer and score by persons not trained in neonatal neurology. In the first phase of test development, all the neurologic items from the existing examination schemes of Ste-Anne Dargassies,[37,96] Prechtl,[32] and Parmelee and Michaelis[97] were tested with 50 full-term infants to determine which items met the aforementioned test purposes. Some Brazelton scale[18] items were selected to reflect "higher" neurologic function. The items selected, accompanied by a comprehensive instructional manual, were then tested with over 500 babies over a 2 year period. The results of this phase showed the test to be useful with full-term infants but not with preterm infants, and to be cumbersome and time-consuming to administer and score. In the second phase of development the scoring system was simplified by modifying each item so that it could be graded from its minimal to its maximal response on a 5-point scale. In addition, the instructions for eliciting items and the definitions for each possible response were transferred to the recording sheet. These two modifications enabled the test to reflect change in premature infants and greatly reduced the time required to administer the items and score the responses.

Evidence of Reliability.   Harris and Brady[36] reported that the interobserver reliability of an earlier form of the tool was examined with 11 infants but that no specific percentage agreement or reliability coefficients were reported. The manual contains the statement that "good interobserver correlation" was obtained in administering a selected group of the items to 100 preterm and full-term infants admitted to intensive care. No reliability data are reported for the final form of the instrument.

Evidence of Validity. Dubowitz et al.[98] examined the correlation of selected item results with results of ultrasound examinations in 100 preterm and full-term infants admitted to intensive care. Decreased muscle tone and mobility, tight popliteal angle, absent visual tracking, and roving eye movements were related to the presence of intraventricular hemorrhage.

Palmer et al.[99] demonstrated that the Dubowitz could discriminate preterm from full-term neonates at the postconceptional age of 40 weeks. The major differentiating signs were that the preterm infants had a more extended posture in supine, decreased arm and leg recoil and arm traction, decreased head control, and weak adduction phase of the Moro response. The preterm infants also, however, had better auditory and visual orientation ability and alertness than did the full-term neonates. The Dubowitz also identified some differences among preterm infants with different gestational ages. The less mature infants had more extended posture, poorer extensor neck muscle control, and increased extension of legs in ventral suspension.

In a more recent study, Murphy et al.[76] examined 19 preterm infants with persistent pulmonary hypertension of the newborn and matched controls with the Dubowitz prior to hospital discharge. Abnormal or borderline Dubowitz results were related to seizures and cerebral infarction.

Dubowitz et al.[100] compared neonatal results with scores on a neurologic examination at 12 months of age in 101 premature infants examined at 40 weeks postmenstrual age. The Dubowitz examination correctly classified 81 percent of the infants as abnormal or normal at one year. The sensitivity was 83 percent and the specificity 80 percent. The false-positive rate was relatively high (36 percent), so the predictive value of a positive test was only 64 percent. The false-negative rate, however, was quite low (only 8 percent), and the predictive value of a negative test was 92 percent.

Qualitative Evaluation

The Dubowitz is quick and simple to administer and to record results. The recording sheet contains the instructions for administration and descriptions and illustrations of the responses. The examiner simply circles the response that most closely resembles that observed. The examination system was developed for use by professionals who are not trained in neonatal neurology. No specific guidelines for examiner training are given in the manual. Most items are within the area of expertise of the developmental therapist.

Summary Evaluation

The fact that the Dubowitz examination is viable with both full-term and premature infants and can be used with sick infants makes this a particularly useful clinical tool for assessing the progress of the high-risk infant. Reliability studies with the revised instrument are needed to evaluate further its clinical usefulness and validity.

Neonatal Neurobehavioral Examination

Brief Description

The Neonatal Neurobehavioral Examination (NNE)[93] is a 27-item, criterion-referenced assessment tool that closely resembles the Dubowitz. It contains nine items in each of three sections: tone and motor patterns, primitive reflexes, and behavioral responses. The purpose of the NNE is to characterize neurobehavioral fitness at given conceptional ages with objective, numerical scores. It can be used with both full-term and preterm infants.

Technical Evaluation

Test Development.   The items for the NNE were selected from existing gestational age scales and neonatal examination systems[15,34,92] for their ability to detect maturational changes in neurobehavioral functions. A 3-point scale was applied to each item. In the tone and motor pattern and reflex sections, the score of 3 indicates performance expected of a full-term infant; 2 represents performance of an infant 32 to 36 weeks gestational age; and 1 the performance of an infant at less than 32 weeks gestational age. Abnormal responses are also scored as 1. The behavioral responses section was subdivided into responsiveness, temperament, and equilibration subsections. Behavioral response items are scored 3 for optimal performance and 1 for deficient response. Scores of the items in each section are summed to provide section scores, and section scores are summed to provide the total score.

The NNE was standardized with a sample of 54 normal full-term infants and 298 high-risk infants. The full-term infants were examined at 48 hours of age. The high-risk infants were examined when they approached term conceptional age or at discharge, whichever came first.

Evidence of Reliability.   Internal consistency was good, with section scores substantially correlated with the total score (at ≥ 0.80). Inter-rater reliability for the full-term infants averaged 88 percent for item agreement and 95 percent for section agreement for 20 infants tested within the same hour by two different examiners. Inter-rater reliability was not reported for a high-risk group.

Evidence of Validity.   Total and section scores of the NNE differentiated the full-term and high-risk infants. Full-term infants had average total scores of 76 and received no total scores below 70 (of a possible 81). They had averages of 25 to 26 on section scores and no section scores below 20 (of a possible 27). High-risk infants tested at 37 weeks or greater conceptional age had average section scores of 21 to 22 and total scores averaging 66. High-risk infants tested at 34 to 36 weeks conceptional age averaged 20 points for sectional scores and 61 points for total scores. High-risk infants tested at less than 34 weeks had the lowest scores, with section scores averaging 16 to 17 and total scores averaging 51 points. Intercorrelations among the three sections were modest, indicating that some overlap was present, but also that a reasonable amount of variance was unique to each section.

Predictive validity of the NNE for performance on the Peabody Developmental Motor Scales (PDMS) was reported by Lee et al.[101] The NNE was given to a sample of 100 high-risk preterm infants at 37 to 41 weeks conceptional age prior to discharge from the NICU. The infants were examined with the PDMS at 6 and 18 months corrected age. Low correlations (figures not given) were noted between NNE subtest scores and PDMS scores and higher correlations (figures not given) when subtest scores were combined (presumably the total score). With multiple regression analysis, the primitive reflex subtest was predictive for infants born between 37 and 42 weeks, and the tone and motor patterns subtest was predictive for infants born with birth weights of 1,500 g or less.

Qualitative Evaluation

In the standardization study, the NNE was completed and scored consistently within 15 minutes, and scorable responses were obtained for each item with every infant. The source article contains the recording/score sheet in an appendix. The sheet is very similar to that of the Dubowitz examination, containing instructions for administration and scoring and descriptions of each response. Six states are defined on the recording sheet, but the source article does not indicate how state is to be incorporated into the examination.

Summary Evaluation

The NNE is similar in format to the Dubowitz and provides similar information. The ability to quantify the responses should be helpful in charting progress of individual infants over time, although that ability has not yet been tested. Further study is also needed of inter-rater reliability with the high-risk group, and more definitive information should be published regarding the predictive validity. Finally, the recording and rules for testing of behavioral state need to be reported.

The last two neurobehavioral assessment systems to be presented here are still in development. The first is for use with preterm infants, and the second is for full-term infants in the first week of life.

Neurobehavioral Assessment for Preterm Infants

Brief Description

The Neurobehavioral Assessment for Preterm Infants (NAPI) is designed to measure the maturity of preterm infant functioning in the age range of 32 to 42 weeks postconceptional age.[94,102–104] The authors suggest that the NAPI can be used to test the effects of intervention and monitor progress, generate normative data, study development and individual differences, and detect neurologically suspect performance in preterm infants.[94,103,104]

Technical Evaluation

Test Development. The NAPI has been extensively piloted, psychometrically tested, and revised over the course of almost a decade since a pilot form was developed to assess the neurobehavioral functioning of premature infants involved in a vestibular-proprioceptive stimulation program.[102] The items were selected from the available examination schemes of Amiel-Tison,[105] Brazelton,[18] Dubowitz and Dubowitz,[92] and Prechtl[32] on the basis of their ability to reflect clear developmental trends.

In the second phase of test development, a revised form of the NAPI was submitted to psychometric analysis in order to select the test items and clusters that would be retained in the examination based on both their conceptual and psychometric soundness.[104] The examination was administered to 179 premature infants between 32 weeks and term gestation, for a total of 354 examinations. Item test–retest reliability coefficients were calculated on two consecutive days at 34 weeks postconceptional age. All items with r less than 0.20 were discarded. Cluster cohesion with 34 weeks data was tested by averaging item scores within each cluster and then discarding the items that were not significantly correlated with the cluster score (in which that test item was not included), or whose reliability coefficient did not fall within the range of correlations for other items in the cluster. Clusters were retained if cluster test–retest r was at least 0.60. Remaining clusters were intercorrelated, and redundant clusters were discarded, with conceptually or clinically more meaningful clusters retained.

The third phase of NAPI development consisted of a replication study with a second cohort and different examiners to determine the psychometric soundness of the items and clusters retained in the second phase.[94] A sample of 290 premature infants was tested (533 examinations) between 32 and 42 weeks of postconceptional age. Infants were excluded who had discrepant gestational age assessments, grade III or IV intraventricular hemorrhage, persistent seizures, herpes, or severe asphyxia. All were breathing room air, off intravenous feeding, and medically stable. Two clusters from the second phase were dropped, one for low test–retest reliability and the other for a skewed distribution of scores. A third cluster was derived from others. The seven retained clusters were then tested for developmental validity. No further deletions were needed. The final form of the test consists of seven neurobehavioral dimensions: motor development/vigor, scarf sign, popliteal angle, alertness/orientation, irritability, vigor of crying, and percent time sleeping.

Evidence of Reliability. Reliability was tested and reported for each version of the test in each phase of the study. Test–retest reliability of the seven final dimensions was calculated using data from 55 infants aged 34 weeks post-conception tested on 2 consecutive days. Reliability coefficients were all statistically significant and ranged from 0.51 to 0.85. Interobserver reliability was calculated with 43 infants between 33 and 36 weeks conceptional age and averaged 0.85 (range of 0.64 to 0.98).[94]

Evidence of Validity. In the second stage of NAPI development, developmental validity was tested via a linear regression model with the eight retained clusters.[104] All retained clusters demonstrated age-related changes that were statistically significant. The seven final dimensions derived in the replication study also had acceptable developmental validity.[94]

Qualitative Evaluation

The NAPI has not yet been published, so little information is available as to its time requirements, standardization, administration and scoring, or examiner qualifications and training requirements. The authors caution that the validation samples did not include infants with problems such as drug addiction, severe intraventricular hemorrhage, severe asphyxia, or who were HIV positive, so that validation of its usefulness with those infants awaits further study.

Summary Evaluation

The strength of this assessment lies in the rigor with which it was developed and validated. One would like to know a bit more about item selection criteria and the items that make up the final dimensions. Until the test is made available through publication, its actual usefulness for its stated purposes remains unknown. If it is sensitive to neurobehavioral change as predicted, it may prove to be a valuable tool to assess the effects of intervention programs for premature infants.

Neonatal Neurological Examination

Brief Description

The Neonatal Neurological Examination (Neoneuro)[95] is a 32-item, criterion-referenced battery of neurologic and behavioral items. The items include observation of posture, muscle tone, reflexes, and orientation to auditory and visual stimuli. The purpose of the Neoneuro is to assess neurologic integrity in full-term neonates. It is appropriate for use with full-term infants, normal and abnormal, but not with infants born at less than 37 weeks of gestation.

Technical Evaluation

Test Construction. The Neoneuro was constructed in a similar way to the INFANIB. A test battery of 44 items was derived from existing examination systems.[32,92] A single examiner administered the items to a sample of normal, neurologically suspect, and abnormal neonates. The examination was performed with 727 neonates between birth and 48 hours of age and again with 510 infants between 72 hours and 7 days of age. Only the first two examinations in infants 37 weeks of gestation or older were analyzed for this study. The examinations were performed in Prechtl states 3 or 4. The examiner also scored muscle tone and movement, reflexes, neurobehavior, and an overall assessment as normal, questionable or abnormal, based on experience. The items were first scored as originally described in their source tests and later were transformed, based on clinical experience of the authors, to progress from abnormal to normal. A correlation matrix was submitted to factor analysis, resulting in the generation of seven factors. Items were retained if their factor loadings were 0.28 or greater. If a factor had more than seven items, the lower loading items were dropped, as were items that did not load consistently on any factor. The result was a 32-item battery with three or more items representing each of the seven factors. The item scores were transformed to a 5-point scale, and items were equally weighted. Factor scores are summed to form subscores, and subscores are summed to form the total score. A 21-item short form to be used for screening was also constructed from the three highest loading items for each factor. The final form was also tested by physicians not acquainted with the test construction, who helped to clarify the scoring sheet.

Evidence of Reliability. The internal consistency of the 32-item test is 0.80 and for the 21-item short form is 0.73. The test–retest reliability coefficient between the first and second tests was 0.73. Further work needs to be done to determine inter-rater reliability.

Evidence of Validity. The intercorrelations among factors ranged from 0.08 to 0.25 indicating that the factors are assessing different aspects of neurologic integrity. Neoneuro total scores discriminated between the classifications of "normal," "suspect," and "abnormal" for tone and movement, reflexes, and neurobehavior. Cut points for abnormality/normality were developed based on extensive clinical experience, but predictive validity based on those cut points awaits further research.

Qualitative Evaluation

The time required to administer and score the Neoneuro was not mentioned in the source article. Examiners can be physicians, nurses, occupational therapists, or physical therapists. The source article contains an appendix in which administration of the 32 items is clearly described. The Neoneuro recording forms are available from the second author. The forms closely resemble those of the INFANIB and are completed in a similar way.

Summary Evaluation

The Neoneuro appears promising, pending evaluation of its inter-rater reliability and predictive validity. It is not applicable for infants over 1 week of age; therefore, it might not be useful for assessing infants at hospital discharge who have had prolonged hospital stays. The authors state that they have future plans to develop the test for administration to infants older than 1 week.

CLINICAL APPLICATION

Formal, standardized, neurobehavioral testing of neonatal behavior that involves handling the infant is best avoided until the infant is judged to be medically stable, e.g., breathing room air, off any life support system and able to be examined without the need for cardiorespiratory monitoring. Prior to that time, the most appropriate means of assessment are (1) observation of the infant's reactions to routine caregiving procedures, as described by Sweeney (Ch. 2) and (2) chart review for documenting perinatal and neonatal risk factors to aid in selection of infants in need of later, more detailed assessment.[5] When the infant becomes medically stabilized but has not yet attained term-equivalent age, he or she can be assessed with one of the systems for preterm infant assessment, the Dubowitz,[92] NNE,[93] or APIB,[17] depending on the level of training of the examiner. Serial examinations are needed to assess the progress of the infant over time and to select those infants in need of close follow-up after discharge. At the time of discharge, if the infant is approaching term-equivalent age, the Neoneuro,[95] INFANIB,[43,44] and BNBAS[15] are also appropriate as they are based on full-term infant behavior.

A highly recommended procedure is to encourage the parents or primary caretakers to observe and participate in at least one of the examinations as discharge time approaches. They should receive information during the examination concerning the infant's behavior, with particular emphasis on the cues the infant gives that are indicative of approach and avoidance. They can be shown ways to minimize stress-related behaviors, to assist the infant in regaining balanced functioning after a disturbing event, and to facilitate their infant's optimal performance. As part of the discharge process, this experience is extremely valuable as parents go through the process described by Als[87] of "regaining their infant" and preparing themselves to take full responsibility as his or her primary caretakers.

ACKNOWLEDGMENTS

Ms. Wilhelm was Research Associate Professor, Department of Medical Allied Health Professions, University of North Carolina at Chapel Hill, when this chapter was written. Her work was supported in part by Maternal and Child Health Training Grant 149, U.S. Department of Health and Human Services.

REFERENCES

1. Goldberg K: The high-risk infant. Phys Ther 55:1092, 1975
2. Dickson JM: A model for the physical therapist in the intensive care nursery. Phys Ther 61:45, 1981
3. Anderson J, Auster-Liebhaber J: Developmental therapy in the neonatal intensive care unit. Phys Occup Ther Pediatr 4(1):89, 1984
4. Sweeney JK: The High-Risk Neonate: Developmental Therapy Perspectives. Haworth Press, New York, 1986
5. Wilhelm IJ: The neurologically suspect neonate. p. 67. In Campbell SK (ed): Pediatric Neurologic Physical Therapy. 2nd Ed. Churchill Livingstone, New York, 1991
6. Sweeney JK: Neonatal physical therapy: medical risks and professional education. Inf Young Child 2(3):59, 1990
7. Scull S, Deitz J: Competencies for the physical therapist in the neonatal intensive care unit (NICU). Pediatr Phys Ther 1:11, 1989
8. Marx J: Predictive value of early neuromotor assessment instruments. Phys Occup Ther Pediatr 9(4):69, 1989
9. Gorski PA, Lewkowicz DJ, Huntington L: Advances in neonatal and infant behavioral assessment: toward a comprehensive evaluation of early patterns of development. J Dev Behav Pediatr 8:39, 1987
10. Thoman EB: Sleeping and waking states in infants: a functional perspective. Neurosci Biobehav Rev 14:93, 1990
11. Prechtl HFB, Akiyama Y, Zinkin P, Grant DK: Polygraphic studies of the full-term newborn: 1. technical aspects and qualitative analysis. p. 1. In MacKeith R, Bax M (eds): Studies in Infancy. Clinics in Developmental Medicine No. 27. Heinemann Medical Books, London, 1968
12. Wolff PH: Observation on newborn infants. Psychosom Med 21:110, 1959
13. Wolff, PH: The causes, controls, and organization of behavior in the neonate. Psychol Iss 5 (Monogr 17):1, 1966
14. Prechtl HFR: The behavioural states of the newborn infant (a review). Brain Res 76:185, 1974
15. Brazelton TB: Neonatal Behavioral Assessment Scale. Clinics in Developmental Medicine No. 68. J.B. Lippincott, Philadelphia, 1984
16. Prechtl HFR, Fargel JW, Weinmann HM, Bakker HH: Postures, motility and respiration of low-risk, preterm infants. Dev Med Child Neurol 21:3, 1979
17. Als H, Lester BM, Tronick EZ, Brazelton TB: Manual for assessment of preterm infants' behavior. p. 65. In Fitzgerald HE, Lester BM, Yogman MW (eds): Theory and Research in Behavioral Pediatrics. Vol 1. Plenum Press, New York, 1982
18. Brazelton TB: Neonatal Behavioral Assessment Scale. Clinics in Developmental Medicine No. 50. J.B. Lippincott, Philadelphia, 1973
19. Prechtl HFR: Assessment methods for the newborn infant: a critical evaluation. p. 21. In Stratton P (ed): Psychobiology of the Human Newborn. J. Wiley & Sons, Chichester, 1982
20. Beintema DJ: A Neurological Study of Newborn Infants. Clinics in Developmental Medicine No. 28. Heinemann Medical Books, London, 1968
21. Prechtl H, Beintema D: The Neurological Examination of the Full-Term Newborn Infant. Clinics in Developmental Medicine No. 12. Heinemann Medical Books, London, 1975

22. Colombo J, Moss M, Horowitz FD: Neonatal state profiles: reliability and short-term prediction of neurobehavioral status. Child Dev 60:1102, 1989
23. Davis DH, Thoman EB: Behavioral states of premature infants: implications for neural and behavioral development. Dev Psychobiol 20:25, 1987
24. Theorell K, Prechtl HFR, Blair AW, Lind J: Behavioral state cycles of normal newborn infants. Dev Med Child Neurol 15:597, 1973
25. Prechtl HFR, Theorell K, Blair AW: Behavioral state cycles in abnormal infants. Dev Med Child Neurol 15:606, 1973
26. Holditch-Davis D: The development of sleeping and waking states in high-risk preterm infants. Inf Behav Dev 13:513, 1990
27. Thoman EB: Sleep and wake behaviors in neonates: consistencies and consequences. Merrill-Palmer Q 21:295, 1975
28. Thoman EB, Denenberg VH, Sievel J et al: State organization in neonates: developmental inconsistency indicates risk for developmental dysfunction. Neuropediatrics 12:45, 1981
29. Moss M, Colombo J, Mitchell DW, Horowitz FD: Neonatal behavioral organization and visual processing at three months. Child Dev 59:1211, 1988
30. Horowitz FD, Sullivan JW, Linn PL: Stability and instability in the newborn infants: the quest for the elusive threads. Monogr Soc Res Child Dev 43(2, Serial No. 177), 1978
31. Korner AF: State as variable, as obstacle, and as mediator of stimulation in infant research. Merrill-Palmer Q 18:77, 1972
32. Prechtl HFR: The Neurological Examination of the Full-Term Newborn Infant. 2nd Ed. Clinics in Developmental Medicine No. 63. J.B. Lippincott, Philadelphia, 1977
33. Palisano RJ, Short MA: Methods for assessing muscle tone and motor functions in the neonate: a review. Phys Occup Ther Pediatr 4(4):43, 1984
34. André-Thomas, Chesny Y, Saint-Anne Dargassies S: The Neurological Examination of the Infant. Little Club Clinics in Developmental Medicine No. 1. National Spastics Society, London, 1960
35. St Clair K: Neonatal assessment procedures: a historical review. Child Dev 49:280, 1978
36. Harris SR, Brady DK: Infant neuromotor assessment instruments: a review. Phys Occup Ther Pediatr 6(3/4):121, 1986
37. Saint-Anne Dargassies S: Neurological Development in the Full-Term and Premature Neonate. Excerpta Medica, New York, 1977
38. Francis PL, Self PA, Horowitz FD: The behavioral assessment of the neonate: an overview. p. 723. In Osofsky J (ed): Handbook of Infant Development. 2nd Ed. John Wiley & Sons, New York, 1987
39. Bierman-van Eendenburg MEC, Jurgens-van der Zee AD, Olinga AA et al: Predictive value of neonatal neurological examination: a follow-up study at 18 months. Dev Med Child Neurol 23:296, 1981
40. Amiel-Tison C, Grenier A: Neurological Assessment During the First Year of Life. Oxford University Press, New York, 1986
41. Amiel-Tison C, Grenier A: Neurological Evaluation of the Newborn and the Infant. Masson, New York, 1983
42. Wetzel AP, Wetzel RC: A review of the Amiel-Tison neurologic evaluation of the newborn and infant. Am J Occup Ther 38:585, 1984
43. Ellison PW, Horn JL, Browning CA: Construction of an Infant Neurological International Battery (INFANIB) for the assessment of neurological integrity in infancy. Phys Ther 65:1326, 1985

44. Ellison PW: Scoring sheet for the Infant Neurological International Battery (INFANIB). Phys Ther 66:548, 1986
45. Milani-Comparetti A, Gidoni EA: Routine developmental examination in normal and retarded children. Dev Med Child Neurol 9:631, 1967
46. Capute AJ, Accardo PJ, Vining E et al: Primitive Reflex Profile. University Park Press, Baltimore, 1978
47. Paine RS, Oppé TE: Neurological Examination of Children. Clinics in Developmental Medicine Nos. 20/21. Heinemann Medical Books, London, 1966
48. Stavrakas PA, Kemmer-Gacura GE, Engelke SC, Chenier TC: Predictive validity of the Infant Neurological International Battery (INFANIB), abstracted. Dev Med Child Neurol 33(Suppl 64):35, 1991
49. Hansen NB, Kopechek J, Miller RR et al: Prognostic significance of cystic intracranial lesions in neonates. J Dev Behav Pediatr 10:129, 1989
50. Ellison PH, Browning CA, Larson B, Denny J: Development of a scoring system for the Milani-Comparetti and Gidoni method of assessing neurologic abnormality in infancy. Phys Ther 63:1414, 1983
51. Als H, Tronick E, Lester BM, Brazelton TB: Specific neonatal measures: the Brazelton Neonatal Behavioral Assessment Scale. p. 185. In Osofsky J (ed): Handbook of Infant Development. John Wiley & Sons, New York, 1979
52. Lester BM: Data analysis and prediction. p. 85. In Brazelton TB: Neonatal Behavioral Assessment Scale. 2nd Ed. Clinics in Developmental Medicine No. 88. JB Lippincott, Philadelphia, 1984
53. Sostek AM, Anders T: Relationships among the Brazelton Neonatal Scale, Bayley Infant Scales and early temperament. Child Dev 48:320, 1977
54. Jacobson JL, Jacobson SW, Fein GG, Schwartz PM: Factors and clusters for the Brazelton Scale: an investigation of the dimensions of neonatal behavior. Dev Psychol 20:339, 1984
55. Horowitz FD, Linn PL: Use of the NBAS in research. p. 97. In Brazelton TB: Neonatal Behavioral Assessment Scale. 2nd Ed. Clinics in Developmental Medicine No. 88. JB Lippincott, Philadelphia, 1984
56. Worobey J: A review of Brazelton-based interventions to enhance parent–infant interaction. J Reprod Inf Psychol 3:64, 1986
57. Nugent JK, Brazelton TB: Preventive intervention with infants and families: the NBAS model. Inf Mental Health J 10(2):84, 1989
58. Nugent JK, Sepkoski C: The training of NBAS examiners. p. 78. In Brazelton TB: Neonatal Behavioral Assessment Scale. 2nd Ed. Clinics in Developmental Medicine No. 88. JB Lippincott, Philadelphia, 1984
59. Clopton N, Martin AS: A criticism of interrater reliability procedures for the Brazelton Neonatal Behavioral Assessment Scale. Phys Occup Ther Pediatr 4(4):55, 1984
60. DiPietro JA, Larson SK: Examiner effects in the administration of the NBAS: the illusion of reliability. Inf Behav Dev 12:119, 1989
61. Linn PL, Horowitz FD: The relationship between infant individual differences and mother–infant interaction during the neonatal period. Inf Behav Dev 6:415, 1983
62. Lester BM, Emory BK, Hoffman SL, Eitzman DV: A multivariate study of the effects of high-risk factors on performance on the Brazelton Neonatal Assessment Scale. Child Dev 47:515, 1976
63. Sameroff AK, Krafchuk EE, Bakow HA: Issues in grouping items from the Neonatal Behavioral Assessment Scale. In Sameroff AJ (ed): Organization and Stability of Newborn Behavior: a Commentary on the Brazelton Neonatal Behavioral Assessment Scale. Monogr Soc Res Child Dev 43(56, Serial No. 177), 1978

64. Gyurke JS, Reich JN, Holmes DH: An examination of the effectiveness of multiple summary scoring procedures of the BNBAS in detecting group differences. Inf Mental Health J 9(3):201, 1988

65. Aleksandrowicz MK, Aleksandrowicz DR: Obstetrical pain-relieving drugs as predictors of infant behavior variability. Child Dev 45:935, 1974

66. Standley K, Soule AB, Copans SA, Duchowny MS: Local–regional anesthesia during childbirth: effect on newborn behaviors. Science 186:634, 1974

67. Horowitz FD, Ashton J, Culp R et al: The effects of obstetrical medication on the behavior of Israeli newborn infants and some comparisons with Uruguayan and American infants. Child Dev 48:1607, 1977

68. Rizzo T, Freinkel N, Metzger BE et al: Correlations between antepartum maternal metabolism and newborn behavior. Am J Obstet Gynecol 163:1458, 1990

69. Coles CD, Smith IE, Lancaster JS, Falek A: Persistence over the first month of neurobehavioral differences in infants exposed to alcohol prenatally. Inf Behav Dev 10:23, 1987

70. Soule B, Standley K, Copans S, Davis M: Clinical uses of the Brazelton Scale. Pediatrics 54:583, 1974

71. Strauss ME, Lessen-Firestone JK, Starr RH, Ostrea EM: Behavior of narcotics-addicted newborns. Child Dev 46:887, 1975

72. Eisen LN, Field TM, Bandstra ES et al: Perinatal cocaine effects on neonatal stress behavior and performance on the Brazelton Scale. Pediatrics 88:477, 1991

73. Stjernqvist K, Svenningsen NW: Neurobehavioural development at term of extremely low-birthweight infants (<901 g). Dev Med Child Neurol 32:679, 1990

74. Als H, Tronick E, Adamson L, Brazelton TB: The behavior of the fullterm but underweight newborn infant. Dev Med Child Neurol 18:590, 1976

75. Telzrow RW, Kang PR, Mitchell SK et al: An assessment of the behavior of the preterm infant at 40 weeks conceptional age. p. 85. In Lipsitt LP, Field TM (eds): Infant Behavior and Development: Perinatal Risk and Newborn Behavior. Ablex, New Jersey, 1982

76. Murphy TF, Scher MS, Klesh KW, Guthrie RD: Early neurobehavioral abnormalities in infants with persistent pulmonary hypertension of the newborn. Inf Behav Dev 11:159, 1988

77. Escher-Graub DC, Fricker HS: Jaundice and behavioral organization in the full-term neonate. Helv Paediatr Acta 41:425, 1986

78. Paludetto R, Rinaldi P, Mansi G et al: Early behavioural development of preterm infants. Dev Med Child Neurol 26:347, 1984

79. Beal JA: The Brazelton Neonatal Behavioral Assessment Scale: a tool to enhance parental attachment. J Pediatr Nurs 1:170, 1986

80. Lester BM: Change and stability in neonatal behavior. p. 51. In Brazelton TB, Lester BM (eds): New Approaches to Developmental Screening of Infants. Elsevier, New York, 1983.

81. Als H, Lester BM, Tronick EZ, Brazelton TB: Toward a research instrument for the assessment of premature infants' behavior (APIB). p. 35. In Fitzgerald H, Lester BM, Yogman MW (eds): Theory and Research in Behavioral Pediatrics. Vol 1. Plenum Press, New York, 1982

82. Als H: Infant individuality: assessing patterns of very early development. p. 363. In Call J, Galenson E, Tyson RL (eds): Frontiers of Infant Psychiatry. Basic Books, New York, 1983

83. Als H, Duffy FH, McAnulty GB: Continuity of neurobehavioral functioning in preterm and full-term newborns. p. 3. In Bornstein MH, Krasnegor NA (eds):

Stability and Continuity in Mental Development. Lawrence Erlbaum, Hillsdale, NJ, 1989

84. Als H: Toward a synactive theory of development: promise for the assessment and support of infant individuality. Inf Mental Health J 3(4):229, 1982

85. Als H: Self-regulation and motor development in preterm infants. p. 63. In Lockman J, Hazen N (eds): Action in Social Context. Perspectives on Early Development. Plenum Press, New York, 1989

86. Als H: Patterns of infant behavior: analogues of later organizational difficulties? p. 67. In Duffy FH, Geschwand N (eds): Dyslexia. Little, Brown, Boston, 1985

87. Als H: A synactive model of neonatal organization: framework for the assessment of neurobehavioral development in the premature infant and for support of infants and parents in the neonatal intensive care environment. Phys Occup Ther Pediatr 6(3/4):3, 1986

88. Als, H, Duffy, FH, McAnulty GB: Behavioral differences between preterm and full-term newborns as measured with the APIB system scores: I. Inf Behav Dev 11:305, 1988

89. Als H: The assessment of preterm infants' behavior (APIB): theoretical base and training. p. 78. In Proceedings of the Sixth Annual Conference, Developmental Interventions in Neonatal Care, Washington, DC, November 1990. Contemporary Forums, Danville, CA, 1990

90. Als H, Duffy, FH, McAnulty GB: The APIB, an assessment of functional competence in preterm and full-term newborns regardless of gestational age at birth: II. Inf Behav Dev 11:319, 1988

91. Culp RE, Culp AM, Harmon RJ: A tool for educating parents about their premature infants. Birth 16(1):23, 1989.

92. Dubowitz L, Dubowitz V: The Neurological Assessment of the Preterm and Full-Term Newborn Infant. Clinics in Developmental Medicine No. 79. JB Lippincott, Philadelphia, 1981

93. Morgan AM, Koch V, Lee V, Aldag J: Neonatal neurobehavioral examination: a new instrument for quantitative analysis of neonatal neurological status. Phys Ther 68:1352, 1988

94. Korner AF, Constantinou J, Dimiceli S, Brown BW Jr: Establishing the reliability and developmental validity of a neurobehavioral assessment for preterm infants: a methodological process. Child Dev 62:1200, 1991

95. Sheridan Pereira M, Ellison PH, Helgeson V: The construction of a scored neonatal neurological examination for assessment of neurologic integrity in full-term neonates. J Dev Behav Pediatr 12:25, 1991

96. Saint-Anne Dargassies S: Neurodevelopmental symptoms during the first year of life. I. Essential landmarks for each key age. Dev Med Child Neurol 14:235, 1972

97. Parmelee AH, Michaelis MD: Neurological examination of the newborn. p. 3. In Hellmuth J (ed): Exceptional Infant. Vol 2. Brunner/Mazel, New York, 1971

98. Dubowitz LMS, Levene MI, Morante A et al: Neurologic signs in neonatal intraventricular hemorrhage: a correlation with real-time ultrasound. J Pediatr 99:127, 1981

99. Palmer PG, Dubowitz LMS, Verghote M, Dubowitz V: Neurological and neurobehavioral differences between preterm infants at term and full-term newborn infants. Neuropediatrics 13:183, 1982

100. Dubowitz LMS, Dubowitz V, Palmer PG et al: Correlation of neurologic assessment in the preterm newborn infant with outcome at 1 year. J Pediatr 105:452, 1984

101. Lee VL, Morgan A, Ling W: Predictability of the neonatal neurobehavioral examination at 6 and 18 months corrected age, abstracted. Phys Ther 69:362, 1989

102. Korner AF, Schneider P, Forrest T: Effects of vestibular-proprioceptive stimulation on the neurobehavioral development of preterm infants: a pilot study. Neuropediatrics 14:170, 1983

103. Korner AF: Neurobehavioral assessment: a new approach in measuring the effects of intervention. p. 71. In Proceedings of Developmental Interventions in Neonatal Care. Contemporary Forums, Danville, CA, 1985

104. Korner AF, Kraemer HC, Reade EP et al: A methodological approach to developing an assessment procedure for testing the neurobehavioral maturity of preterm infants. Child Dev 58:1478, 1987

105. Amiel-Tison C: Neurological evaluation of the maturity of newborn infants. Arch Dis Child 43:89, 1968

4 | Assessment of Family Resources and Needs

Joyce W. Sparling

One could argue as to whose claims were greater, God's, the church's or the king's, but any sensible man would have to admit that first came his family's.[1]

The first requirement of the assessment process is to know what you are attempting to assess. This first requirement is not clear when assessing families of special needs infants and toddlers. Repeatedly we hear the question, "Who is in this family?" and "What aspects of this family should we be assessing?" To clarify the developmental therapist's role in family assessment, a definition of family is needed that is consistent with the diverse compositions of contemporary families and recognizes the family as the critical health and educational environment of the infant. The family consists of "those significant others who profoundly influence the personal life and health of the individual over time".[2] Building on this definition, the purpose of this chapter will be to describe the way in which therapists interested in various aspects of motor development may assess the family to benefit the infant and to respond to the mandate of PL 99-457.[3]

REASONS FOR FAMILY ASSESSMENT

The Law

Physical and occupational therapists and speech and language pathologists have been trained to assess and intervene with motor delay and impairment. Assessment of families is thought by some to be beyond the purview of these disciplines and appropriate for social workers and psychologists. According to the Part H reauthorization of PL 99-457,[4] however, developmental therapists are now required to assess families. This mandate exists even though most developmental therapists have not participated directly in the process of establishing it. Several critical factors of the Public Law that relate to assessment are

  1. "Assessment must be family-directed and may, with the concurrence of the family, include an assessment of the family's resources, priorities and concerns."
  2. Assessment may "identify family preferences, supports, and services necessary to enhance the parents' and siblings' capacity to meet the developmental needs of their infant or toddler with a disability."
  3. Early intervention services, which may include assessment, must be provided in the natural environment of the infant or toddler.

A number of profound factors support these mandates and suggest the need for disciplinary preservice and inservice education on families and family assessment.

Family Influence on Infant

Whatever their composition and whatever the direction of their effect, families provide a major learning environment for their infants. That learning environment can relate directly to the infant's achievement of his or her learning potential.[4] The importance of family influence is supported by research from a number of fronts. For example, the authors of one follow-up study of 82 newborn infants weighing less than 1,500 g at birth[5] reported that parent–child behaviors and the quality of the home environment are the most predictive variables of the intellectual development of the child at age 36 months. Another investigator suggested that the relationship between the toddler and a parent is associated with motor performance in terms of the way the toddler negotiates his or her environment.[6] Competence in negotiating the environment is defined largely as maintaining balance in standing, sitting, crawling and squatting, and maintaining a grasp on toys and using them appropriately. Results of this study show a significant positive relationship between the quality of attachment of 18-month-old toddlers and their mothers and the toddlers' competence in adapting to their environment.

Family Diversity

Underlying the influence of family on the infant is the family's understanding of the unique characteristics of the infant. Most frequently, parents know their infant best[7] and understand the family environmental and cultural factors that exist for the infant. These factors are vastly different from those of just 10 years ago.[8] No longer is the average family nuclear in its composition, consisting of mother, father, and children. Instead, approximately one-fourth of contemporary families are single-parent families, with the parent being the mother in 21 percent, the father in 3 percent, and the step-parent or foster-parent in 3 percent of the families.[8] The diversity of the contemporary U.S. family obfuscates any attempts at categorization and necessitates a sensitive, knowledgable, and thoughtful approach to learning each family's perceptions and priorities.

Family Potential for Involvement

Coupling any of the dimensions of contemporary families with a special needs infant suggests an added expenditure of energy just to maintain the family unit. For example, Breslau and her colleagues[9] described the plight of low-income mothers of special needs children in contrast to middle-income mothers in terms of the remuneration they can expect from employment outside the home. Child care costs and low-paying jobs necessitate long working hours for low-income mothers, a fact that further depletes their energies and decreases their capability for involvement in the health and education of their infants and toddlers. Discrepancies in parental involvement, however, are not limited to socioeconomic factors; they include a unique complexity of family characteristics that require further identification and study.[10]

Healthy Family Variables

By appropriate assessment of families, common variables can be identified that support healthy family functioning and foster the development of competent infants and toddlers. Cowan and Hetherington[11] suggest that previous family research has been too concerned with crisis events and not sufficiently concerned with reorganization as a result of a critical life event. A corollary of this statement is that assessment should occur over time to guide families in their reorganization efforts and to record their progress toward this goal. Recent reports suggest that family progress may be the most important result of intervention with infants and their families.[12,13]

Program Evaluation

Family assessment can also be used to evaluate early intervention regimens and programs. By showing family support for program innovations,[14] a public statement is made about program purposes and future needs. Family advocacy originates in infant and toddler needs and in programmatic identification of ways to meet those needs. Scales have been developed to assess parent satisfaction with medical services,[15] and several State Interagency Coordinating Councils have established statewide assessment of parental satisfaction. Follow-up assessment and evaluation have resulted in positive outcomes for infants and their families. In a study of very-low-birth-weight infants,[5] those families who were not monitored over the 3 years after hospital discharge were more rigid and less well integrated, showed a higher psychosocial risk, and accessed needed services less readily than monitored families.

Information about infants and their developmental tasks, about parents and their energy resources, and about families and their home environment is pertinent to appropriate infant assessment. Requesting information and priorities from families during the assessment process can facilitate infant assessment, family involvement in intervention, and understanding of adaptive family functioning, while providing a mechanism for program evaluation.

DEVELOPMENTAL THERAPISTS' KNOWLEDGE OF FAMILY ASSESSMENT

Preservice Training

Recognizing the importance of family assessment is only the initial step in assessing families. Knowledge is needed about the structure, function, and development of families of special needs infants.[16-18] In the traditional preservice training of personnel, however, little information is given about contemporary families, about normative and nonnormative stressors experienced by families, or about appropriate assessment and effective intervention techniques to be used with families.[19-21] Preservice training in family dynamics as well as infant motor development might better prepare developmental therapists to individualize assessment and treatment. In some cases, to enhance an infant's motor development, an assessment of the family's daily tasks, the environments in which these tasks are conducted, and suggestions for task or environmental modification would be sufficient intervention. Preservice instructional information is becoming available to assist in educating entry-level students in family assessment.[2,22-24] Enthusiasm for including this material into an already replete curriculum is undetermined, but evaluation of these curricular materials is in progress.

Inservice Training

Continuing education has been one of the major formats through which family material has been shared. During a 5-year training period, organizations receiving U.S. Department of Education Infant Personnel Preparation Grants have developed materials and conducted training for professional personnel.[25] Written procedures related to the Individualized Family Service Plan (IFSP)[26] have provided critical material for implementing specifics of the regulations. With effective dissemination and utilization of this information and with increased efforts at disciplinary training related to families, interventionists may become adequately prepared to meet the mandate expressed in PL 99-457 and the competencies of their disciplines.[27]

Transfer of Authority

Not only must interventionists learn to assess families' resources, priorities, and concerns, but, based on this information, therapists must attempt to empower families to act on behalf of their infants in programming and advocacy roles.[28] In some cases, parents may want to become the service coordinators for their infant.[29] Additional skill in assessment of family interaction is required if developmental therapists are to modify their roles in relation to parents and permit parents to become service coordinators.[30] Attending to parental, in concert with therapeutic, prescriptions will be critical to this process.

Constraints to Involvement

Ironically, educational and legal enthusiasm for family involvement in establishing goals for the special needs infant is occurring simultaneously with the apparent dissolution of the family as a social unit.[31] At the same time that professionals are trying to learn about families, the family unit is being redefined by major cultural changes.[32] The family in the United States today has fewer children, more single parents, more mobility, more women employed outside of the home, and an increasing minority representation. Without definitive preservice and inservice instruction in the tasks, environments, and control variables that occur in these families, adequate assessment of the contemporary family is a major challenge. In addition, developmental therapists may themselves represent a biased sample of the population, a fact that, without training, may limit their effectiveness with diverse family structures.

Developmental therapists need preservice and inservice education about families and their assessment. Understanding that the stereotypical U.S. family no longer exists is preliminary to addressing families as unique systems that differentially affect infant development. Developmental therapists' assessments of families therefore may be guided by principles that incorporate individuality and by a framework for selecting family assessment instruments.

PRINCIPLES OF ASSESSMENT

Theory-based practice characterizes the "reflective practitioner",[33] guides decision-making, and directs assessment. One of the most widely accepted and used theories related to individuals is General Systems Theory. Bronfenbrenner[34] established the basic elements of systems theory that have permitted other investigators to develop models grounded in this theory. According to the systems perspective, the individual is a microsystem embedded within the family or sociocultural unit, that in turn is embedded within a still larger system—the community or sociopolitical system. Assessment of any one of these systems necessarily includes assessment of the others, for the systems are interactive. A number of principles have been derived from the systems perspective to guide the assessment of families.

1. Families have a right and a need to choose the kind and amount of external involvement they want in their infant's health and education. For assessment, this means parents may select and prioritize the areas to be assessed, which means parents must be interviewed.[35]

2. Screening is critical for determining the parents' perceptions, knowledge, vulnerabilities, energy, and motivation related to intervention.[36] Appropriate screening enables therapists to refer the family to another team member or assess the family themselves.

3. Developmental therapists should have knowledge of a broad array of family assessments.[37] For example, a developmental therapist trained in methods of family assessment could assess motor skills of the infant, locus of control of the parent, or the parent at play with his or her infant. For the family to be assessed on these dimensions by members of three different disciplines may fractionate the assessment process and the parents' understanding of intervention.

4. Assessment of special needs infants is a reciprocal analytical process including at least three interacting systems of infant, caretaker, and assessor.[11] Different types of assessment are therefore required to obtain information about or from these three perspectives.

5. Families need to be assessed over time,[38] because they and their special needs infants and toddlers change over time.[39] This necessitates assessment in a developmental framework related to family factors supporting functional adaptations over time.[11]

In this chapter we will use these principles as a basis for selecting assessments and conducting the assessment process. To understand the dimensions of family assessment, trends in family assessment will first be explored.

TRENDS IN FAMILY ASSESSMENT

Using a family assessment paradigm that supports the intent of PL 99-457 is a challenge for developmental therapists trained only in motor assessment. Numerous approaches have been suggested, however, and range from assessing parents directly, to asking parental perceptions of infant and toddler behaviors, to requesting parental needs. Current assessments that represent these three approaches are described.

Direct Assessment

A number of investigators have proposed models for assessing specific family elements. Three major family dimensions are described in the Circumplex Model[40] as cohesion, adaptability, and communication. *Cohesion* refers to "the emotional bonding that family members have toward one another''; *adaptability* focuses on ''the extent to which the family system [is] flexible and able to change . . . its power structure, role relationships, and relationship rules in response to situational and developmental stress''; and *communication* refers to the potential for sharing ''changing needs and preferences as they relate to cohesion and adaptability''. From various combinations of these factors, 16 types of family interaction can be described. As with neonatal state, access to the total range of behaviors is healthy, but continual behavior at the extremes of the ranges is usually not conducive to healthy family functioning. Healthy families are able to modify their behavior along the cohesion and adaptability dimensions across the life span. Family members are able to express clear messages, offer support, and use problem-solving skills when confronted with stressors. Based on the Circumplex Model, a series of assessment instruments have been developed. The most recent is the Family Adaptability and Cohesion Evaluation Scales (FACES III), [41] a self-report measure to assess the insider's perspective on his or her family.

Although the FACES III information is useful for an understanding of family function, assessments related to this and other similar models[38,42–45] appear to be within the domain of psychology, for they require skilled psychological interpretation. The widely used Family Environment Scale[46] (FES) and the Family Assessment Device[47] (FAD) are also included in this category. The FAD is a self-report standardized screening assessment that includes a ''general functioning'' category and six specific dimensions of family functioning: problem solving, communication, roles, affective responsiveness, affective involvement, and behavior control. The FES measures the social environment of all types of families. Its 10 subscales form three dimensions of relationship, personal growth, and system maintenance. Recent studies using the FAD and the FES question their reliability when used with different social[46] and cultural[47] groups. Because of the multicultural nature of contemporary society and the psychological nature of these assessments, these instruments are not recommended for use by developmental therapists.

Parental Perceptions

Traditionally, therapists have requested parental input for completing standardized developmental assessments. Obtaining these perceptions met the program needs for family involvement and provided information about the child that was difficult to obtain in any other way. The Battelle Developmental Inventory[48] and the Alpern-Boll Developmental Profile[49] have parent-interview sections through which parental descriptions of observed or perceived child behavior can be obtained. The Minnesota Child Development Inventory[50] has a section completed by parents for identifying physical and adjustment problems of their child.

A new assessment, which stands within the same model, is directed at facilitating parent awareness of infant needs. The TOLL Control System[51] consists of a series of seven developmental checklists for use with children with chronic illnesses. The checklists were developed based on the authors' wide experience with children aged 6 to 60 months who have chronic disorders such as juvenile rheumatoid arthritis, epilepsy, and sickle cell disease and who may experience delays in emerging developmental and behavioral skills. "Concerns" related to the child's performance are obtained through specific questions for the parent and direct observation by the examiner. An intervention plan is formulated directly from that summary for any level of concern about the child's performance. The 100 items on the checklists were derived mostly from standardized assessments. Content validity was developed with six experts in early childhood development who achieved an 83 percent agreement on all but three items. This system is being pilot tested, and inter-rater and test–retest reliability are being established.

Another new assessment is the Pediatric Evaluation of Disability Inventory,[52] which permits functional assessment of the infant and toddler through interview with the parent. This has been well constructed by a physical therapist (see Ch. 10). This type of assessment is consistent with our renewed interest in function, and it permits parents and other family members to interact with the team and share information about which they are experts.

Family Needs Assessment

Rather than simply accessing parent information about infant and toddler behaviors, some clinicians have described infant assessment as a broad family process. To support this process, The Family-Focused Intervention Model[16] was developed. It contains three assessment steps, including the initial assessment of family needs, strengths, and characteristics; a focused interview with the caretakers to verify the initial assessment and determine the need for further assessment; and follow-up assessments, which can include factors related to developmental transitions for family and child, parent–child interaction, home environment, child characteristics, or family support. Based on this series of assessments, IFSP goals can be prioritized.

A number of clinically developed assessments are associated with the Family-Focused Intervention Model. The Family Needs Survey[16] consists of 35 items that are separated into six categories of family needs: information and support, explaining infant status to other persons, community services, finances, family functioning, and communication. A similar assessment has been developed by Turnbull and Turnbull[35] for their work with families of mentally retarded children. These forms have shown clinical utility, but their psychometric properties have not been established.

PROCESS OF FAMILY ASSESSMENT

Although many families are able to voice their needs directly and participate vigorously in establishing priorities, the changing demographics of Western society suggest that many families do not readily do so. Families may require guidance in the expression of their rights and unique family needs. To comprehend these needs as they influence child development, the developmental therapist may require information on the family's cultural and social structure, its functional needs, goals and aspirations, and the way in which these factors change over time.[53] The complexity of these factors suggests the wisdom of using a systems perspective to direct the selection of instruments. Assessments that are based on systems principles and have some established psychometric properties will be described in detail. In addition, a sequential list of questions (Fig. 4-1) will be used to guide therapists in test selection as they initiate the family assessment process. This list is only a suggested guide and includes some of the most relevant assessments available to address these questions. Additional assessments applicable in unique settings are described in the narrative of this chapter.

Within the family system, six elements require evaluation: the individual child, the caregivers' relationship, the parent–child relationship, sibling relationships, intergenerational relationships, and community relationships.[11] The developmental therapist assesses the infant's functional level and may identify some of these other areas for additional assessment. For example, emphasis could be placed on the family's sense of mastery, its locus of control, or the division of labor within the family. To understand role relationships, parent–child or sibling–child interaction might provide useful information, as would the role characteristics of grandparents or significant extended family members. Knowledge about other community social support might also provide useful information and could be ascertained from an interview with personnel in community agencies. Given the constraints on clinical time, an extensive assessment package is impractical, but assessments in one or two of these areas could augment understanding of the help the family provides to facilitate the motor development of the infant.

In selecting the most appropriate assessment tools for any child and family, developmental therapists could ask the caregivers a series of questions as shown in the decision tree in Figure 4-1. Progressing through this decision tree, family concerns related to the child's participation in functional activities may be identified, and the family's influence on the motor development of the child may be clarified. The list of instruments noted in Figure 4-1 is not inclusive. These assessments are simply those thought to meet some psychometric standards and to be the most appropriate and relevant to therapeutic intervention for physical therapists, occupational therapists, and speech and language pathologists. Other assessments will be briefly discussed in the text for those practicing in different arenas requiring different assessments.

Does This At-Risk Child Need Assessment?

The Infant Monitoring Questionnaire

Brief Description. The Infant Monitoring Questionnaire[53] (IMQ) was designed by a team from the Center on Human Development at the University of Oregon as a screening instrument that enables parents to monitor their at-risk

Questions	Type of Assessment	Instrument	Results
1. Does this at risk child need assessment? ──→ Yes ↓ No	Screening by parent	Infant Monitoring Questionnaire (IMQ)	Refer for further testing
2. Does the family choose to be involved? ──→ Yes ↓ No (if no, go to #8)	Initial Interview with parent	Process described by Winton, or Wright & Leahy	Further family Assessment
3. Are you concerned about family membership and intergenerational factors: ──→ Yes ↓ No	Interview	Genogram	
4. Are you concerned about family routines, roles, and resources? ──→ Yes ↓ No	Checklist Interview Rating Scale	Family Routines Inventory (FRI) ECOMAP Family Inventory of Resources for Management (FIRM)	
5. Are you concerned about family environments? ──→ Yes ↓ No	Checklist	Home Observation for Measurement of the Environment (HOME)	

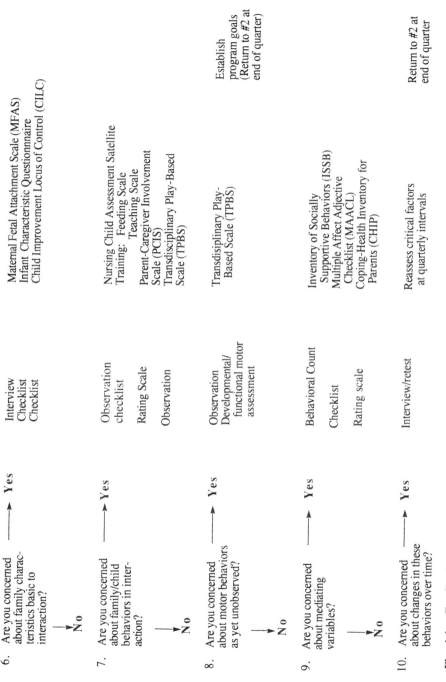

Fig. 4-1. Family Assessment Selection Guide. Arrows indicate direction therapist takes after making an assessment decision.

6. Are you concerned about family characteristics basic to interaction? ———→ Yes → Interview → Maternal Fetal Attachment Scale (MFAS)
Checklist → Infant Characteristic Questionnaire
Checklist → Child Improvement Locus of Control (CILC)
↓ No

7. Are you concerned about family/child behaviors in interaction? ———→ Yes → Observation checklist → Nursing Child Assessment Satellite Training: Feeding Scale / Teaching Scale
Rating Scale → Parent-Caregiver Involvement Scale (PCIS)
Observation → Transdisciplinary Play-Based Scale (TPBS)
↓ No

8. Are you concerned about motor behaviors as yet unobserved? ———→ Yes → Observation → Transdisiplinary Play-Based Scale (TPBS)
Developmental/ functional motor assessment
Establish program goals (Return to #2 at end of quarter)

9. Are you concerned about mediating variables? ———→ Yes → Behavioral Count → Inventory of Socially Supportive Behaviors (ISSB)
Checklist → Multiple Affect Adjective Checklist (MAACL)
Rating scale → Coping-Health Inventory for Parents (CHIP)
↓ No

10. Are you concerned about changes in these behaviors over time? ———→ Yes → Interview/retest → Reassess critical factors at quarterly intervals
Return to #2 at end of quarter

81

infants and toddlers at home. The Manual includes procedures for following children aged 4 to 36 months with eight age-appropriate questionnaires. Each of the eight assessments consists of a cover sheet for demographic data, four sheets with items in the five major behavioral categories, and one sheet for general impression items and comments. The five categories are communication, gross motor, fine motor, adaptive, and personal–social. Each of these five categories consists of six scored items, and the overall category consists of five items. These categories can be assessed at eight corrected ages of 4, 8, 12, 16, 20, 24, 30, and 36 months. The assessment items have been taken from developmentally based, norm-referenced tests and do not exceed the 75 to 100 developmental quotient range for each age level. Pictures accompany some of the items for clarification. The eight 6-page assessments are color coded according to gender, with items reflecting the gender of the child to be assessed. For research purposes the questionnaires can be photocopied, and a program disk is included for computerized filing of data.

Procedure.   Using the correct score sheet for gender and corrected age, the parent checks one of three responses to each item: "Yes," "Sometimes," or "Not Yet." Scores of "1," "0.05," and "0" are given for these responses with the higher total score indicating the greatest developmental achievement. The "overall" category consists of five problem-related questions requiring a "No" or "Yes" response. Additional space is allotted for an explanation of these responses that do not receive a score but are individually evaluated. Based on 3,300 questionnaires, mean scores and standard deviations are provided, and two standard deviations or more from the mean suggest abnormal development. In cases in which the child's score is abnormal, the parent is contacted and further testing is suggested. A 6-step follow-up procedure in these cases is described in the Manual.

Technical Evaluation.   The items for each test were drawn from a number of developmentally based, norm-referenced tests, including the Bayley Scales of Infant Development, the Revised Gesell Developmental Schedules, and the Ordinal Scales of Psychological Development. Through two separate studies reliability and validity were determined.[54,55] Inter-observer reliability of 112 parents and two professional testers ranged from 87 to 97 percent. Test–retest reliability with 175 parents over a 2- to 3-week period ranged from 91 to 99 percent.

Concurrent validity of the IMQ with the Revised Gesell Developmental Schedules ranged from 79 percent at 4 months to 94 percent at 16 months, with an overall agreement of 88 percent. Concurrent validity with the Bayley Scales of Infant Development and the Stanford-Binet Intelligence Scale ranged from a low of 85 percent at 30 months to a high of 91 percent at 12, 20, and 36 months, with an overall agreement of 89 percent. Using the Gesell, Bayley, and Stanford-Binet as criterion measures, the overall underscreening rate was 2 to 7 percent, while the overall overscreening rate was 5 to 8 percent. The proportion of infants correctly identified as delayed (sensitivity) was best at higher ages (and ranged from 0.43 to 0.94, while the proportion of infants correctly rated within normal limits (specificity) ranged from 0.83 to 0.94.

Qualitative Evaluation.   The clinical utility of the IMQ rests on the professional time saved, the appropriateness of using parents as a referral source, and the test's low cost. The items do not include any professional jargon, are on a sixth-grade or lower reading level, and are accompanied by examples or pictures to assist in understanding the item. This is a well-developed instrument, especially appropriate for toddlers, and meets the demands of identification of special needs children and at the same time educates parents to the normal developmental progression.

The Family APGAR

Another screening approach is suggested by the Family APGAR,[56] which was developed as a 5-item screening instrument to determine family functioning. One of the five questions of this quick screening device is "I am satisfied with the way my family talks over things with me and shares problems with me." Three responses can be scored on a scale of 0, 1, or 2, giving a possible total score of 10. Concurrent validity with the Pless-Satterwhite Family Function Index was 0.80. Discriminate validity was established by differentiating married graduate students from mental health clinic patients. A number of studies have been conducted that indicate psychometric support for the use of this instrument. In one study with pregnant women,[57] the Family APGAR was used as the measure of family function and was shown to be the best psychosocial predictor of pregnancy complications. Family function interacted with biomedical risk to explain 11 percent of the variance in postpartum complications. This assessment may be appropriate in some nursery settings, but the use of one assessment so early in life as a predictor for later development is questionable. Evaluation during the process of pregnancy or during development in infancy may prove to be more beneficial than at any one point in time.

Screening initiates the assessment process and permits identification of infants who are in need of further evaluation or who will self-right and not need intervention. Involvement of parents at the screening level appears to facilitate reliable and cost-effective identification of at-risk infants while educating parents in the developmental process. The selection of a screening instrument and the time at which it is used are the essential factors in reliable screening.

Does the Family Choose To Be Involved?

With parents who have an infant known to be impaired or at significant risk, a more interactive approach using established interviewing techniques is suggested. A high level of skill in interviewing is required to share potential dimensions of involvement with the parent, gain rapport with the parent, and ascertain the parent's or caregiver's preferences.[58] Winton[59] has established a model for conducting a family-focused interview. The first step is to prepare for the interview by summarizing any data available from screening. With this background information, the first interview is initiated with a clear explanation to the parent of its purpose, the time allotted for discussion, and the maintenance of confidentiality. In this interview the therapist transfers authority to the parent in terms of encouraging the parent to voice opinions and ask questions. The summary section of the interview permits the therapist and the family to specify family priorities and collaboratively to set goals. The final step in the interview process permits closure in which the therapist voices appreciation for parental involvement and requests any further concerns. Although this final step may sound redundant, critical information often surfaces at this time. For instructional purposes, an interview evaluation tool has been developed[60] and has proven useful for students in critiquing their own performance. Additional guidance for interviewing families of special needs children is contained within the Calgary Family Assessment Model.[18]

Based on the success of the interview, the family may feel empowered to pursue the remaining assessment process as described in Figure 4-1. The purpose of this process is to establish a foundation for the longitudinal involvement of parents in the education of their child. Responses to many of these questions will be negative, necessitating only a functional motor assessment of the infant. For some families, however, evaluation of the structure, function, and developmental course of the family will augment the establishment and implementation of an appropriate program for the infant.

Are You Concerned About Family Membership and Intergenerational Factors?

Family structure has been defined as "the relationships among family members and the extent to which those relationships determine how the family deals with daily tasks."[16] The first factor in this definition requires an understanding of the actual membership or degrees of freedom of the family, for example the number, age, and gender of family members. The second factor requires an understanding of the rules and tasks related to the interaction of these participants (e.g., routines, roles, and resources). A third element of family structure is the environment that family members create and in which they live and perform.

An accepted interviewing practice is to request the number, age, and gender of children living in the home and the number of family members living nearby. If we extend our interviewing only slightly beyond this point, we can rather rapidly establish a genogram for a child and family.[61] This form of assessment depicts several generations of a family, showing their ages, relationships, roles and occupations, causes of death, infirmities, or responses to life transitions (as

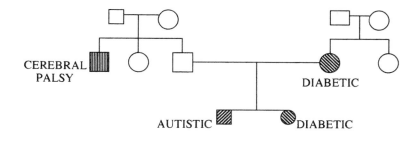

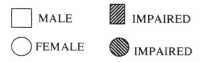

Fig. 4-2. Genogram.

shown in Fig. 4-2). Members of numerous disciplines[16,18,59] have suggested the use of this kind of structural assessment for clarifying the dimensions of a family. Not only does the interviewer gain a better understanding of the family through the reciprocal process of creating the genogram, but family members gain a better understanding of the characteristics of their intergenerational family.

Are You Concerned About Family Routines, Roles, and Resources?

Once the family composition has been determined, the rules that organize a family can be delineated in terms of family routines, roles, and resources.

Routines

Obtaining a family's daily schedule permits parent involvement in the assessment process, identification of periods in which successful family interaction occurs, and an understanding of family priorities.

The Family Routines Inventory

Brief Description. The Family Routines Inventory[62] (FRI) measures 28 common observable behaviors that occur within the typical day of a family with at least one child aged 16 years or younger. The purpose of developing the scale was to identify consistent and stable routines that support a family during times of clear stress. These routines comprise 10 categories: workday, weekend and leisure time, children's routines, parental routines, bedtime, meals, extended family, leaving and homecoming, disciplinary routines, and household chores.

Procedure.   The 28 items are presented in a paper and pencil checklist to the respondent. For each routine, two response categories exist: frequency of occurrence of the routine and importance to the family. A sample item is "Family eats at the same time each night." If this routine occurs every day, a score of 3 is given; if it occurs three to five times per week, a score of 2 is given; if it occurs from one to two times per week, a score of 1 is given; and "almost never" is scored 0.

Technical Evaluation.   To diminish the effects of race and social class differences, 52 families were identified according to a stratified sampling procedure. This procedure identified 26 black and 26 white families who were interviewed for 60 to 90 minutes about their typical daily routines. The resultant 104 routines were weighted for importance by a second sample of 260 women of mixed race, age, marital status, education, and income. To be included in the final test, an item had to receive a median 6.5 rating on an 11-point scale, the range of scores on each item could not exceed 5.5 on the 11-point scale, and no significant differences were noted according to race or social class. Twenty-eight routines were identified. The test–retest realiability coefficient for frequency scores was 0.79. Using the FES, the frequency score of the FRI was a significant predictor of family cohesion, solidarity, order, and satisfaction with family life.

Qualitative Assessment.   The scale is useful to determine the regulated flow of the day as might be interpreted by an infant or toddler. Frequency scores on specific items could suggest modifications in daily routines and the provision of greater family stability and consistency for the infant. Four of the 28 behaviors relate to school-aged children so are not appropriate for families with infants. Further study of the psychometric properties of this assessment is warranted, although initial results suggest its validity.

Roles

Family roles provide additional information about family structure. The ecomap[63] is a pictorial diagram of family members and the way in which they interact with systems external to the family (e.g., health care, work, and church). As with the genogram, the ecomap can be constructed through an interview. A systems diagram is drawn, as shown in Figure 4-3, which depicts not only the important systems related to an infant and family but also the strengths and directions of influence of those relationships[18] and important allegiances within and external to the family.

More formal assesments have been developed to determine roles of family members. The Role Checklist[64] was developed to assess an adult's value of 10 roles in the past, present, and future. Initial work indicates that the instrument has good test–retest reliability. The Child Care Role Scale[65] is a clinical research tool designed to identify what family member "feeds the child" or "puts the

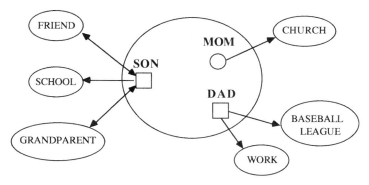

Fig. 4-3. Ecomap. Arrows indicate the direction of the interaction: no interaction among family members, but much interaction of members with external activities.

child to sleep." Another instrument, The Family Role Scale,[66] can be used by family members themselves or as the basis for a family interview that extends discussion initiated with the development of the ecomap.

Resources

Fundamental to roles and rules and their enactment is an analysis of the wide range of resources available to a family. One model describes the family's resources, both financial and psychological, and the family's perception of the gravity of any stressor. When perceptions of stress increase, a "pile up" of stressors occurs and stretches the family's resources, making coping and adaptation more of a challenge. It is not the stressor or "life event" itself that is important for the interventionist to understand, but the pile up of stressors and the resources available to help families cope with them. Therefore, life event scales will not be described.[67,68] The family's sense of mastery and of competence in meeting these life events appear to be critical factors, however, and have been reliably assessed by the Family Inventory of Resources for Management (FIRM).[69]

Family Inventory of Resources for Management

Brief Description. The FIRM was developed at the University of Wisconsin–Madison to assess the social and psychological resources that help the family adapt to stressful situations. It operationalizes the resources element of the double ABC-X model of stress. The 69-item scale contains five subscales: esteem and communication, mastery and health, extended family social support, financial well-being, and resource strains.

Procedure. The FIRM is a self-report, paper and pencil measure that requires the respondent to circle one of four responses of "Not At All," "Minimally,'' ''Moderately,'' or ''Very Well''. This format permits manual or computer scoring of the responses on a 0 to 3 scale. ''Very Well'' receives a 3, while ''Not At All'' receives a 0. The assessment usually takes 10 to 15 minutes to complete.

Technical Evaluation.   Internal consistency (Cronbach's alpha) of the five scales was 0.85 except for the subscale of "extended family support," which was 0.62. On initial assessment of 322 families with a child with either myelomeningocele or cerebral palsy, the scales were highly intercorrelated ($p < 0.001$). Concurrent validity was determined using the FES and showed high positive correlations with the cohesion, expressiveness, and organization subscales and a high negative correlation with the conflict subscale of the FES.

High- and low-conflict families could be differentiated on mastery and health for families with children with myelomeningocele and families with children with cerebral palsy. High- and low-conflict families with children with cerebral palsy could be differentiated on esteem and communication. In a recent study[70] of single- and two-parent families with a child with cerebral palsy, no differences were noted between the two groups in all but the financial well-being subscale. Single-parent families reported a lower level of financial well-being than did two-parent families.

Clinical Utility.   The FIRM has a Profile of Family Resources based on normative data that can be used as a summary sheet to assist in consultation with family members. The FIRM can be used as a pre- and a post-test to evaluate an intervention program if a goal has been increasing social support or a sense of mastery.

Other types of resources include a parent's understanding of human development. Determining parental knowledge of fetal, infant, and toddler development could foster more effective parenting.[71] The Knowledge of Infant Development[72] is a 75-item paper and pencil assessment of the parent's current understanding of aspects of infant development. These aspects include infant norms and milestones, health care and safety, principles and processes of development, and parent responsibilities and strategies. Most of the items are responded to by selecting "Agree," "Disagree," or "Not Sure" responses. The assessment has been carefully developed and could be used to direct parent education related to infant development.

Are You Concerned About Family Environments?

Assessment of the environment that the family creates, in which family members live and work, and in which children move can provide information critical to the implementation of intervention regimens. The most widely used assessment of the home environment is the Home Observation for Measurement of the Environment (HOME).[73]

Home Observation for Measurement of the Environment

Brief Description. The infant version of the HOME assessment measures the "stimulation potential" of the environment that is created by the family to facilitate infant development from birth to age 3 years. The 45-item scale includes six factors: emotional and verbal responsivity of parents, acceptance of child, organization of physical and temporal environment, provision of appropriate play materials, parental involvement with child, and opportunities for variety in daily stimulation. These six factors were determined by a 0.34 or higher factor loading.

Procedure. The 1 hour assessment is administered in the infant's home while the infant is playing with the caregiver. Using a binary scale with "Yes" and "No" as the responses, one-third of the items (n = 15) are scored by parent report, and two-thirds of the items (n = 30) are observed and scored later by the clinician.

Technical Evaluation. Inter-rater reliability of 90 percent can be achieved with brief training. Internal consistency measured by the Kuder-Richardson 20 coefficients ranged from 0.44 to 0.89 for the subscales and were 0.89 for the total scale. Stability ranged from a low of 0.20 to a moderate 0.60. The issue of validity was addressed with 77 persons of diverse socioeconomic status. Of them, 65 percent were black, and 35 percent were white. Predictive validity from ages 6 months to 3, 4, and 7 years ranged from 0.38 to 0.50. Concurrent validity was assessed using the subscales of positive orientation, enthusiasm, alertness, and activity level of the Bayley Infant Behavior Record. Scores on all subscales correlated with six socioeconomic factors except maternal occupation. Discriminant validity existed between the designations of "adequate" and "inadequate" home environment, but not as clearly between "adequate" and "above adequate" home environment.

Clinical Utility. The HOME is easy for nonprofessionals as well as professionals to learn (10 home visits and scale scorings are required). Its items are clearly written, and only 3 out of the 45 items require direct questioning of the parent. It can be used with a variety of learning environments for an infant. Clinical research with low-birth-weight infants has suggested that HOME assessments in the first year of life were a better predictor of general development at age 4 years than were demographic and medical variables.[74] In addition, the HOME can be used effectively to instruct parents in developing a learning environment for their infants. Some items on this assessment are culturally biased, requiring modification for use with a broader segment of the population.

A working knowledge of family membership, rules, resources, and the environments in which children perform permits the developmental therapist to identify the uniqueness of each child and family unit. Use of any one of these assessments may be suggested to and endorsed by a family, but determining the way in which family members function through interaction may be a more sensitive area of assessment.

Are You Concerned About Family Characteristics Basic to Interaction?

The way in which family members perform interactively can affect the child's development and is therefore of interest to developmental therapists. Several parental characteristics are fundamental to the way in which parents interact and may need to be assessed first. These prefunctional determinants of interaction include early parental attachment, parental perception of infant temperament, and parental locus of control.

Attachment

Parental attachment is characterized by parental observation of the fetus' or infant's activities and safety and by demonstration of alarm when danger or uncertainty occurs in relation to the fetus or infant. The Maternal–Fetal Attachment Scale and the Paternal–Fetal Attachment Scale[75] can determine the degrees to which parents are affiliated with or engaged in interaction with their unborn child. Each form has five subscales: role taking, differentiating self from fetus, giving of self, interacting with fetus, and attributing characteristics to the fetus. The assessments are administered as paper and pencil checklists with a five-point response scale from "Definitely Yes" to "Definitely No." Internal consistency on the maternal scale gave an alpha coefficient of 0.85 and on the paternal scale gave a Cronbach's alpha coefficient of 0.80. The scale was developed for use with 30 mothers of all five Hollingshead socioeconomic groups with mixed parity and types of delivery. All infants were within normal limits. The assessment can be used from early in the second trimester and with primary caregivers to determine the relationship between early attachment and parental perceptions of their newborn and infant.

To assess attachment, Bretherton et al.[76] developed The Parent Attachment Interview. Five components of this interview were revealed by content analysis: mother's feelings at the infant's birth, baby as a person, parental and child responses to nightime waking, maternal feelings about separations, and maternal responses when a child wants to perform an unmastered activity unaided. A sensitivity/insight scale used to score the texts of these interviews was significantly correlated with five other attachment scales, suggesting its valid use with parents of infants.

Temperament

A discrepancy exists in the literature as to whether temperament is a stable trait[77] or a parental perception.[78] The Bates Infant Characteristic Questionnaire[78] differentiates infants according to parental perceptions of temperament on four variables: fussy-difficult, unadaptable, dull, and unpredictable. In a study of behavioral responsiveness of preterm infants with intraventricular hemorrhage,[79] the preterm infants were rated by the parents as more fussy-difficult and harder to soothe than the full-term infants. Whether temperament is a trait or a state, interventionists need to recognize that this factor can modify family dynamics and may need assessment.

Locus of Control

Individuals and families develop expectations of behavior. When a person's behavior in a specific situation is consistently thwarted, that person begins to expect that control comes from external forces (i.e., an external locus of control). When persons have success in goal achievement through their efforts, they come to believe that they are in control of their destiny and thus develop an internal locus of control.[80] When a personal experience, such as the birth of a premature or impaired infant, threatens an established internal locus of control, the individual or family may resort to an external belief system temporarily, but their internal locus will still determine their coping ability to a large degree. When a person with an external locus of control is challenged, factors external to the individual often are "blamed" for the event.

The Child Improvement Locus of Control (CILC) Scale[81] is a 27-item assessment used in studies with autistic and physically handicapped children. Factor analyses have identified five factors that influence an improvement in child health: chance, divine influence, parents, professionals, and the child. Using the CILC scale with a younger sample of children with cerebral palsy, Phillips, Campbell, and Wilhelm (presented at the Society for Research in Child Development, April, 1987) determined that difficult caregiving was associated with the parent's belief in chance and with the parent's ability level. Severity of cerebral palsy was associated with a belief in the relationship with professionals, with older mothers having a greater belief in professionals than younger mothers. Studies of parents of different ethnicities have associated an internal locus of control with best parenting practice[82] and self-esteem[83].

Are You Concerned About Family–Child Behaviors in Interaction?

With some understanding of prefunctional determinants of interaction, caregiver–child interaction can be more readily assessed. Barnard and Eyres[84] have developed an integrated model of caregiver–infant interaction in which the infant gives cues that are readable by the parent, the parent recognizes and responds to these cues, and the infant in turn responds to the parent. In this reciprocal interaction, the parent alleviates the infant's distress when possible and presents learning experiences for the infant. To support her view of development, Barnard has developed a series of assessments that are clearly documented, relatively short and easy to administer, and have been shown to be valid and reliable.

Nursing Child Assessment Satellite Training Teaching and Feeding Scales

Brief Description. The Nursing Child Assessment Scales were developed at the University of Washington to assess parent responsiveness to infant cues given in specific circumstances. The development of these scales is based on the Child Health Assessment Interaction Model, which describes the interaction of the mother and the infant within a supportive environment. The Teaching Scale consists of 73 items appropriate for use from birth to age 3 years. The Feeding Scale consists of 76 items and is used with infants from birth to age 1 year. Each scale consists of six subscales: sensitivity to cues, response to distress, social–emotional growth fostering, cognitive growth fostering, clarity of cues, and responsiveness to parent.

Procedure. The two assessments are on color-coded single sheets. To each item a "Yes" or "No" response is required. A subscale score is determined by summing the number of Yes responses in each of the six categories. A total score is formulated by adding all the subtotal scores. The respondent is asked whether this was a typical feeding or if the respondent was uncomfortable due to the presence of the tester. Space is provided for an explanatory narrative, including parental concerns or the observer's comments.

Technical Evaluation. Every seventh subject from the Nursing Child Assessment Project was used to describe the normative sample of 14 female and 18 male infants. Their mothers were white, married, had a mean of 14.5 years of education (SD = 2.4), and were on average 25.4 years old (SD = 3.4). Items on each scale were "positively correlated" and items between scales "not as strongly correlated." When establishing test–retest reliability, test intervals of at least 3 months were used (i.e., 1 to 4, 4 to 8, and 8 to 12 months). Correlations of scores at these two testing times were positive but not significant. Discriminant validity was determined in a study with 95 infants, in which premature (n = 28) and abused (n = 22) scored lower than normal controls (n = 45). In another sample, premature infants (n = 39) and failure-to-thrive infants (n = 9) scored a low of 51.3 compared with controls (n = 342), who scored 61.8.

Predictive validity of the Feeding Scale is suggested with results at 8 months correlating at 0.72 with results on the 24-month HOME and at 12 months correlating at 0.79 with the 35-month results on the HOME. The Teaching Scale at 1 month positively correlates with expressive language at 36 months (0.71); at 4 months correlates with expressive language at 36 months (0.76); at 8 months correlates with Bayley 12-month Mental Development Index (MDI) and Psychomotor Development Index (PDI) (0.66); and at 12 months correlates with Bayley MDI (0.67).

Clinical Utility. The Teaching and Feeding Scales are easy to use and provide a wealth of information about the way in which parents interact with their infants in specific situations. With the scales, the clinician can determine the educational needs of the parent. Unlike observation of spontaneous play behavior, however, these scales place restrictions on the parent and infant, challenging them to perform in ways that are not necessarily their most characteristic or their best. In addition, the wording and content of the items appear to be culturally biased, as the normative sample was based on highly educated, two-parent, white families.

Numerous parent–child interaction scales have been developed to assess spontaneous behavior in interaction (for review, see Comfort[85]). One of these, the Parent Behavior Progression,[86] was developed for clinical use to enhance the interaction of the parent with the infant through an increased sensitivity on the part of the clinical staff to parent issues. A form exists for observation of parents of 0- to 9-month old infants and 9- to 36-month old toddlers. No reliability or formal validity reports accompany the scale. One parent–infant interaction assessment that has some psychometric data available is the The Parent–Caregiver Involvement Scale (PCIS).[87]

Parent–Caregiver Involvement Scale

Brief Description. The PCIS was initially developed at the University of North Carolina at Chapel Hill to assess the quality, quantity, and appropriateness of a caregiver's interaction with a 2- to 57-month-old child. The test is composed of 11 subscales: physical, verbal, responsiveness, teaching, play, control, goal orientation, positive and negative affects, directives, and relationship among activities. A manual and videotape are available and contain detailed descriptions of each item in terms of quantity, quality, and appropriateness.

Procedure. The PCIS is scored after a 20 minute observation of parent and child playing in a naturalistic environment. The rater uses a 5-point anchored scale to score the quantity, quality, and appropriateness of the caregiver's behaviors on the 11 items. A videotape of instructions assists in the training of examiners, a process that requires a minimum of 3 hours.

Technical Evaluation. Inter-rater reliability on the subscales was determined on scores from home observation (0.77 to 0.87) and on scores made from videotaped play sessions (0.54 to 0.93). The videotape prevented some behaviors from being heard or seen, but permitted replay to clarify other behaviors. Intra-rater reliability of 21 videotapes of fathers in interaction with their children was 0.92 to 0.95. Moderately high correlations have been reported in the manual with behavioral counts of parental interactive behaviors. Ratings of mothers have been moderately correlated with infant temperament. The lack of independence of categories and the difficulty in achieving reliability using exact scores rather than scores within 1 point suggest the need for further psychometric definition.

Clinical Utility. The PCIS can be used to assess the spontaneous behavior of either a parent or a caregiver in a natural environment. With a standardized set of toys and a clear description of how they are commonly used, the scale provides a reliable framework for clinical assessment and intervention. Because the 11 categories are not independent, using total scores on these items for research purposes is questionnable.

Are You Concerned About Motor Behaviors as Yet Unobserved?

Interaction of an infant with peers and siblings as well as with parents has been assessed by intervention teams. One example of a team assessment that includes parents as full participants is the Transdisciplinary Play-Based Assessment.[88] In this process, the toddler is observed for 60 to 90 minutes in six settings: unstructured facilitation, structured facilitation, toddler–toddler interaction, parent–toddler interaction with an attachment sequence included, motor play both structured and unstructured, and snack time. Observation guidelines for sensorimotor development and worksheets on which to record observations are included. A summary sheet permits the observer to record both the toddler's strengths and developmental age in eight gross and fine motor activities and positions and the family's "needs" and their justification. Follow-up team meetings including the parent enable all participants to have a voice in development of the program plan.

Assessment of family function can be an invasive process or one in which the individual family comes to perceive its needs more clearly. The developmental therapist is uniquely challenged in learning about the interactive characteristics and needs of the family in order to provide more appropriate information to and support for the family teaching and caring for the child.

Are You Concerned About Mediating Variables?

Social Support

Many special needs families experiencing a number of stressors have a diminished ability to "self soothe or to soothe other family members."[89] This diminished ability to provide social support for its members is a limiting factor in a family's process of adapting to changing circumstances. Social support has been shown to be a critical factor in alleviating stress during pregnancy and early parenting.[90,91] The Inventory of Socially Supportive Behaviors (ISSB)[91] has been used to ascertain which behaviors are supportive and who provides them during these periods. As a relatively short assessment, it can be used effectively during any life span transitions.

Inventory of Socially Supportive Behaviors

Brief Description. The ISSB was developed to determine the relationship between social support and adjustment. It is a 40-item paper and pencil test consisting of objective behaviors that were thought to help others master "emotional distress, sharing tasks, giving advice, teaching skills and providing material aid."[91] A sample item from the inventory is: During the last 4 weeks, someone "Expressed interest and concern in your well-being."

Procedure. Responders are asked to think about the past 4 weeks as they determine how often specific activities were done for, to, or with them. Responses are given by a 5-point Likert-type scale, providing a frequency of occurrence of activities ranging from "Not at all" to "About every day" over the past 4 weeks.

Technical Evaluation. Internal consistency of the scale using coefficient alphas was 0.93 and 0.94 on two testings separated by 2 days. Because of the high internal consistency, the total score of the ISSB is used rather than any item or factor score. Test–retest reliability for 71 university students with the 2-day interval was 0.88 and for individual items ranged from 0.44 to 0.91. Concurrent validity was determined with 43 university students using the FES cohesion subscale and a test of perceived social support (0.36, $p < 0.01$). For 86 pregnant women, stressful life events were positively correlated with results on the ISSB (0.41, $p < 0.001$), indicating the greater the number of stressful events, the greater the social support.

Clinical Utility. The ISSB provides a brief (5 to 10 minutes) multimethod approach to assessing social support by asking which people supply behaviors as well as what behaviors are supplied. A third aspect of social support, satisfaction or perceived adequacy of support, can also be asked for each behavior through interviewing the responder. The scale can be used in clinical research as a pre- and postmeasure to determine the role of social support as a mediator of stressful events or as an evaluation of one aspect of an intervention program.

Anxiety

Parental anxiety has been associated with parental perceptions of and behaviors with their child.[92] Assessment of anxiety in a simple and direct way can act as a preventive measure by keeping parents informed of their emotional state at any one point in time. This can be done simply while the therapist is recording data on the child or demographics of the family, using the Multiple Affect Adjective Checklist.[93] This 1-page assessment consists of 132 eighth-grade-level adjectives that describe the way in which the responder feels at one time. In previous work with this scale,[94] the interviewers recognized its therapeutic value for assisting patients in tracking their emotional state as they went through the stress of a high-risk pregnancy.

Coping

Combrinck-Graham[95] has described a system oscillation model in which family members or elements are brought together at several times in the life course, such as birth, adolescence, middle adulthood reevaluation, and retirement. This recycling through life events enables family members to practice earlier coping behaviors and to become more competent in their expression. Over the life spiral these coming together or centripetal periods are interspersed with periods of autonomy and disengagement, or centrifugal periods. Change during these times (e.g., starting work) can add to the stress level, causing a "pile up" of stress. McCubbin and co-workers[96] have developed an instrument with which to understand the way families cope with this pile up of stressors.

Coping-Health Inventory for Parents

Brief Description. The Coping-Health Inventory for Parents (CHIP) was initially designed at the University of Minnesota to assess parents' perceptions of their response to managing family life with a seriously or chronically ill child. *Coping,* according to these investigators, refers to "personal or collective efforts to manage the hardships associated with health problems in the family."[68] According to the ABC-X Model underlying this scale, the greater the variety of coping behaviors, the more effective the family coping in relation to a chronically ill child. The scale was developed as part of The Family Stress Project, and its selection of items was based on previous study of family response to stress; theories of social support, family stress, and coping; and experience with medical support offered families. The CHIP contains 45 items within three scales: maintaining family integration, cooperation, and an optimistic definition of the situation (19 items); maintaining social support, self-esteem, and psychological stability (18 items); and understanding the medical situation through communication with other parents and consultation with medical staff (8 items). A sample item is "Believing that my child is getting the best medical care possible."

Procedure. A computer-scoreable form is provided for the parent rater, who responds to the 45 items by circling with a pencil one of four responses from "Extremely helpful" to "Not helpful." Scores are given each response, with 3 given to "Extremely helpful" and 0 to "Not helpful." In addition, the parent may select two other responses of "Choose not to" or "Not possible" if the parent does not cope as described in the item. After rating the items, the tester may wish to score the items manually and discuss the family member's response by means of a profile with means and standard deviations derived from the normative data.

Technical Evaluation. The 45 items and three factors that comprise the CHIP were developed from an original 80 items used with a sample of 185 parents who had a child with cystic fibrosis. Factor loadings for the three categories ranged from 0.48 to 0.74, with the three factors explaining 71 percent of the variance. Moderate intercorrelations of the factors are reported, but no supportive data are given. Internal reliabilities (Cronbach's alpha) of 0.79, 0.79, and 0.71 are given, respectively, on the three factors. Using a sample of 308 mothers and fathers with a chronically ill child, means and standard deviations were established for the CHIP.

Concurrent validity was determined with parents of children with cystic fibrosis using the FES and two child measures of the child's height/weight and pulmonary function index. The mother's use of all three coping measures was associated with cohesiveness and expressiveness on the FES. The father's use of two coping strategies was significantly associated with cohesiveness, conflict, organization, and control on the FES. Discriminant validity was achieved with high and low conflict families. High versus low coping families used all coping patterns ($p < 0.05$), supporting the concept of coping as a response to stress and conflict.

Clinical Utility.   The scale was developed based on responses from an equal number of fathers and mothers and therefore appears to be appropriate for the increasing number of single parents. A profile based on normative data from parents of chronically ill children can be used for comparative purposes. The CHIP can be adapted for use with any ill family member, not simply an ill child. The scale is one page long and easy to read and score.

Are You Concerned About Changes in Parental Behaviors Over Time?

Theoretical models and the assessments supporting them have been used to attempt to predict behavior. These models may not have extended systems theory sufficiently to address the dimension of change and how families restructure themselves to cope with change. Dynamic Systems Theory[97] and the Theory of Chaos[89] are grounded in change, however, and focus on transitions within development in order to understand the variables that control system elements, to describe the properties of family transitions, and to facilitate the emergence of new behaviors. They are concerned with processes rather than outcomes and therefore offer guidance in assessing the changes experienced by families over time.

In addressing change and family assessment, we may need to recognize that some families are regulated in their behaviors and some families exhibit characteristics of chaos, as Gottman[89] has suggested. The regulated family system moves in and out of a stable state of equilibrium during transitions by the ability to draw on energy stored to cope and regain a more steady state. The regulated system, in times of crisis or transition, will order change and adjust.

In contrast, the chaotic family system is extremely sensitive to small perturbations and does not appear to have the stored energy reserves required to address change. Chaotic families are not predictable and might describe some of the more contemporary families. For the chaotic system, the process of change and adaptation may involve withdrawal, aggression, decreased ability to use new information and to concentrate on tasks, use of overlearned behaviors, loneliness, and a hypervigilance "to potentially threatening and escalating interactions."[89] Small changes that do not affect regulated families can, however, thrust chaotic families into enormous long-term upheavals. At such times, the potential for therapists to increase family disequilibrium is real. Awareness of the characteristics of regulated and chaotic families can enhance therapists' interactions during assessment, especially during the infant's transition periods such as independent eating, walking, or initial language expression.

NEW DIRECTIONS FOR FAMILY ASSESSMENT

Transitions

Two of the most exciting new sources of information that are relevant to assessment of motor development within the family context come from the field of developmental psychology. Thelan and Ulrich[97] have written a short but classic monograph, entitled *Hidden Skills*, in which they describe development in terms of self-organizing behavior and spontaneous pattern generation as the results of dynamic interaction of internal and external systems. These investigators speak of motor milestones as having limited developmental significance, while behavioral transitions and context-related performance are developmentally more relevant. Their concepts suggest that process variables rather than motor milestones should be the focus of assessments.

Cowan and Hetherington[11] have made a similar leap into a productive area of research in their work *Family Transitions*. They believe that psychosocial adaptation to life events and the pile up of stressors should be assessed rather than the crisis events themselves. These can best be assessed during developmental transitions in which families are in disequilibrium and vulnerable to modification. For assessment purposes, parent interviews[59,89] conducted over a period of time (i.e., 4 to 36 months) and during transitional times (i.e., during pregnancy through birthing) may be the most appropriate and productive assessment techniques to ascertain concerns and priorities. Further training in interviewing is required if developmental therapists are to achieve a higher level of skill in this area.

Tasks

Because the nature of tasks determines the way in which systems will perform, parents of special needs infants might well be most effectively assessed through their handling and caregiving tasks. This is the basis of Barnard and Eyres' assessments,[84] with the Teaching Scale creating more of a unique challenge for the parent, whereas the Feeding Scale is used to assess a more practiced set of behaviors. Observation of the child in interaction with the parent using an established format as described with the Transdisciplinary Play-Based Scale[88] may provide some of the most relevant information for an educational plan.

Environment

The present federal law supports family participation in the development and education of the special needs infant and toddler. In so doing, responsibility for the infant is extended beyond the maternal caretaker to any involved member of the family unit. Members of the family who surround the infant and provide daily experiences for and with the infant can add to the developmental therapist's understanding of that infant. In addition, the actual educational environment created by all family members will continue to be an important variable of the assessment process. Instruments such as the HOME[73] will be especially useful when made more applicable to contemporary diverse populations.

Evaluation

Program evaluation is an area of assessment that has been referred to only briefly. A number of the assessments described, however, could be used to evaluate different aspects of programs. Use of the ecomap, for example, provides information about interaction of family members with systems outside the family and can help one gain a perspective on which groups are supportive of the complex needs of the infant and family. In turn, parental assessment of the learning environment of the infant is conducted informally at present. Through assessments such as the Early Childhood Environment Rating Scale[98] more formal assessment may become a reality. Used to evaluate daycare settings, this scale may provide an opportunity for parents to assess the environment into which they are entrusting their child and thus act as a program evaluation tool.

THE NEED FOR FAMILY ASSESSMENT

A multitude of assessments have been reviewed. These assessments have been determined to be appropriate based on their focus, their psychometric properties, and the relevancy of their information to therapeutic intervention. The realities of practice are such, however, that time becomes a major factor in provision of care. Developmental therapists have numerous responsibilities that consume their time:

1. Providing direct infant intervention
2. Writing clinical objectives
3. Writing progress notes
4. Writing reimbursement claims
5. Consulting with team members
6. Determining need for and ordering equipment

In light of these demands, the only way developmental therapists can consider asking the questions presented in Figure 4-1 is to understand the long-term effect of a belief in the family as the unit of health care and educational need. This is not only a philosophical perspective removed some distance from the reality of the clinic but also a practical necessity.

The demand for developmental therapists continues. Financial concerns remain and limit the ability to educate sufficient professionals to meet these demands. Rather than "using" parents or caretakers,[99] developmental therapists may need to educate and support them in providing appropriate learning experiences for their infants. The family assessments suggested in this chapter not only access family information for the intervention team but also educate and support the family and its concerns and priorities.

REFERENCES

1. Michener JA: Caribbean. Fawcett Crest, New York, 1989, p. 109
2. Sparling JW: Embedding Family Information Into an Entry-Level Physical Therapy Curriculum. Frank Porter Graham Child Development Center, Chapel Hill, NC, 1992
3. House of Representatives, 99th Congress; Education of the Handicapped Act Amendments of 1986 (Public Law 99-457). Report 99-860, S.1106. Washington, DC, 1986
4. Senate, 102nd Congress: Individuals With Disabilities Education Act Amendments, Report 102-84, H.R.5520. Washington, DC, 1991 pp 16, 25
5. Slater MA, Maqvi M, Andrew L, Haynes K: Neurodevelopment of monitored versus nonmonitored very low birth weight infants: the importance of family influences. J Dev Behav Pediatr 8:278, 1987
6. Cassidy J: The ability to negotiate the environment: an aspect of infant competence as related to quality of attachment. Child Dev 57:331, 1986
7. Squires JK, Nickel R, Bricker D: Use of parent-completed developmental questionnaires for child-find and screening. Inf Young Child 3(2):46, 1990
8. House of Representatives: U.S. Children and Their Families: Current Conditions and Recent Trends, 1989. U.S. Government Printing Office, Washington, DC, 1989
9. Breslau N, Salkever D, Staruch KS: Women's labor force activity and responsibilities for disabled dependents: a study of families with disabled children. J Health Soc Behav 23:169, 1982
10. Gajdosik CG, Campbell SK: Effects of weekly review, socioeconomic status and maternal belief on mothers' compliance with their disabled children's home exercise program. Phys Occup Ther Pediatr 11(2):47, 1991
11. Cowan PA, Hetherington M (eds): Family Transitions. Lawrence Erlbaum Associates, Hillsdale, NJ, 1991
12. Bailey DB, Simeonsson RJ, Winton PJ et al: Family-focused intervention: a functional model for planning, implementing, and evaluating individualized family services in early intervention. J Div Early Child 10:156, 1986
13. Harris SR: Efficacy of physical therapy in promoting family functioning and functional independence for children with cerebral palsy. Pediatr Phys Ther 2:160, 1990
14. Gillette Y, Hansen NB, Robinson JL et al: Hospital-based case management for medically fragile infants: results of a randomized trial. Patient Educ Counsel 17:59, 1990
15. Lewis CC, Scott DE, Pantell RH, Wolf MH: Parent satisfaction with children's medical care: development, field test, and validation of a questionnaire. Med Care 24:209, 1986
16. Bailey DB, Simeonsson RJ: Family Assessment in Early Intervention. Merrill Publishing, Columbus, OH, 1988, pp. 29, 105

17. Dunst CJ, Trivette CM: A family systems model of early intervention with handicapped and developmentally at-risk children. p. 131. In Powell DR (ed): Parent Education as Early Childhood Intervention: Emerging Directions in Theory, Research, and Practice. Ablex Publishing Corporation, Norwood, NJ, 1988
18. Wright LM, Leahey M: Nurses and Families: a Guide to Family Assessment and Intervention. FA Davis, Philadelphia, 1989
19. Cochrane CG, Farley BG, Wilhelm IJ: Preparation of physical therapists to work with handicapped infants and their families: current status and training needs. Phys Ther 70:372, 1990
20. Crais ER, Leonard CR: PL 99-457: are speech–language pathologists prepared for the challenge? ASHA 32:57, 1990
21. Humphry R, Link S: Entry level preparation of occupational therapists to work in early intervention programs. Am J Occup Ther 44:828, 1990
22. Crais ER: A Practical Guide to Embedding Family-Centered Content Into Existing Speech–Language Pathology Coursework. Frank Porter Graham Child Development Center, Chapel Hill, NC, 1991
23. Winton P: Working With Families in Early Intervention: an Interdiscplinary Preservice Curriculum. Carolina Institute for Research on Infant Personnel Preparation, Chapel Hill, NC, 1991
24. Nover AR, Timberlake EM: Meeting the challenge: the educational preparation of social workers for practice with at-risk children (0–3) and their families. Inf Young Child 2:59, 1989
25. Bailey DB, McWilliam PJ, Winton PJ, Simeonsson RJ: Implementing Family-Centered Services in Early Intervention: a Team-Based Model for Change. Frank Porter Graham Child Development Center, Chapel Hill, NC, 1991
26. McGonigel MJ, Kaufman RK, Johnson BH (eds): Guidelines and Recommended Practices for the Individualized Family Service Plan. 2nd Ed. American Association for the Care of Children's Health, Bethesda, MD, 1991
27. APTA Task Force on Early Intervention, Section on Pediatrics: Competencies for physical therapists in early intervention. Pediatr Phys Ther 3:77, 1991
28. Dunst C, Trivette C, Deal A (eds): Enabling and Empowering Families. Brookline Books, Cambridge, MA, 1988
29. Crutcher DM: Family support in the home: home visiting and Public Law 99-457. Am Psychol 46:138, 1991
30. Case-Smith J: Occupational and physical therapists as case managers in early intervention. Phys Occup Ther Pediatr 11(1):53, 1991
31. Masnick G, Bane MJ: The Nation's Families: 1960–1990. Auburn House Publishing Co., Boston, 1980
32. Sparling JW: The cultural definition of the family. Phys Occup Ther Pediatr 11(4):17 1991
33. Shepard KF, Jensen GM: Physical therapist curricula for the 1990's: educating the reflective practitioner. Phys Ther 70:566, 1990
34. Bronfenbrenner U: The Ecology of Human Development. Harvard University Press, Cambridge, MA, 1979
35. Turnbull AP, Turnbull HR: Families, Professionals, and Exceptionality: a Special Partnership. Merrill, Columbus, OH, 1986
36. Knobloch H, Stevens F, Malone A et al: The validity of parental reporting of infant development. Pediatrics 63(6):873, 1979
37. Sluzki CE: Process, structure and world views: toward an integrated view of systemic models in family therapy. Fam Process 22:469, 1983

38. Perosa LM, Perosa L: The use of a bipolar item format for FACES III: a reconsideration. J Marital Fam Ther 16(2):187, 1990
39. Minuchin P: Families and individual development: provocations from the field of family therapy. Child Dev 56:289, 1985
40. Olson DH, Russell CS, Sprenkle DH: Circumplex model of marital and family systems: VI. Theoretical update. Fam Process 22:69, 70, 71, 1983
41. Olson DH: Circumplex model VII: validation studies and FACES III. Fam Process 25:337, 1986
42. Beavers R, Hampson R, Hulgus Y: Commentary: the Beavers' system approach to family assessment. Fam Process 24:398, 1985
43. Reiss D: The Family's Construction of Reality. Harvard University Press, Cambridge, MA, 1981, p. 35
44. Epstein NB, Baldwin LM, Bishop DS: The McMaster Family Assessment Device. J Marital Fam Ther 9:171, 1983
45. Moos RH, Moos BS: Family Environment Scale, Manual. 2nd Ed. Consulting Psychologists Press, Palo Alto, CA, 1986
46. Roosa MW, Beals J: Measurement issues in family assessment: the case of the family environment scale. Fam Process 29:191, 1990
47. Morris TM: Culturally sensitive family assessment: an evaluation of the Family Assessment Device used with Hawaiian-American and Japanese-American families. Fam Process 29:105, 1990
48. Newborg J, Stock JR, Wnek L: Battelle Developmental Inventory-Motor Domain. DLM Teaching Resources, Allen, TX, 1984
49. Alpern G, Boll T: Developmental Profile. Psychological Development Publications, Indianapolis, IN, 1972
50. Ireton H, Thwing E, Currier SK: Minnesota Child Development Inventory: identification of children with developmental disorders. J Pediatr Psychol 2:18, 1977
51. Brandon DH, Frauman AC, Huber CJ et al: Toll Control System Manual. University of North Carolina, Chapel Hill, NC, 1989
52. Haley SM, Fass RM, Coster WJ et al: Pediatric Evaluation of Disability Inventory: Examiner's Manual. New England Medical Center, Boston, 1989
53. Squires J, Bricker D, Potter L: Infant/Child Monitoring Questionnaires Procedures Manual. Center on Human Development, University of Oregon, Eugene, 1990
54. Bricker D, Squires J, Kaminski R, Mounts L: The validity, reliability, and cost of a parent-completed questionnaire system to evaluate at-risk infants. J Pediatr Psychol 13:55, 1988
55. Bricker D, Squires J. The effectiveness of parental screening of at-risk infants: the infant monitoring questionnaires. Top Early Child Spec Educ 9(3):67, 1989
56. Smilkstein G, Ashworth C, Montano D: Validity and reliability of the family APGAR as a test of family function. J Fam Pract 15:303, 1982
57. Smilkstein G, Helsper-Lucas A, Ashworth C et al: Prediction of pregnancy complications: an application of the biopsychosocial model, Soc Sci Med 18:315, 1984
58. Kolobe THA: Family-focused early intervention. p. 397. In Campbell SK (ed): Pediatric Neurologic Physical Therapy. 2nd Ed. Churchill Livingstone, New York, 1991
59. Winton PJ: The family-focused interview: an assessment measure and goal-setting mechanism. p. 185. In Bailey DB, Simeonsson RJ (eds): Family Assessment in Early Intervention. Merrill, Columbus, OH, 1988
60. Blow C: Family Interview Performance Rating Scale. Frank Porter Graham Child Development Center, University of North Carolina, Chapel Hill, NC, 1990
61. Hartman A: Diagramming assessment of family relationships. Soc Casework 59:465, 1978

62. Boyce WT, Jensen EW, James SA et al: The Family Routines Inventory: theoretical origins. Soc Sci Med 17:193, 1983
63. McPhatter AR: Assessment revisited: a comprehensive approach to understanding family dynamics. Fam Society 72:11, 1991
64. Oakley F, Kielhofner G, Barris R et al: The Role Checklist: development and empirical assessment of reliability. Occup Ther J Res 6:157, 1986
65. Parent Child Reciprocity Project: The Child Care Role Scale. Carolina Institute for Research on Early Education of the Handicapped, Chapel Hill, NC, 1983
66. Gallagher JJ, Beckman P, Cross AH: Families of handicapped children: sources of stress and its amelioration. Except Child 50:10, 1983
67. Abidin RR: Parenting Stress Index. 2nd Ed. Pediatric Psychology Press, Charlottesville, VA, 1986
68. McCubbin HI, Patterson JM: Systematic Assessment of Family Stress, Resources and Coping. University of Minnesota, St. Paul, 1981
69. McCubbin H, Comeau J: FIRM: Family Inventory of Resources for Management. p. 145. In McCubbin H, Thompson A (eds): Family Assessment Inventories for Research and Practice. University of Wisconsin, Madison, 1987
70. McCubbin MA: Family stress and family strengths: a comparison of single- and two-parent families with handicapped children. Res Nurs Health 12:101, 1989
71. Giblin PT, Poland ML, Waller JB et al: Correlates of parenting on a neonatal intensive care unit: maternal characteristics and family resources. J Genet Psychol 149:505, 1988
72. MacPhee D: The pediatrician as a source of information about child development. J Pediatr Psychol 9(1):87, 1984
73. Caldwell B, Bradley RH: Home Observation for Measurement of the Environment (birth to three years). University of Arkansas, Little Rock, 1984
74. Schraeder BD, Heverly MA, Rappaport J: The value of early home assessment in identifying risk in children who were very low birth weight. Pediatr Nurs 16:268, 1990
75. Cranley MS: Roots of attachment: the relationship of parents with their unborn. Birth Defects 27:59, 1981
76. Bretherton I, Biringen Z, Ridgeway D et al: Attachment: the parental perspective. Inf Ment Health J 10:203, 1989
77. Carey WB, McDevitt SC: Revision of the Infant Temperament Questionnaire. Pediatrics 61:735, 1978
78. Bates JE, Freeland CAB, Lounsbury ML: Measurement of infant difficultness. Child Dev 50:794, 1979
79. Garcia Coll CT, Emmons L, Vohr BR, Ward AM et al: Behavioral responsiveness in preterm infants with intraventricular hemorrhage. Pediatrics 81:412, 1988
80. Schroeder MA: Development and testing of a scale to measure locus of control prior to and following childbirth. Maternal Child Nurs J: 14(2):111, 1985
81. deVellis RF, deVellis BM, Revicki DA et al: Development and validation of the Child Improvement Locus of Control Scales. J Soc Clin Psychol 3:307, 1985
82. Galejs I, Pease D: Parenting beliefs and locus of control orientation. J Psychol 120:501, 1986
83. Hendrix-Wright B: Influence on self esteem: internal versus external control and racial group identification. J Soc Behav Sci 27:12, 1981
84. Barnard KE, Eyres SJ: Child Health Assessment, Part 2: The First Year of Life. DHEW Publ No. HRA 79-25. U.S. Department of Health, Education, and Welfare, Hyattsville, MD, 1979
85. Comfort M: Assessing parent–child interaction. p. 65. In Bailey DB, Simeonsson RJ (eds): Family Assessment in Early Intervention. Merrill, Columbus, OH, 1988

86. Bromwich RM: Working with Parents and Infants: an Interactional Approach. University Park Press, Baltimore, 1981
87. Farran DC, Kasari C, Comfort M et al: Parent/Caregiver Involvement Scale. Department of Child Development and Family Relations, University of North Carolina, Greensboro, 1986
88. Linder TW: Transdisciplinary Play-Based Assessment: a Functional Approach to Working With Young Children. Paul H. Brookes, Baltimore, 1990
89. Gottman JM: Chaos and regulated change in families: a metaphor for the study of transitions. p. 247. In Cowan P, Hetherington M (eds): Family Transitions. Lawrence Erlbaum Associates, Hillsdale, NJ, 1991
90. Sosa R, Kennell J, Klaus M et al: The effect of a supportive companion on perinatal problems, length of labor, and mother–infant interaction. N Engl J Med 303:597, 1980
91. Berrera M: Social support in the adjustment of pregnant adolescents: adjustment issues. p. 69. In Gottlieb BH (ed): Social Networks and Social Support. Sage, Beverly Hills, CA, 1981
92. Culley BS, Perrin EC, Chaberski MJ: Parental perceptions of vulnerability of formerly premature infants. J Pediatr Health Care 3:237, 1989
93. Zuckerman M, Lubin B: Manual for the Multiple Affect Adjective Checklist. Educational and Industrial Training Service, San Diego, 1965
94. Sparling JW, Seeds JW, Farran DC: The relationship of obstetric ultrasound to parent and infant behavior. Obstet Gynecol 72:902, 1988
95. Combrinck-Graham L: A developmental model for family systems. Fam Process 24:139, 1985
96. McCubbin M: Coping Health Inventory for Parents—CHIP. p. 175. In McCubbin H, Thompson A (eds): Family Assessment Inventories for Research and Practice. University of Wisconsin, Madison, 1987
97. Thelen E, Ulrich BD: Hidden Skills. Monogr Soc Res Child Dev 56(1), Serial no.223, 1991
98. Harms T, Clifford RM: Early Childhood Environment Rating Scale. Teachers College Press, New York, 1980
99. Farber B, Lewis M: The symbolic use of parents: a sociological critique of educational practice. J Res Dev Educ 8(2):34, 1975

5 | Musculoskeletal and Growth Measures

Nancy Clopton

This chapter covers a number of different measures of infant growth and development that may be viewed as the "old standbys": tests and measures that have been available for many years and have been retained because their usefulness has been proven over time. These are simple evaluation procedures, most of which require minimal training and equipment for correct performance and are relatively straightforward to interpret.

Growth measures are compared with normative data by plotting the measure (length, weight, head circumference) on graphs of normal age distributions for the particular measure or comparing the infant's measure with standards of typical growth. Growth measures are routinely performed on all newborn infants and, because of their very simplicity, may at times be administered in a hurried or imprecise manner. Errors in measurement of growth may lead to more serious problems, since medication dosages are often calculated according to the infant's weight. In addition, the data are frequently used as evidence in cases of child neglect by documenting failure to grow and catch-up growth following intervention or placement in foster care situations. Care must be exercised in choosing the charts to plot growth data, because norms developed in other countries or for different racial groups may be inadequate.[1] Differences in growth patterns between racial groups may be partially caused by differences in socioeconomic status, but also result from differences in frequency of premature delivery, rates of smoking, and probably from differences in body proportions.[2]

Gestational age assessment measures are administered to neonates to assess relative maturity at birth. Gestational age assessment tools may require the observation of external characteristics of the infant, the administration of simple manipulations to test the infant's resistance to movement, or an attempt to elicit reflexive responses. The exact requirements depend on which tool is chosen. Each of the items on a gestational age assessment demonstrates developmental change correlated with gestational age. By assessing several such items, gestational age can be estimated accurately.

Musculoskeletal measures such as range of motion, bony alignment, and manual muscle testing are familiar to physical therapists from their didactic training. Like growth measures, musculoskeletal measures have broad application as general indicators of the patient's present status. Only screening for hip stability is performed routinely on newborn infants. Although musculoskeletal measures are not administered routinely to all newborn infants, as is the case with growth measures, most infants referred to a physical therapist will require musculoskeletal assessment. Whenever muscle tone or joint range of motion appears to be abnormal, paralysis is suspected, or deformity is noted, musculoskeletal assessment should be performed to provide baseline information and to monitor progress.

GROWTH MEASURES

Length

Length measurements are typically taken on each visit to the physician or at regular intervals during a hospital stay. With infants under age 2 years, recumbent length is measured as a substitute for height. The two measures are not interchangeable, as recumbent length is usually greater than standing height. The recommended procedure is to use a measuring table with movable perpendicular head and footboards and two persons to help hold the infant. One person places the supine infant's head against the headboard with the head in the Frankfurt position in the vertical plane. The other person straightens the infant's hips and knees, places the footboard against the sole of the infant's foot, and reads the length measure. The infant is then repositioned and the entire process repeated. Length is reported to the nearest 0.25 inch or 0.5 cm. If the two measures differ, a third measure should be taken and so on until two measures agree.

Using alternative methods or having only one person take the measurement may reduce accuracy. For an alternative method, the child may be positioned supine on a table on a piece of paper with the head in the Frankfurt position, knees straight, and ankles at 90 degrees. The infant is measured by marking the top of the head and the bottom of the heel on the paper, then measuring the distance between the two marks after removing the child. A second alternative is to stretch a tape measure beside or under the properly positioned infant and read the length directly from the tape.[1,3] Infants whose hips or knees cannot be completely extended are difficult to measure. In such cases, a flexible tape measure is placed along the midline of the limb and the infant's trunk, bending the tape to follow the limb and trunk as necessary at each joint.[1]

Crown-rump length is a standard measure of the fetus and can be used with infants or older children. This measure may give more useful information than length measures in children with congenital limb deficiencies, severe contractures or deformities, or disproportionate growth syndromes. Crown-rump length is measured with the child supine, head positioned as above, and hips flexed to 90 degrees. The measure is taken from the top of the head to the bottom of the buttocks.[1,3]

Length measures have traditionally been considered the most reliable of the external measures of growth[4] and are most useful as nonspecific indicators of an infant's overall general health and nutritional history. Length measures are plotted on a chart[3] that indicates length percentiles for male or female infants of various gestational and postnatal ages. The infant's absolute position on the chart is not nearly as important as a change in position over time. For instance, an infant who remains below the 5th percentile on the chart but whose growth over time follows the normal curve is probably healthier than an infant who starts out at the 95th percentile and falls to the 50th percentile over a few months, even though the second infant is still within the typical range of length measures and the first is not. Parental heights are important in interpreting single measures and trends, since infants of short parents will tend to be short and vice versa.[1]

A collaborative multiple site study of 985 infants who were both premature and low birth weight[5] indicates that such infants have growth curves for length, weight, and head circumference that do not follow the standard pattern even when the infant's age is corrected for prematurity. Length and weight measures corrected for gestational age tended to remain below standard curves throughout the follow up period of 36 months, although catch-up growth in length tends to occur in the first year for both boys and girls. Head circumference adjusted for gestational age actually starts out larger than the standards for term infants for all but the smallest preterm low-birth-weight infants. The rate of head circumference growth, however, is much less in the preterm low-birth-weight group; thus they lose ground throughout the first 36 months according to standards developed for term infants. The results of this study suggest that these infants may require specialized norms that reflect their atypical growth patterns.

Weight

As with length, weight is also typically measured during each visit to a physician or at regular, usually daily, intervals if the infant is in the hospital. All clothing, including the diaper and any blankets, should be removed prior to weighing. The infant is weighed by being placed in an infant scale and is not allowed to touch or grasp anything except the scale. A standing scale can be used by having an adult hold the infant and weighing the infant and adult together. The adult is then weighed alone and the adult's weight is subtracted from the total. Weight is reported to the nearest half ounce or gram in infancy. Weights should be measured again to ensure accuracy.[1,3] If the two weights differ, a third weight should be taken and so on until two results agree.

During the first 3 days after birth, infants normally lose up to about 10 to 15 percent of their birth weight. This loss is mostly due to less fluid and can be minimized by adequate hydration.[4] Infant weights can also be affected by recent feeding or bowel movements. For that reason, information about time of the most recent bowel movement and most recent feeding must be gathered to interpret longitudinal measures of weight. In the absence of one or more limbs, weight by height charts should be adjusted by 11 percent for an upper extremity and 20 percent for a lower extremity.[1]

Weight data are plotted on graphs similar to those for length and may also be indexed with height to determine proportionality.[3] Weight is used for determining recent nutritional status, in counseling the parents concerning the infant's dietary needs, and in selecting dosages for medication. Weight measures, particularly longitudinal ones, may also be important evidence in cases of physical neglect.

Head Circumference

Head circumference may be measured once or a few times in the newborn nursery as standard procedure. If hydrocephalus is suspected, serial daily measurements of head circumference will be taken. Measurements may also be repeated if the head is unusually small or large for reasons unrelated to hydrocephalus, as may happen in the case of congenital anomalies.

Head circumference is measured at the maximum skull circumference. The measure should be taken using a flexible tape placed just above the glabella horizontally and extended to the top of the occipital bone. The tape should be moved around, however, to ensure that this is indeed the largest circumference for the particular infant being measured. The measure is plotted on a graph of normal head circumference measurements.[3]

Craniostenosis and other cranial deformities are usually poorly represented by simple head circumference measures. In such cases width, length, and height measures should be plotted on x-ray.[1,3] Microcephaly, the condition in which the head is atypically small, should be interpreted in relation to total body size. The condition in which the head is small in comparison to body size has more serious implications for predicted intelligence than when head and body are both small.[1]

In hydrocephalus, the head size is not only large, but changing. The change is more significant than the absolute size in determining whether the hydrocephalus is resolving spontaneously, remaining stable, or increasing. Other signs of increased intracranial pressure such as bulging of the fontanelle, separation of cranial sutures, seizures, lethargy, or irritability should be monitored. A parent should be taught to take accurate daily measurements of head circumference and to recognize signs of increased intracranial pressure in order to continue to monitor hydrocephalus after shunt placement or hydrocephalus that has apparently arrested spontaneously.

Skinfold Thickness

Skinfold thickness in infants is measured at three sites: triceps, subscapular, and suprailiac. The calipers must be carefully calibrated to exert a pressure of 10 g/mm³ and allow accurate readings to 0.1 mm. Standard procedure is to use the left side for all measures. The triceps skinfold is measured halfway down the skin overlying the triceps with the arm relaxed. The skin pinch is vertical. The subscapular skinfold is measured just below the inferior angle of the scapula. The suprailiac fold is measured just above the iliac crest in the midaxillary line. Compression should be for less than 3 seconds and should not be immediately repeated, because the tissues may have become compressed and the measurement will thus be falsely low.[1,3]

Each measure may be plotted separately on charts of normal skinfold measures or may be summed and plotted (Fig. 5-1). Measures from multiple sites tend to be more accurate than single measures because of variations in body shape and proportions.[1] Skinfold measures are used to estimate body composition and can be useful in interpreting discordant height and length data.

Anthropometric Measures

Other anthropometric measures can be taken to assess the presence of congenital syndromes. These include hand length, palm length, middle finger length, foot length, outer canthal distance, inner canthal distance, interpupillary distance, palpebral fissure length, ear length, fontanelle size, penile length, and testicular size. Proportional measures such as upper to lower torso length may also be useful. Normal standards for each measure are available in a number of standard references.[3,6–8] Marked variation in proportions of body parts may assist the physician to diagnose a particular syndrome. Apparent variations in proportion should be assessed by careful measurement and compared to established norms because the initial impression from visual inspection may be misleading.

GESTATIONAL AGE ASSESSMENT

Significance

Until the 1960s, birth weight alone was often used to classify infants as premature, and all infants weighing 2,500 g or less were identified as premature. Full-term infants, however, sometimes weigh less than 2,500 g. Such infants are now referred to as *low-birth-weight infants*.[9] More importantly, infants are classified by gestational age (GA) as well as by weight. Simultaneous consideration of gestational age and birth weight has allowed more specific prediction of the complications that should be anticipated for the infant at risk.

GA is most commonly estimated prenatally from last menstrual period (LMP), from ultrasound examination, or from observations of fundal height and other developmental observations made by the physician and mother during antenatal visits.[10] Infants are considered "full-term" when between 37 and 42 weeks GA. They are considered preterm or premature before 37 weeks and postterm after 42 weeks. Calculation of GA from reliable LMP data is considered the most accurate, but may be complicated by a number of factors, including

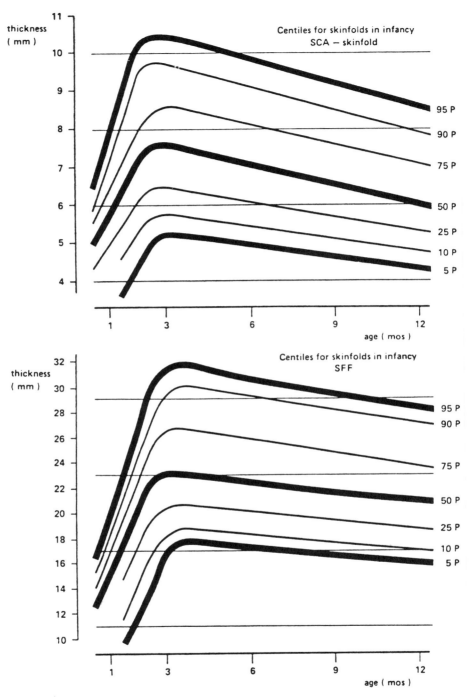

Fig. 5-1. Skinfold thickness percentiles for triceps (TRI), suprailiac (SIL), and subscapular (SCA) sites and for the sum of all three sites (SFF). (From Schluter et al.,[56] with permission.)

variability of menstrual flow and poor record-keeping by many women. Ultra-sound estimation from crown-rump length is accurate within 4 to 7 days in the first trimester, and biparietal diameter on ultrasound correlates well with GA from 12 to 18 weeks.[10] Many women, however, do not have ultrasound examination or have the examination too late for optimal assessment of GA. Assessment of GA from physician examinations is also more accurate in early pregnancy than late pregnancy.[10] Complications that can affect the accuracy of the prenatal physician's examination include poor or no prenatal care, previous cesarean section, race, maternal height, intrauterine growth retardation, and variability in the physician's skill.[4,10]

Calculation of GA from observation of the characteristics of the newborn infant was developed because of the need for a method of evaluating gestational maturity in cases with no prenatal care or in which the prenatal assessment of GA was inadequate or suspect. GA assessment is used in conjunction with routine weighing and GA norms for weight.[9] By plotting weight and GA an infant may be accurately classified as *small for gestational age* (SGA), *appropriate for gestational age* (AGA), or *large for gestational age* (LGA). The SGA infants will be further classified as symmetrically or asymmetrically growth retarded. Infants who are symmetrically growth retarded appear old for their size and seem to have been undergrown for a long time. Their head circumference, length, and weight are all proportionally small. Infants who are asymmetrically undergrown are thin but their length and head size are near normal. Symmetrically undergrown infants tend to exhibit genetic syndromes, while asymmetrically undergrown infants often have survived intrauterine stress or malnourishment.[9] Macrosomia in infants of diabetic mothers (IDMs) is the most common etiology for LGA infants,[11] although IDMs are not always large for dates but are, in fact, often undergrown.[9]

Each separate classification regarding GA and weight implies a spectrum of specific risk factors. Additionally, mortality rates for premature SGA infants are higher than those for premature LGA infants, and premature LGA infants carry increased mortality risk over AGA premature infants. The mortality rate for SGA term infants is slightly increased over that for AGA or LGA term infants, but the risk for term LGA infants is not increased over that for term AGA infants.[9]

Factors Used To Assess GA

Premature, term, and post-term infants differ in several observable characteristics that can be used to assess GA. Those differences are outlined below.

Presence and Strength of "Primitive" Reflexes

Reflex withdrawal responses to oral stimulation begin to appear as early as 8 weeks of fetal life. The so-called primitive reflexes (such as Moro, grasp, rooting, crossed extension, sucking, and automatic walking) develop prenatally and become gradually better organized as GA approaches full term. Amiel-Tison[12] suggests that observation of the presence and strength of primitive reflexes may be used to assess GA in combination with measures of active and passive muscle tone.

Physiologic Flexion

As the fetus approaches term, its increasing size leads to crowding within the uterus. The fetus must assume and maintain a tightly flexed position, which leads to passive shortening of many of the flexor muscle groups. The term infant's resting posture is markedly more flexed than that of a premature infant. This "physiological flexion" can be tested most readily in the lower extremities by attempting to take the limb through the full range of extension and assessing the limitation in range of motion. The hip and knee flexors become progressively more resistant to passive extension in the term infant than in the premature infant. Another way to assess physiological flexion is to take the upper or lower extremities into extension and suddenly release them. The limbs will rebound to the flexed position with more force and speed in the infant of greater GA.[9]

Increased Muscle Tone

General muscle tone increases as the infant approaches term. The premature infant usually appears hypotonic compared with the term infant. Passive shoulder adduction and internal rotation is one maneuver used to quantify this passive tone. This maneuver is referred to as the *scarf* sign, because the premature infant's arm may be brought across the neck like a scarf, with the elbow past midline. In the term infant, increased muscle tone prevents the elbow from reaching midline in the scarf sign. Increased muscle tone also decreases the amount of head lag observed in the pull-to-sit maneuver, so that less head lag is seen in the more mature infant. When suspended prone, decreased muscle tone causes the preterm infant to droop over the examiner's hand, while the term infant maintains a straighter back and may even lift the head slightly.[4]

Active antigravity axial extension also increases as the infant approaches term. The preterm infant is rarely able to lift the head from the prone position, while the term infant frequently has this ability. Placed in a supported standing position, the preterm infant may actively extend only the lower extremities, while the term infant often straightens the trunk and head as well.[4]

Ligamentous Laxity

The ankle and wrist joints show the opposite effect of other joints in that their range of motion increases with maturity while the range of motion of hips, knees, and shoulders decreases with maturity. The wrist shows increased flexion, so that the palm can be flexed against the forearm in the term infant. The ankle shows increased dorsiflexion so that the dorsal aspect of the foot may often be brought into contact with the anterior tibia. Increased range in these two joints, which are both much less mobile in early gestation, is probably due to the transplacental effect of the maternal hormones relaxin and extrogen, which prepare the mother's pelvis for delivery by relaxation of ligamentous structures. These hormones are thought to relax the mother's symphysis pubis to allow a slight increase in the diameter of the pelvic outlet so that the infant's head can more easily pass through in a vaginal delivery. The infant's ankle dorsiflexion range of motion may also have been affected by crowding against the uterine wall in late pregnancy.[4]

External Appearance

Various traits of appearance may be used as indicators of GA. The amount of vernix, the number and depth of creases on the sole of the foot, skin thickness, breast and genital development, ear formation and stiffness, and length of the nails all increase with GA. Skin color becomes less red and more pink. The skull sutures become firmer. Lanugo first appears at 20 weeks gestation and decreases after 28 weeks. The appearance of the hair changes toward term to become less curly, except in black infants.[4] External characteristics are incorporated in several of the tools used to assess GA.

Standardized Tools for Assessment of GA

Farr et al.[13] produced a tool for the assessment of GA based entirely on external criteria. The criteria include edema, skin texture, skin color, skin opacity, lanugo, plantar creases, nipple formation, breast size, ear form, ear firmness, and development of the genitalia. Farr et al. also presented a chart that shows conversion of the total score to GA, but the derivation of the infant's score from criteria is not explained.

Amiel-Tison[12] presented an assessment of GA in three parts: passive tone, active tone, and reflexes. Passive tone is assessed by six items:

1. The overall amount of flexion in the infant's resting posture. Flexion increases with gestational age.
2. The heel-to-ear maneuver. The infant's heel is drawn toward the ear. Toward term, the heel cannot be drawn as close to the ear as it could be earlier in gestation because of increasing muscle tone and knee flexion limitation.
3. Popliteal angle. The infant's thigh is flexed against the abdomen, and the knee is straightened. With increasing GA, the angle of the knee becomes more acute because of increased tone and decreased range of motion.
4. Dorsiflexion. Near term, the angle becomes more acute because maternal hormones have relaxed the ligamentous structures of the ankle.

5. The scarf sign. The infant's arm is adducted and internally rotated across the chest. As GA increases, the arm increasingly resists being drawn across the chest because muscle tone is higher.
6. Return to flexion of forearms. The arms are drawn down straight beside the infant's trunk and released. In the premature infant, the arms may remain at the side, but in the term infant, the arms will spring into flexion promptly when released because of increased muscle tone.

Active tone is assessed by four items:

1. The supporting reaction of the lower extremities in standing, which increases with GA.
2. Vertical trunk righting, which increases late in gestation.
3. Neck extension in supported sitting, which increases with GA.
4. Neck flexion when pulled to sit, which increases with GA.

Finally, six reflex items are assessed that all increase in strength with increasing GA: the sucking, rooting, grasp, Moro, crossed extension, and automatic walking reflexes.

Descriptions and pictures of the expected results for each test item at specified GAs are arranged on a chart.[12] No guidance is offered about how to reconcile discrepant results for the various test items. No reliability information is provided for the assessment.

Dubowitz et al.[14] offered an assessment based on 10 neurologic and 11 external criteria. Among the neurologic criteria, posture, ankle dorsiflexion, popliteal angle, and the heel-to-ear maneuver are performed in the same manner as in the Amiel-Tison[12] assessment. The "head lag" item on the Dubowitz assessment is equivalent to the "neck flexion" item on the Amiel-Tison, and the "arm recoil" on the Dubowitz is identical to the "return to flexion" item on the Amiel-Tison. New items are the "square window," an assessment of the increase in flexion of the wrist, "leg recoil," similar to "arm recoil," and ventral suspension in which the infant is suspended prone over the examiner's hand to assess neck and truck extension and extremity flexion against gravity. Neck and trunk extension and extremity flexion should increase with increased GA. External criteria were adapted from Farr et al.[13] and scoring criteria are fully defined.

Each neurologic and external criterion is scored on a scale from 0 for the most immature characteristic to 2, 3, or 4 for the most mature. The scores are added, and the total score is plotted on a regression line derived by Dubowitz et al.[14] from testing 167 infants with dependable maternal menstrual data. According to the authors, serial assessments showed that the score was reliable from 24 hours to 4 days but reliability figures were not reported. Intrarater reliability was determined for four testers. The Student's *t* test showed no significant difference among three of the raters, but values and significance levels of the *t* tests were not reported. One of the raters was consistently 5 points higher than the others.

Several reliability studies of the Dubowitz examination have been conducted cross-culturally, with low birth-weight infants, and with infants who have low Apgar scores. In each population, the results were found to be acceptably accurate and reliable.[15] Interestingly, skin color and opacity are useful criteria even among African infants.[16] The Dubowitz examination, however, appears to overestimate GA by about 2 weeks for low-birth-weight infants[17,18] and for preterm infants.[19] This 2 week discrepancy caused 24 percent of the low-birth-weight infants to be reclassified into a different growth category (SGA, AGA, LGA) than would have been the case using alternative methods of estimating GA.[17]

Ballard et al.[20] simplified the Dubowitz et al. assessment by eliminating some of the items that they believed were either difficult to administer to ill infants or less reliable for other reasons. Dorsiflexion was eliminated and wrist angle ("square window") was retained, because the authors believed that dorsiflexion might vary according to intrauterine position or congenital deformity but that wrist angle would be less variable. Arm recoil was retained, but leg recoil was eliminated because it may be difficult to administer or less reliable in an infant born breech. Head lag and ventral suspension were also considered difficult to administer to an ill infant and were therefore eliminated. Edema and skin color were judged to be too variable and were eliminated. Skin opacity and texture were combined to produce one item, "skin." Nipple formation and breast size were combined into one item, "breast."

The Dubowitz et al.[14] and Ballard et al.[20] examinations were both administered to 252 infants. The correlation between the two examinations for these infants was 0.969 ($p = 0.00001$). The correlation of the Ballard examination with menstrual dates was 0.852 (probability not reported); the correlation was 0.848 for the Dubowitz. Ballard et al. stated that their examination will be more accurate than the Dubowitz with ill infants, because the pull-to-sit and ventral suspension items may be omitted in clinical practice, requiring the examiner to estimate the results of those two items. They found that the examination correlated at the 0.05 level of significance with maternal menstrual dates in ill infants.

The Ballard examination is most accurate when administered between 30 and 42 hours of age. Prior to 30 hours, the examination is slightly less accurate, but the accuracy drops precipitously after 42 hours, which is also the case for the Dubowitz examination. The Ballard may be slightly more reliable than the Dubowitz in the infant who is 18 to 30 hours old. The time saved by using the new examination instead of the Dubowitz averages less than 40 seconds. The Ballard examination is currently the most commonly used GA assessment tool.[3,10] It is simple to administer, and its reliability appears to be comparable to that of the Dubowitz. The Ballard, however, appears to overestimate maturity of low-birth-weight infants (under 1,500 g) about 2 weeks, as does the Dubowitz examination,[18] and thus poses similar problems.

Disagreement of GA Measures

The various estimates of GA can at times disagree. For instance, LMP estimates may disagree with fundal height estimates, and both estimates may disagree with the examination of the newborn. Prenatal ultrasound provides yet another GA estimate. In these cases, each separate estimate should be reported along with the method of estimation. Averaging of different estimates is not recommended. Instead, DiPietro and Allen[10] suggest that the best available single estimate as determined for each case should be used. They recommend that LMP should be used if available and if the mother provides a single date, rather than a range of dates. Second choice would be the date from a sonogram before 19 weeks. Third choice would be a fundal height examination before 13 weeks, and the postnatal examination would be fourth choice. DiPietro and Allen admitted that their system introduces problems in that different maturity standards will be used for each infant, but they argue that universal use of the postnatal examination estimates introduces nonrandom error that distorts data analysis.

Correction for GA

Evaluations of growth measures are routinely adjusted for prematurity by subtracting the appropriate number of weeks from the child's chronologic age. There is general agreement that giving full correction for prematurity in growth measures is appropriate,[21] but there is less agreement about whether full correction, partial correction, or no correction at all is appropriate for other measures of developmental status. Based on his review of the literature, Blasco[21] found support for separating the evaluation of motor and mental functions, half correction for both types of evaluation until 4 months of chronologic age, partial or full correction for motor skills until at least 4 to 6 months, and no need to correct either type of assessment after 18 or 24 months of chronologic age. He suggested the convention of half correction at all ages be adopted. The proposed convention would avoid the extremes of no correction, which may overestimate the infant's problems, and full correction, which may cause infants who need intervention to be missed. Half correction would have the great advantage of allowing consistency from one age to the next and across types of evaluations. Palisano (see Ch. 9) discusses correction for GA in interpreting the results of norm-referenced testing of premature infants.

MUSCULOSKELETAL MEASURES

Range of Motion

For most infants referred to physical therapy, range of motion (ROM) measures will be part of the assessment procedure. ROM measures can be used to document objectively the manifestation of deformity, tone abnormality, or joint restriction. In many cases, physical therapy intervention may have a goal of increasing ROM. In such cases, goniometric measurements may be required to assess the effect of intervention on joint range.

Newborn infants often exhibit ligmentous laxity because of the transplacental transfer of relaxin and estrogen from the mother.[22] For a therapist who is knowledgable in arthrokinematics, this transient laxity can be utilized to correct mild deformity or to decrease the severity of marked deformity. Positioning, splinting, or taping[22] may produce marked improvement in a relatively short period of time compared with the difficulty that will be encountered in correcting the same problems when the infant is just a few months older.

The difficulties of measuring ROM in infants, especially premature infants, have been noted by Harris et al.[23] and by Katz et al.[24] Difficulties include palpating bony landmarks, stabilizing the infant, the small size of body segments, the lack of appropriately sized goniometers, the fact that verbal instructions will not be obeyed by the infant, and the occasional need to work within the confines of an incubator. In some cases, body proportions may contribute to difficulty in obtaining precise measures. For example, a protuberant abdomen may limit full hip flexion, or plump thighs may cause problems in measuring hip adduction.

The therapist will need to modify the ROM administration as well as interpretation. Usually only passive ROM measures can be obtained with accuracy. Transitory ligamentous laxity in the newborn infant requires the therapist to exercise care not to overestimate joint ROM by overstretching. The infant's head will need to be positioned in midline during goniometric measurements to avoid influence from the asymmetric tonic neck reflex. In determining whether measured ROM is normal for the infant, adult values for normal range are inappropriate.

Nine studies of normative infant goniometric ROM measures obtained with clearly described methodologies have been published.[23–31] Two other studies suggesting normal values for ROM[32,33] appear to have been conducted without benefit of goniometry, and methodology is only briefly described [33] or not described at all.[32] Finally, Alston[34] contributed ROM measures of healthy preterm infants from an unpublished study. She replicated the study by Waugh et al.[30] with preterm infants instead of full-term infants.

The number of infants examined at each age in each of the studies ranged from a high of 400[27] to a low of 4 in the Katz et al.[24] study that had 12 GA groups. Variation among the studies in methods for positioning the infant and aligning the goniometer makes comparisons difficult. Only two of the studies[23,32] included upper extremity measures. Two included only the right [28,31] and four only the left side,[24,26,29,30] all relying on an earlier report[27] of no difference in ROM between the two sides of the body. Harris et al.[23] also reported a high correlation between measures on the two sides of the body, and Alston[34] reported no significant difference between the two sides. Drews et al.[25] recorded small differences between the two sides of the body in hip abduction and external rotation and ankle inversion, but did not report whether the differences were statistically significant.

Breech presentation can affect the shape and position of the lower extremities.[20] Four of the studies[26,28,30,31] of hip ROM excluded infants who were delivered breech. Drews et al.[25] reported no correlation of ROM measures with delivery information.

Reliability

Inter-rater reliability was reported in four of the studies of infant ROM and intrarater reliability in three. Amiel-Tison[12] claimed 50 to 90 percent interobserver agreement within 10 degrees for "eyeball" estimates and 90 percent intraobserver agreement within 10 degrees. She believed a measuring device to be unnecessary for estimating ROM accurately enough for GA assessment. In a longitudinal study of premature infants, Harris et al.[23] assessed inter-rater reliability of joint ROM measurements for six infants at birth and at 4, 8, and 12 months. Interclass correlation coefficients ranged from a low of 0.59 for wrist extension to perfect agreement for elbow extension. Other measures included ankle dorsiflexion (0.87), hip extension (0.72), hip abduction (0.85), scarf sign (0.84), and popliteal angle (0.83). Correlation coefficients for inter-rater reliability in the study by Drews et al.[25] varied from a low of 0.33 for ankle eversion to a high of 0.97 for hip abduction in extension. The mean correlation coefficient for all ranges was 0.71. Katz et al.[24] reported a mean overall intrarater standard deviation of 3.23 degrees and a mean error of 0.75 degrees for hip ranges in premature infants. Forero et al.[31] reported only the investigator with the highest intratester ($r = 0.99$, $p < 0.05$) and intertester ($r = 0.98$, $p < 0.05$) reliability.

Intrarater reliability is usually assumed to be higher than inter-rater reliability. One person should therefore be responsible for serial ROM measures whenever possible. Inter-rater reliability figures presented for these studies, while acceptable for clinical practice, suggest caution in interpreting goniometric data from infants. Use of a goniometer is recommended because accuracy within 10 degrees would not be sufficient for monitoring joint ROM in physical therapy.

Hip Extension Limitation

Limitation of hip extension is reported in nine studies of newborn infants.[23–27,30–32,34] These limitations are produced by the infant's cramped intrauterine position of marked hip flexion. The term *hip flexion contracture* is avoided because of its implication of abnormality, and the term *hip extension limitation* is used.

The Thomas test, in which the infant is positioned supine and the lumbar spine is flattened by flexing the contralateral extremity to the infant's abdomen, was used in six studies.[23,24,26,27,30,31] Hip extension limitation is then measured by allowing the hip to extend as far as possible before the pelvis rocks forward and determining the angle of the thigh with the flat surface. In the term newborn infant, findings for average hip extension limitations measured by the Thomas test were 28 (SD = 8)[27] and 46 (*SD* = 8)[30] degrees. Drews et al.[25] used a similar procedure, but positioned the infant sidelying, and reported the mean extension limitation to be 28 (*SD* = 6) degrees. Hoffer[32] reported comparatively high figures (50 to 120 degrees) at birth, decreasing by 15 months of age to 10 to 25 degrees. Since he failed to report methodology, one cannot determine why his figures are higher than in other studies.

In three studies the Thomas test was performed on premature infants: by Katz et al.[24] and Alston[34] within 1 week after birth and by Harris et al.[23] at discharge from the hospital (approximately 40 weeks of GA). Average hip extension limitations were 11 (*SD* = 5) degrees for infants 33 to 36 weeks of GA in the Alston[34] study and 13 (*SD* = 6) degrees for infants under 35 weeks gestation in the Harris et al.[23] study. Katz et al.[24] reported hip extension limitations by GA group from 25 to 36 weeks gestation. Average limitations between 25 and 28 weeks were 13 to 19 (*SD* = 8 to 15) degrees. From 29 to 36 weeks average limitations were 28 to 33 (*SD* = 10 to 29) degrees. Because the premature infant spends less time in utero and is less crowded, these results are in the expected direction, showing less limitation than those found in studies of term infants. Caution must be exercised when comparing studies, because methodological or population differences other than GA may have caused differences in measured hip extension limitation.

The hip flexors tend to remain relatively shortened for several months after birth, causing the lordotic posture so often seen in toddlers and promoting the development of the lumbar curve. Coon et al.[26] studied older infants using the Thomas test. They reported hip extension limitations of 19 degrees at 6 weeks and 7 degrees at 3 and 6 months. Hoffer[32] reported limitation of hip extension of 10 to 25 degrees at 15 months, but did not report his method of measurement. Phelps et al.[28] used the Staheli test,[35] in which the infant is positioned prone for better control of pelvic position, instead of the Thomas test. Phelps et al.[28] reported average limitations of 10 degrees at 9 months, 9 degrees at 12 months, decreasing to 4 degrees at 18 months, and 3 degrees at 24 months. Using the Thomas test with infants who had been premature at birth, Harris et al.[23] measured hip extension limitations of 19 degrees at 4 months, 17 degrees at 8 months, and 16 degrees at 12 months (adjusted ages). Again, comparisons among the various studies should be made with the knowledge that factors other than GA may have contributed to differences in results.

Hip Flexion

Hip flexion is measured with the same landmarks and position as for the Thomas test, but the hip and knee are flexed fully to the point just before the pelvis rocks into posterior tilt. Forero et al.[31] report average hip flexion of 128 (*SD* = 5) degrees in term infants. Katz et al.[24] reported averages for premature infants grouped by GA of 129 to 137 (*SD* = 5 to 12) degrees.

Hip Abduction

Hip abduction, especially when measured with the hip and knee flexed, is influenced by intrauterine position that typically involves marked hip abduction with hip and knee flexion in vertex presentation in late pregnancy. To measure hip abduction, the infant is positioned supine with the hips and knees flexed to 90 degrees or as straight as possible. If hips and knees are flexed, the angle of the thigh with the vertical axis or the horizontal surface is measured. If the horizontal axis is used, the angle with the vertical axis is computed by subtracting 90 degrees. If the hips and knees are extended, the angle of the thigh with the midline trunk axis is measured.

In studies[25,27,31] in which abduction was measured in full-term infants with the knees flexed, average values ranged from 69 to 79 (SD = 4 to 12) degrees. Katz et al.[24] found average values of 70 to 84 (SD = 0 to 28) degrees in preterm infants measured in flexion. When the hips and knees were extended, average values for term infants were 56 (SD = 10)[25] or 39 (SD = 5) degrees.[31] Amiel-Tison[33] suggested that normal hip abduction at term birth ranges between 40 and 80 degrees in extension. Katz et al.[24] and Harris et al.[23] reported average ranges of 49 to 63 (SD = 8 to 26) degrees in preterm infants measured in extension. Phelps et al[28] reported average hip abduction varying between 54 and 60 (SD = 5 to 8) degrees in term infants 9,12,18, and 24 months old. They did not report whether hip abduction was measured with the hips and knees flexed or extended. In premature infants, Harris et al.[23] reported that abduction range in extension remained about the same at 4 and 8 months of age, then increased to about 68 (SD = 26) degrees at 12 months.

Hip Rotation

Hip internal and external rotation may be affected by intrauterine position, particularly shortening of the psoas major, which will limit internal rotation. Rotatory motions of the hip are also affected by the fact that the infant's femoral neck is in approximately 25 to 30 degrees of anteversion, which will not reduce to adult values of 8 to 16 degrees until normal compression and tension loading occurs as the infant stands and walks.[36] Anteversion is disguised by the soft tissue limitation of internal rotation.

Internal and external rotation of the hip may be measured supine with one hip and knee flexed to 90 degrees by aligning one arm of the goniometer with the trunk axis and one arm with the tibia. In prone, with hips in neutral and one knee flexed to 90 degrees, internal and external rotations are measured by aligning one arm of the goniometer with the tibial crest and one arm vertical to the surface.

Investigators of full-term infants report means of 62 to 89 (SD = 6 to 13) degrees of internal rotation and 89 to 114 (SD = 3 to 14) degrees of external rotation measured supine.[25,27,31] Hoffer,[32] whose methodology is not described, reported 40 to 80 degrees of external rotation and internal rotation "contractures'' of 30 degrees. Katz et al.,[24] in their study of preterm infants grouped by GA, reported mean internal rotation measures of 0 to 4 ($SD = 0$ to 12) degrees and external rotation of 49 to 63 ($SD = 8$ to 23) degrees in prone.

Measures of hip internal and external rotation in older infants[26,28] were obtained prone. Coon et al.[26] reported relatively stable measures of prone hip internal rotation of 21 to 26 ($SD = 3$ to 5) degrees at 6 weeks, 3 months, and 6 months. Phelps et al.[28] reported that prone hip internal rotation gradually increased from 41 ($SD = 8$) degrees at 9 months to 52 ($SD = 10$) degrees at 24 months. Hoffer [32] reported that internal rotation is 40 to 70 degrees at 15 months of age. Coon et al.[26] reported prone external rotation values between 45 and 48 ($SD = 5$ to 11) degrees at 6 weeks, 3 months, and 6 months. Phelps et al.[28] reported that prone external rotation decreased from 56 ($SD = 7$) degrees at 9 months to 47 ($SD = 9$) degrees at 24 months.

Knee Extension

Popliteal angle is measured with the thigh fully flexed against the infant's abdomen. The knee is extended as far as possible, and the angle at the knee is measured with the greater trochanter, the lateral femoral condyle, and the lateral malleolus used to align the arms of the goniometer. Mean popliteal angle measures of 150 to 153 ($SD = 6$ to 13) degrees have been reported in term [29,30] and premature[23] infants. Amiel-Tison[33] described normal popliteal angles in term newborn infants of 80 to 100 degrees. Waugh et al.[30] suggested that Amiel-Tison's much lower figures may have reflected less time allowed for the infant to accommodate to the stretching procedure. Harris et al.[23] reported little change in popliteal angle among premature infants from birth to 12 months adjusted age.

In three studies[25,29,30] knee extension was measured with the hip positioned in as much extension as possible (HEKE position). In the HEKE position, average knee extension was 159 to 165 ($SD = 5$ to 10) degrees. The HEKE is thought to reflect posterior capsule tightness, whereas the popliteal angle reflects hamstring tightness.

Ankle Ranges

Ankle dorsiflexion in the term newborn infant is frequently limited only by contact of the dorsum of the foot with the anterior shin. Intrauterine crowding and ligamentous laxity produces increased dorsiflexion in term infants compared with premature infants. To measure ankle dorsiflexion, the infant is positioned supine with hip and knee flexed. The lateral aspect of the fifth metatarsal and the fibular head are used as reference points for alignment of the goniometer. Waugh et al.[30] reported an average of 59 ($SD = 8$) degrees of dorsiflexion in term infants. Amiel-Tison[33] suggested that 60 to 70 degrees of dorsiflexion is normal in a term infant, while Hoffer[32] suggested that as much as 80 degrees of dorsiflexion may exist. Harris et al.[23] reported average dorsiflexion ranges of 38 ($SD = 11$) degrees in premature infants at hospital discharge.

Positioning and alignment of the goniometer for measuring plantar flexion are the same as for measuring dorsiflexion. Plantar flexion may be limited because of relative shortening of the anterior compartment of the leg. Waugh et al.[30] reported an average of 26 ($SD = 6$) degrees in term infants, and Hoffer[32] reported plantar flexion of "no more than 30 degrees."

Upper Extremity Ranges

ROM data are not readily available for upper extremities, probably reflecting the fact that infant ROM values for upper extremities more closely approximate those for adults. Hoffer[32] reported that elbow extension is limited as much as 30 degrees in term infants, but Harris et al.[23] measured average elbow extension of 179 ($SD = 3$) degrees in premature infants at hospital discharge. This comparison may reflect the increased "physiological flexion" of the term infant compared with the premature infant. Hoffer[32] reported that hand, wrist, and forearm motions are comparable to adult values. Harris et al.[23] reported 98 ($SD = 9$) degrees of wrist extension in premature infants. Dubowitz et al.[14] reported the "square window" in which the wrist becomes increasingly flexible during gestation so that it can be flexed with the palm contacting the forearm in a full-term infant.

Clinical Significance

Amiel-Tison[33] suggested that hip abduction, popliteal angle, dorsiflexion, and the scarf sign may be useful tools in the assessment of potential neurologic involvement in infancy. Harris et al.[23] reported that ankle dorsiflexion at 8 months was reduced an average of 38 degrees for premature infants with known neurologic damage compared with premature infants with no known neurologic damage. Hip abduction ranges were comparable in the two groups at discharge, but did not increase in those infants with known neurologic damage as they grew older. Hip abduction did increase with age in those infants with no known neurologic damage so that at 12 months mean abduction values were 58 degrees for the former group and 72 for the latter.

Reade et al.[29] showed that the popliteal angle and the HEKE both decrease steadily to zero by 12 months of age in term newborn infants. They suggested that HEKE and popliteal angle measures may be useful to clinicians as a quick assessment tool in examining infants for neuromuscular problems. Johnson and Ashhurst[37] reported a prospective investigation of the usefulness of popliteal angle measurement in predicting cerebral palsy. The measure had limited predictive value, as the subjective judgment of the health visitor about the child's status was more predictive than the popliteal angle measure. Furthermore, many of the health visitors did not perform the test, perhaps because they were unsure about how to administer it.

Bony Alignment

At birth, the spine demonstrates a kyphotic total "C" curve from the coccyx to the thorax. A secondary lordotic cervical curve is present in 83 percent of fetuses at 9.5 weeks of gestation. The cervical curve is believed to result from the action of the capital neck extensors in the "gasp" reflex, which is present at 6.5 weeks of gestation. The gasp reflex may also be responsible for stimulating early ossification of the occipital bone.[38] The scapulae ride relatively high on the rib cage, elevating the shoulder girdle and creating the impression that the infant has no neck. The thoracic area of the infant spine is relatively inflexible. As the infant lifts the head in prone position, cervical lordosis is accentuated, forming the normal cervical curve of adulthood within the first few months. Weight bearing in prone-on-elbows, prone-on-hands, and creeping positions protracts the scapulae and separate the shoulders from the head so that the head no longer appears to sit directly on the shoulders.[39] Normal lumbar lordosis begins to develop as the infant pulls to stand. Tightness in the iliopsoas pulls the lumbar spine anteriorly as the infant fully extends the hip to stand. Tightness of the hip flexors and relatively weak abdominals combine to allow anterior pelvic tilt, which produces a lordotic, pot-bellied posture in early standing.[39,40,41] Ribs are positioned more nearly perpendicular to the spine in the neonate,[42] causing a proportionally larger anteroposterior chest diameter than that found in adults, and the chest wall is more compliant.

The angle of the neck of the femur with the shaft is about 130 to 150 degrees (coxa valga) compared with the adult values of about 125 degrees.[36,40,41,43,44] Anteversion is greater in the infant hip than will be the case after weight bearing is established. The femoral shaft of the infant shows increased medial twisting (antetorsion) of about 25 to 40 degrees.[36,40,43] Within the first 2 years of life, antetorsion will decrease to 30 degrees. In the newborn infant, antetorsion does not present as a "knock knee" appearance, because the hips are held in external rotation by the shortened psoas. External rotation of the hip positions the distal femoral condyles in external rotation relative to the frontal plane obscuring the effect of the femoral antetorsion.[41]

Even slight flexion of the knee causes the tibia to rotate internally on the femur. Intrauterine confinement with the knee in sharp flexion causes the heads of the tibia and fibula to rotate internally on the femoral condyles, producing the internal genicular position. The internal genicular position should be distinguished from internal tibial torsion, which affects the shaft of the tibia. The typical newborn tibia exhibits no torsion, whereas the normal adult tibia exhibits about 25 degrees of external torsion. The tibia often appears bowed distally (tibia varum); however, it is actually not bowed. The bowed appearance results from lateral displacement of the posterior leg muscles and from the medial rotation of the tibia on the femur. The appearance of medial rotation of the tibia on the femur is masked, because the shortened hamstrings and psoas place the hip in external rotation and the knee in flexion.[41]

The infant foot is very long in proportion to the rest of the body. It is flexible and exhibits no longitudinal arch.[36,40] The forefoot is in varus. The talus and calcaneous both exhibit torsion compared with adult alignments. The torsion causes calcaneal eversion and weight bearing on the first metatarsal in early relaxed stance at about 1 year. This "flat foot" will often resolve with continued weight bearing and growth. The lateral four metatarsals of the newborn are adducted, and the toes are often tight in flexion.[41]

Management of bony malalignment in infancy is complex but may be efficient and effective. The newborn infant is much more pliable than will be the case later. Aggressive splinting, taping, and positioning in infancy can correct severe joint malalignment much more simply than will be possible later. These interventions apply corrective forces to take advantage of the rapid growth during infancy. Deformities in spina bifida or arthrogryposis may be improved to the point that later surgery may be avoided. Aggressive management of malalignment requires intimate knowledge of normal bony alignment in infancy and careful attention to alignment of articular surfaces during the application of corrective forces.[22]

Hip Instability

Congenital hip dislocation is common among otherwise normal children, affecting approximately 1 per 300 to 600 female infants and 1 per 2,000 to 4,000 male infants. The etiology of congenital hip dislocation is multifactorial. Causative factors include breech positioning, ligamentous laxity, postnatal positioning in hip and knee extension, and genetic influences.[45,46] The value of routine screening for hip instability in newborn infants is controversial, because a high false-positive rate exposes a large number of infants to unnecessary radiation, but early detection and treatment of an unstable hip is definitely advantageous for the infant who does have one.[45]

In nearly all neonatal hip dislocations the head of the femur will dislocate posteriorly and superiorly to the hip socket. To examine the infant for potential hip dislocation, the first step is to suspend the infant and examine the thighs to determine whether the thigh creases are symmetric (Fig. 5-2A). Asymmetry indicates potential hip dislocation. The infant is then positioned supine on a firm surface. The infant must be relaxed, as crying will make the examination nearly impossible. With hips and knees flexed, the hips are checked for restricted range in abduction (Fig. 5-2B) and length of thighs is compared (Fig. 5-2C). Restricted hip abduction may indicate hip dislocation on the restricted side, and unequal thigh length may indicate dislocation on the short side (Galeazzi sign).[47] For the final portion of the examination, the knees and hips are flexed as much as possible, and the contralateral hip and thigh are stabilized with one hand.

The rest of examination is administered in two steps (Fig. 5-2D). In the first step, the thigh of the side that is being examined is grasped by the examiner

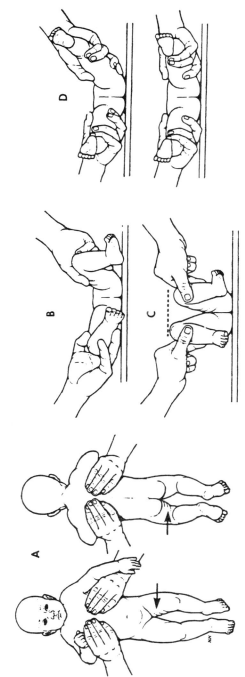

Fig. 5-2. Signs of hip dislocation. (**A**) Asymmetrical skin folds. (**B**) Limited abduction. (**C**) Apparent shortening of one thigh. (**D**) Examination to elicit relocation or dislocation. (From Wong and Whaley,[3] with permission.)

with the infant's knee cradled in the web space of the examiner's thumb and the examiner's thumb pad on the infant's medial thigh midway between the knee and hip. The third and fourth fingers are placed superior to the greater tubercle. The infant's thigh is adducted slightly, and the examiner applies gentle longitudinal pressure toward the surface. If the hip is dislocatable, a "clunk" or jerk is often palpable, audible, and visible when the head of the femur slips over the labrum out of the acetabulum. This portion of the test is often referred to as the *Barlow test* and indicates that the hip is dislocatable.

In the second step, the examiner slides the thumb pad distally to about the level of the adductor tubercle. The infant's leg is then abducted, and slight traction is applied while the examiner's fingers lift the head of the femur toward the hip socket. If the test is positive, resistance to abduction may be felt at about 30 to 40 degrees of abduction. The dislocated head of the femur will be felt to reduce, slipping over the posterior labrum into the acetabulum. A "clunk" or jerk may be felt, seen, or heard as the head of the femur slides over the labrum and into the acetabulum. After reduction, the hip may be taken into full normal abduction of 70 to 90 degrees. This second portion of the test is usually referred to as the *Ortolani maneuver* and indicates that dislocation has already occurred.[45–47]

The sound of the dislocated or dislocatable hip should be differentiated from the "click" sound, which can be produced by nonpathologic enlargements of the ligamentum teres or the iliopectineal bursa.[45] The Baby Hippy[48] is a teaching model that reproduces the positive examination for hip instability (Medical Plastics Laboratory, Gatesville, TX).

If the infant's acetabulum is malformed or very shallow, the two-part test may be inconclusive or misleading because no jerk or "clunk" may be produced. The child should also be examined for signs of adduction contracture on the contralateral side.[49] To conduct this investigation, the examiner places the infant prone and adducts each of the hips observing symmetry. Adduction contracture on one side indicates that hip dislocation of the contralateral side should be ruled out.

Bilateral dislocation is more difficult to detect. Signs may include bilateral limitation of abduction, "clunks" or jerks may be present on the Barlow or Ortolani maneuver, but asymmetric signs will be absent. Herring[45] reported an additional test that was taught to him by Klisik. The examiner places one finger tip on the anterior superior iliac spine and one finger on the greater trochanter. In a normal hip, a line drawn between the two finger tips will point toward the umbilicus. If the hip is dislocated, the line will point well below the umbilicus.

In an older infant, the telescoping sign may be used.[45] To perform this examination, the infant is placed supine on a firm, flat surface. The hip and knee on one side are flexed to 90 degrees. The examiner applies compressive force through the infant's knee perpendicularly toward the table. The examiner then grasps the upper tibia and pulls perpendicularly away from the table. In a dislocated hip, pistoning or telescoping will be observed or felt.

Ando and Gotoh[50] suggest that inguinal skin folds (groin creases) may be the most sensitive test for hip dislocation in infants 3 to 4 months of age. Inguinal

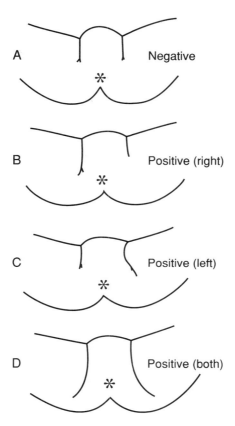

Fig. 5-3.   Detection of hip dislocation by inguinal folds. (From Ando and Gotoh,[50] with permisison.)

folds are inspected by positioning the infant with pelvis symmetrical on a firm, flat surface, hips and knees in 90 degrees of flexion, and hips abducted as far as possible (Fig. 5-3A). The inguinal folds are just lateral to the genital area and medial to the thigh, marking the boundary between the two. They are inspected from a caudal viewing position, looking toward the infant's perineum. Folds that are asymmetrical indicate potential hip dislocation on the longer side (Fig. 5-3B,C). Especially long folds extending symmetrically posterior to the anus indicate the likelihood of bilateral dislocation (Fig. 5-3D).

STRENGTH

Manual muscle testing (MMT), a staple in the armament of pediatric and adult therapists, when it must be performed on an infant, is time consuming and inexact. The infant cannot respond to directions. The infant must be patiently observed and gently stimulated over several sessions, and testing must fre-

quently be limited to major muscle groups because of the excessive time requirements of detailed muscle testing. When determining muscle innervation is important, as in brachial palsies or spina bifida, the information gained is probably
worth the time investment of performing as thorough an assessment as possible.
Because MMT is usually employed to help determine innervation patterns in
infancy, it will typically be used in association with careful testing of segmental
sensory responses.

Procedures for MMT must be highly modified from those used in older
children and adults[51] because of the infant's inability to cooperate. In addition,
the infant's medical condition may require further modification of the procedure,
as in the case of spina bifida, in which supine positioning may be impossible
because of the defect. The infant must be warm and awake for testing. The
testing should be done long enough after birth that any medications given to the
mother during labor have worn off and the infant is fully recovered from the
effects of labor.

The infant can be stimulated to move by use of primitive reflexive responses. Primitive reflexes that may be useful for MMT purposes include flexor
withdrawal, primitive positive support, primitive stepping, plantar grasp, placing, Babinski, and crossed extension. Reflexive responses vary according to
the infant's state and age, so interpretation of absence of response to stimulation
of reflexive muscle contraction can be problematic. Responses to spinal level
reflexes such as the crossed extension and withdrawal reflexes may indicate
only segmental innervation.

Deep tendon reflexes may be used during muscle testing; these stretch
responses can remain intact distal to a severed spinal cord, and stretch itself
tends to facilitate muscle contraction. Muscle contraction that has been stimulated by stretch or other facilitative techniques may be somewhat stronger
than the infant's muscle contraction in more typical situations and does not
necessarily indicate voluntary control of the muscle. Tactile stimulation of the
skin over hip and knee flexors and over ankle and toe muscles may also stimulate
movement even when only segmental spinal cord innervation is present.[52]

General stimulation such as excited talk or gently bouncing may elicit
movement, as may more specific stimulation such as tickling. Holding the limbs
in extreme positions may also stimulate movement. For instance, holding the
lower extremities in extreme abduction may stimulate hip adduction. Sometimes
the "hold everything else" technique may successfully elicit contractions.

In myelodysplasia, reflexive segmental spinal responses must be differentiated from muscle contractions that indicate voluntary control. Lower extremity
movement in response to stimulation of the upper body is good evidence of
intact voluntary control.[52] A response that is highly stimulus dependent is likely
to be reflexive in nature, although the response does not have to follow the
stimulus immediately. The time from stimulus to response can vary widely.[52]
One or two beats of ankle clonus is expected in a normal newborn infant,
but more sustained ankle clonus or clonus in muscle groups other than the
gastrocnemius-soleus may indicate spinal cord damage. Spinal crossed extension responses may produce movement in the contralateral extremity from the
one being stimulated. Finally, reflexive withdrawal responses may be jerky and

quick, but may also appear smooth and coordinated. For that reason, the coordination and speed of the withdrawal response indicate little about intactness of the spinal cord.[52]

In infants, the effect of body proportions on apparent strength should always be considered. Because the head is relatively large in comparison to the trunk and extremities, the neck and trunk flexors and extensors will appear weak compared with adult standards even though such apparent "weakness" is typical for an infant. MMT results for the muscles that are normal for the child's age but appear weak by adult standards can be recorded with the notation NFA, indicating that they are *normal for age.*

The effect of range of motion deficits, such as the typical hip and knee extension limitations of the lower extremity, on muscle contraction should be considered. All substitutions of muscle contraction should be carefully observed for what they reveal about patterns of muscle weakness and strength. The limb should be carefully stabilized so that substitutions can be eliminated and individual muscle contraction can be observed. Muscle contractions should be observed and palpated both with stimulation and during normal movement.

The infant may be positioned so as to test muscle strength against gravity, allowing determination of muscle grades up to "fair," but the infant can only rarely be enticed to contract or hold against resistance to determine higher grades. Tappit-Emas[53] suggests that muscle testing results in infants be recorded as "X" if the contraction is present and strong, "O" if the contraction is absent, "T" if the contraction can be palpated but no movement results, and "R" if the contraction appears to be reflexive in nature. Sheperd[54] recommends "0" for absent, "1" for present but lacking full range of movement, and "2" for present through full range of movement. In both cases, the MMT scale has been greatly simplified to focus testing on essential information and eliminate laborious differentiation of muscle grades.

In spina bifida, MMT should be performed before surgery, then repeated about 10 days after surgery.[53] The MMT results, in combination with results from segmental sensory testing, will be used to determine the level of the lesion. Parents will need to be carefully counseled about the meaning of reflexive muscle contractions so that they will understand that the reflex movements do not necessarily indicate that the spinal cord is intact. The MMT should be used to identify areas where muscle strength is unbalanced and therefore likely to cause deformity. Early intervention through positioning, orthotics, or surgical tendon transfers may be planned. The MMT should not be relied on to predict future function. Other variables such as motivation and intellect will also have a major impact on the child's future attempts to move so that early MMT results correlate only poorly with later functional abilities.[55]

SENSORY TESTING

Sensory testing in infancy is limited to determination of intact sensation, because the infant cannot report quality or intensity of sensation. When the infant is drowsy or quiet, a noxious stimulus such as a pin prick is administered.

The testing proceeds from distally innervated dermatomes to more proximally innervated dermatomes. Withdrawal responses of the lower extremity may indicate only segmental innervation, but crying, grimacing, or a startle response probably indicates intact sensation in the dermatome. Information from sensory testing is usually used in conjunction with MMT results to determine the level of intact innervation in cases of spinal cord or peripheral nerve injury or defect.

SUMMARY

Pediatric physical therapists working with infants must be familiar with growth measures, whether to obtain the measures personally or to interpret growth information in the medical record. Since growth is an important indicator of a child's health status, such information is a critical component of a complete assessment of an infant. Formal GA assessment by a standardized tool may not be performed on term infants if the obstetric record agrees with the infant's general appearance. GA assessment is, however, a vital element for evaluation of an infant whose mother had no prenatal care or when prematurity is suspected. ROM records will be required when joint range appears limited or excessive, conditions that affect most infants referred for physical therapy. Specific MMT and sensory testing will usually be undertaken only in cases of spinal cord or peripheral nerve injury because of the difficulties in performing MMT and sensory testing of infants. In such cases, the information to be gained about the severity and extent of the paralysis and sensory loss is so critical that the extensive investment of time in discriminative testing is well justified. In summary, the tests and measures covered in this chapter often form the critical basis for a complete physical therapy evaluation.

REFERENCES

1. Hall JG, Froster-Iskenius UG, Allanson JE: Handbook of Normal Physical Measurements. Oxford University Press, Oxford, 1989
2. Goldenberg RL, Cliver SP, Cutter GR et al: Black–white differences in newborn anthropometric measurements. Obstet Gynecol 78(5):782, 1991
3. Wong DL, Whaley LF: Clinical Manual of Pediatric Nursing. 3rd Ed. CV Mosby, St. Louis, 1990
4. Lubchenco LO: The High Risk Infant. WB Saunders, Philadelphia, 1976
5. Casey PH, Kraemer HC, Bernbaum J et al: Growth status and growth rates of a varied sample of low birth weight, preterm infants: a longitudinal cohort from birth to three years of age. J Pediatr 119(4):599, 1991
6. Jones KL: Smith's Recognizable Patterns of Human Malformation. 4th Ed. WB Saunders, Philadelphia, 1988
7. Hensinger RN: Standards in Pediatric Orthopedics: Tables, Charts, and Graphs Illustrating Growth. Raven Press, New York, 1986
8. Roche AF, Malina RM: Manual of Physical Status and Performance in Childhood. Plenum Press, New York, 1983

9. Sweet AY: Classification of the low birthweight infant. p. 69. In Klaus MH, Fanaroff AA (eds): Care of the High Risk Neonate. 3rd Ed. WB Saunders, Philadelphia, 1986

10. DiPietro JA, Allen MC: Estimation of gestational age: implications for developmental research. Child Dev 62:1184, 1991

11. Kliegman RM, Wald MK: Problems in metabolic adaptation: glucose, calcium, and magnesium. p. 229. In Klaus MH, Fanaroff AA (eds): Care of the High Risk Neonate. 3rd Ed. WB Saunders, Philadelphia, 1986

12. Amiel-Tison C: Neurological evaluation of the maturity of newborn infants. Arch Dis Child 43:89, 1968

13. Farr V, Mitchell RG, Neligan GA, Parkin JM: The definition of some external characteristics used in the newborn infant. Dev Med Child Neurol 8:657, 1966

14. Dubowitz LMS, Dubowitz V, Goldberg C: Clinical assessment of gestational age in the newborn infant. J Pediatr 77(1):1, 1970

15. Clopton N: The Dubowitz assessment of gestational age. Phys Occup Ther Pediatr 3(3):75, 1983

16. Brueton MJ, Palit A, Prosser R: Gestational age assessment in Nigerian newborn infants. Arch Dis Child 48:318, 1973

17. Spinnato JA, Sibai BM, Shaver DC, Anderson GD: Inaccuracy of Dubowitz gestational age in low birth weight infants. Obstet Gynecol 63(4):491, 1984

18. Sanders M, Allen M, Alexander GR et al: Gestational age assessment in preterm neonates weighing less than 1500 grams. Pediatrics 88(3):542, 1991

19. Shukla H, Atakent YS, Ferrara A et al: Postnatal overestimation of gestational age in preterm infants. Am J Dis Child 141:1106, 1987

20. Ballard JL, Novak KK, Driver M: A simplified score for assessment of fetal maturation of newly born infants. J Pediatr 95(5):769, 1979

21. Blasco PA: Preterm birth: to correct or not to correct. Dev Med Child Neurol 31:816, 1989

22. Sweeney JK, Swanson MW: At-risk neonates and infants: NICU management and follow-up. p. 183. In Umphred DA (ed): Neurological Rehabilitation. 2nd Ed. CV Mosby, St. Louis, 1990

23. Harris MB, Simons CJR, Ritchie SK et al: Joint range of motion development in premature infants. Pediatr Phys Ther 1:185, 1990

24. Katz K, Davidson S, Dulitsky F et al: Normal ranges of hip motion of preterm infants. Dev Med Child Neurol 33:993, 1991

25. Drews JE, Vraciu JK, Pellino G: Range of motion of the joints of the lower extremities of newborns. Phys Occup Ther Pediatr 4(2):49, 1984

26. Coon V, Donato G, Houser C, Bleck EE: Normal ranges of hip motion in infants six weeks, three months and six months of age. Clin Orthop Rel Res 110:256, 1975

27. Haas SS, Epps CH, Adam JP: Normal ranges of hip motion in the newborn. Clin Orthop Rel Res 91:114, 1973

28. Phelps E, Smith LJ, Hallum A: Normal ranges of hip motion of infants between nine and 24 months. Dev Med Child Neurol 27:785, 1985

29. Reade E, Ham L, Hallum A, Lopopolo R: Changes in popliteal angle measurement in infants up to one year of age. Dev Med Child Neurol 26:774, 1984

30. Waugh KG, Minkel JL, Parker R, Coon VA: Measurement of selected hip, knee, and ankle joint motions in newborns. Phys Ther 63(10):1616, 1983

31. Forero N, Okamura LA, Larson MA: Normal ranges of hip motion in neonates. J Pediatr Orthop 9(4):391, 1989

32. Hoffer MM: Joint motion limitation in newborns. Clin Orthop Rel Res 148:94, 1980

33. Amiel-Tison C: A method for neurologic evaluation within the first year of life. Curr Prob Pediatr 7:3, 1976

34. Alston M: Passive range of motion measurements of the ankle, knee, and hip of healthy, preterm infants. Phys Ther [suppl] 71(6):S56, 1991

35. Staheli LT: The prone hip extension test: a method of measuring hip flexion deformity. Clin Orthop Rel Res 123:12, 1977

36. Bernhardt DB: Prenatal and postnatal growth and development of the foot and ankle. Phys Ther 68(12):1831, 1988

37. Johnson A, Ashurst H: Is popliteal angle measurement useful in early identification of cerebral palsy? Dev Med Child Neurol 31:457, 1989

38. Bagnall KM, Harris PF, Jones PRM: A radiographic study of the human fetal spine. 1. The development of the secondary cervical curvature. J Anat 123(3):777, 1977

39. Bly L: Components of Normal Movement During the First Year of Life and Abnormal Development. Neurodevelopmental Treatment Association, Oak Park, IL, 1983

40. LeVeau BF, Bernhardt DB: Developmental biomechanics: effect of forces on the growth, development, and maintenance of the human body. Phys Ther 64:1874, 1984

41. Cusick CD: Progressive Casting and Splinting for Lower Extremity Deformities in Children With Neuromotor Dysfunction. Therapy Skill Builders, Tucson, 1990

42. Crane L: Physical therapy for neonates with respiratory dysfunction. Phys Ther 61:1764, 1981

43. Watanabe RS: Embryology of the human hip. Clin Orthop Rel Res 98:8, 1974

44. Walker JM, Goldsmith CH: Morphometric study of the fetal development of the human hip joint: significance for congenital hip disease. Yale J Biol Med 54:411, 1981

45. Herring JA: Congenital dislocation of the hip. p. 815. In Morrissy RT (ed): Lovell and Winter's Pediatric Orthopedics. 3rd Ed. JB Lippincott, Philadelphia, 1990

46. Lloyd-Roberts GC, Fixsen J: Orthopedics in Infancy and Childhood. 2nd Ed. Butterworth-Heinemann, London, 1990

47. Palmer ML, Epler ME: Clinical Assessment Procedures in Physical Therapy. JB Lippincott, Philadelphia, 1990

48. Cole WG: Evaluation of a teaching model for the early diagnosis of congenital dislocation of the hip. J Pediatr Orthop 3:223, 1983

49. Greene NE, Griffin PP: Hip dysplasia associated with abduction contracture of the contralateral hip. J Bone Joint Surg 64:1273, 1982

50. Ando M, Gotoh E: Significance of inguinal folds for diagnosis of congenital dislocation of the hip in infants aged three to four months. J Pediatr Orthop 10:331, 1990

51. Schneider JW, Gabriel KL: Congenital spinal cord injury. p. 397. In Umphred DA (ed): Neurological Rehabilitation. 2nd Ed. CV Mosby, St. Louis, 1990

52. Garber JB: Myelodysplasia. p. 169. In Campbell SK (ed): Pediatric Neurologic Physical Therapy. 2nd Ed. Churchill Livingstone, New York, 1991

53. Tappit-Emas E: Spina bifida. p. 106. In Tecklin JS (ed): Pediatric Physical Therapy. JB Lippincott, Philadelphia, 1989

54. Sheperd RB: Brachial plexus injury. p. 101. In Campbell SK (ed): Pediatric Neurologic Physical Therapy. 2nd Ed. Churchill Livingstone, New York, 1991

55. Murdoch A: How valuable is muscle charting? Physiotherapy 66(7):221, 1980

56. Schluter K, Funfack W, Pachaly J, Weber B: Development of subcutaneous fat in infancy: standards for tricipital, subscapular, and suprailiac skinfolds in German infants. Eur J Pediatr 123:255, 1976

6 | Evaluation of the Cardiopulmonary System in the Neonate

Jan Stephen Tecklin

Cardiopulmonary evaluation of the neonate differs from assessment of the neonate with neuromuscular or musculoskeletal dysfunction insofar as virtually no published or standardized assessments for the cardiopulmonary system exist that employ either quantitative or qualitative measurements. Evaluation of the cardiopulmonary system is based almost entirely on a medical model of examination for clinical signs that provide information that, when considered in combination with laboratory values and radiologic procedures, can result in a physical therapy diagnosis.

The adult patient with myocardial disease may benefit from an exericse regimen with goals of improving cardiopulmonary endurance, reducing myocardial oxygen demand, and increasing functional work capacity.[1] Although cardiopulmonary evaluation is the intended focus of this chapter, direct physical therapy is not likely to improve the cardiac status of the neonate or young infant with cardiac disease. Because treatment of neonates with cardiac disease is not encountered in contemporary physical therapy, evaluation of the cardiac system will not be discussed. Rather, I will carefully examine the neonatal pulmonary system by briefly reviewing its development, the ways in which it differs from that of the older child or adult, and the standard clinical tools and techniques for its evaluation.

PULMONARY DEVELOPMENT

Development of the pulmonary tract in the fetus is commonly divided into four stages: embryonic, pseudoglandular, canalicular, and alveolar. The embryonic stage of lung development begins around day 24 of gestation and is heralded by division of the primitive foregut into an anterior pouchlike projection that will ultimately become the pulmonary system. The pouchlike projection is the rudimentary trachea, while the posterior foregut section will become the esophagus. About 4 days later, the lung pouch divides into left and right sections. These sections begin to invade surrounding mesenchymal tissue that will differentiate into bronchial structures, including cartilage, smooth muscle, and connective tissue, both elastic and collagen fibers.

During weeks 5 through 16, which demarcate the pseudoglandular period, subsequent subdivisions of the right and left lung buds continue, and smaller airways are formed. A primitive form of bronchial epithelium lines these early airways, although the bronchial mucous glands and supportive bronchial cartilage do not appear until very late in the pseudoglandular period. The pseudoglandular period is so named because a histologic section taken at this time closely resembles one of glandular tissue. A burst of growth occurs during weeks 10 to 14 of gestation. The active branching and subdividing of the airways continues during this period until up to 32 generations of branching are present in those lung segments most distant from the hilum of the lungs. By the end of the pseudoglandular period, the bronchopulmonary tree is complete from the glottis through the terminal bronchioles.[2]

Two major events occur during the canalicular period of lung development, weeks 16 to 24. The synergistic effects of the two events provide for the possibility of gas exchange between the as yet unaerated alveoli and the pulmonary capillaries. The first event involves the epithelial cells in distal airways that will ultimately become respiratory bronchioles and alveoli. The epithelial cells, which have been cuboidal in character, begin to flatten toward a more squamous-like appearance. The second event involves the development of the vascular system. The pulmonary arteries are formed from the inferior surface of the sixth pharyngeal arch arteries and course into the developing lung tissue to divide congruently with the airways. The pulmonary veins develop from the posterior surface of the left atrium and extend into the developing lung tissue.[3] As the vascular system develops, endothelial cells of the developing capillary network move closer to the epithelial layer and, by the end of the canalicular period, begin to protrude or invaginate into the epithelial lining. This close proximity of the blood-carrying endothelial cell system and the air-carrying respiratory bronchioles and alveoli provides for the air–blood interface necessary for gas exchange. Some degree of gas exchange is possible by week 24, the end of the canalicular period.

The final major period of development, the terminal sac or alveolar period, begins at about 25 weeks of gestation and continues until approximately ages 8 to 10 years. During this period the energy of lung development is aimed at expansion of the terminal bronchioles into a multitude of out-pouchings that become gas exchange units: respiratory bronchioles and alveoli. Each terminal bronchiole will give rise to numerous gas exchange units, which maintain their close physical proximity to the developing endothelial cell and capillary network. When a sufficient number of gas exchange units is present, adequate oxygen uptake and carbon dioxide removal may occur to support life, pending one additional biochemical event. The development of pulmonary surfactant—a phospholipid liquid secreted by type II pneumocytes—at a level indicative of lung maturity is considered one of the most critical features of lung development in the fetus. Lecithin and sphingomyelin (L:S) are the major components of surfactant, and an L:S ratio of 2.0 or greater often reflects lung maturity.[4] Pulmonary surfactant reduces the surface tension within alveoli, thereby diminishing the physical work needed to produce negative inspiratory pressures to inflate the lungs in a continuous mode. When immature L:S ratios exist, the lungs of the neonate cannot easily be kept inflated and alveoli collapse, resulting in atelectasis. The presence of mature L:S ratios, the branching of terminal bronchioles into gas exchange units, and the movement of capillaries adjacent to the gas exchange units will usually provide for functional lung activity in the neonate.[2] During the 10 years within the alveolar period, lung growth is almost entirely devoted to an increase in the number of alveoli and the resultant increase in surface area for gas exchange. Weibel,[5] in his classic text, described the quantitative increase in numbers of alveoli from birth, approximately 25 million, to adulthood with approximately 300 million alveoli. The majority of this 12-fold increase in alveolar number occurs during the first several years of extrauterine life. In addition to alveolar number, alveolar size increases significantly between neonatal life and adulthood. When alveolar size and number are considered together, surface area for gas exchange increases approximately 25-fold between neonatal and adult life.[5]

ANATOMIC AND PHYSIOLOGIC DIFFERENCES—NEONATES VS. ADULTS

Significant differences between the neonatal and adult respiratory systems result in the greater likelihood of respiratory difficulties for the neonate. These characteristics, although normal, will often predispose the neonate to airways obstruction, respiratory distress, and respiratory failure.

Anatomic Factors

The neonate is thought to be an obligate nose-breather. As a result of this feature, any complication that reduces the patency of the nasal airway can have a severe effect on breathing.

The previous discussion about numbers of alveoli and cross section of gas exchange area should be recalled. The potential for alveolar growth assumes that healthy lung tissue exists throughout childhood. Any major destructive process to the lungs can reduce the potential both for alveolar growth and for gas exchange surface.[6]

The bronchi and bronchioles in the neonate are, naturally, much smaller than in adults and have less structural support. Their small lumen makes possible obstruction by intraluminal material (e.g., secretions) and by increased resistance to airflow (e.g., bronchospasm or edema).[7] The lack of strong cartilaginous support within the airways makes possible their collapse due to various physiological challenges.

Channels that provide for collateral ventilation between alveoli (pores of Kohn) and between alveoli and respiratory bronchioles (canals of Lambert) are less prevalent in the lungs of neonates than of older children or adults.[8] Given a pathologic challenge, this normal characteristic increases the likelihood of atelectasis or lack of lung expansion in an area.

The diaphragm of the neonate has a relatively high percentage of white, nonoxidative, fast twitch, fatiguable muscle fibers.[9] These fibers cannot provide the fatigue-resistant effects seen in the adult diaphragm, which has a greater percentage of red, high oxidative, slow twitch, fatigue-resistant fibers. The resultant potential for diaphragmatic fatigue and failure is greater in the neonate than in an older child.

In addition to the disadvantage caused by nonfatigue-resistant fiber types in the neonatal diaphragm, mechanical disadvantage can also be found in the neonate thorax. The (well-documented) configuration of the rib cage in neonates plays a disadvantageous role in efficiency of breathing. The neonatal thorax is rounded, with a greater relative anteroposterior dimension, and the ribs are more horizontally situated than in an adult thorax. These normal anatomic factors result in a greater horizontal pull to the diaphragm[10] and less mechanical advantage to the intercostal muscles,[11] each of which results in reduced muscular efficiency and effectiveness of breathing.

The potential of muscular inefficiency combined with a rib cage that is almost entirely cartilaginous, and therefore highly compliant, increases the potential for wasted muscular effort. A neonate's increased inspiratory effort may cause deformation of the thorax. The resultant indrawing or retractions can be of such severity that the inspiratory effort decreases rather than increases thoracic volume.[12]

Physiologic Factors

Neonatal control of ventilation is immature. This lack of maturity causes irregularities in the respiratory cycle and may cause apnea. Although short periods of apnea—several seconds—are common, longer periods can cause bradycardia and diminution of cardiac output.[13]

Several physiologic factors result in greater relative work of breathing in the neonate. During early extrauterine life, lung tissue has diminished compliance, which requires greater inspiratory effort to expand the lungs.[12] Neonatal respiratory rate and minute ventilation per unit of body weight are both much greater than those of adults. Each of these factors results in a greater need for respiratory work and increased metabolic demand. Finally, the small airways of the neonate offer a tubular system of relatively poor conductance through which to provide air to the alveoli. Working against this relatively poor conductance, which does not increase until around age 5 years, the inspiratory muscles must exert greater relative pressures than in an older child.[14] The net effect of these factors is to cause a normal, but significantly greater, demand on the respiratory system than exists in an older child or adult.

The increased need for muscular effort is clear. One of the major fuels for this effort, glycogen stores in the muscle, is very low and will be depleted very rapidly with muscular activity.[15] With the many anatomic and physiologic pulmonary factors in neonates, the fact that many develop respiratory diseases and disorders is not surprising. The physical therapist has a clear role in evaluating neonates with respiratory disorders, and the basis for this evaluation follows. Treatment techniques and their effects are not the focus of this book and have been fully described elsewhere.[13,16–20] The purpose of the remainder of this chapter is to provide a scheme with which to evaluate the neonate with questionable respiratory function. Much of the information is adapted from Crane.[13]

PATIENT EVALUATION

History

Before evaluating the neonate, the therapist must obtain a complete history. The history should include a description of labor and delivery, with careful attention to detect any circumstances that could have had an impact on respiratory development.

Immediate postpartum assessments of the neonate often include the Apgar score and, in the case of premature delivery, a determination of gestational age. The Apgar score is a well-known method of evaluation of general status by examining heart rate, respiratory effort, muscle tone, response to stimulation, and color.[21] The Apgar score has been shown to be a strong predictor of respiratory disturbances in term neonates and in those vaginally delivered from 33 to 36 weeks of gestation. For these infants, a 1 minute Apgar score of less than 7 of a possible 10 points was a powerful risk factor for respiratory disturbances.[22] The Dubowitz Scale, used to determine gestational age, is based on 10 neurologic criteria and 11 external characteristics.[23] The general clinical course of the baby must be evaluated in addition to the specific respiratory history. The latter may include a history of respiratory symptoms and distress, the pattern of arterial blood gas measurements and other laboratory tests, and reports from a series of chest x-rays. Other aspects of care must be considered, such as the specific equipment required for the neonate, the mode of nutrition being employed, and any other care that could affect the respiratory system. Because of the stress induced by virtually all handling and other medical procedures, the baby should not be evaluated when other procedures have immediately preceded.[24,25]

Chest Evaluation

Inspection

Careful inspection of the neonate's thorax can offer useful information. In fact, because the neonate cannot actively participate in the evaluation, inspection becomes one of the most important tools for the therapist.

General Appearance. Note the general state of consciousness, any wounds or scars, obvious skeletal abnormalities, and the presence of edema. Identification of the various pieces of equipment being used can fall into this area.

Head and Neck. Signs of respiratory distress can often be identified in the head and neck. Flaring of the alae nasae is an almost universal sign of respiratory distress in the neonate. Because the infant is an obligate nose-breather, flaring may be a reflex attempt to widen the airways to reduce the resistance to airflow. Head bobbing, which coincides with the respiratory cycle, is an attempt to increase ventilation by using the accessory muscles of inspiration. Head bobbing occurs because the infant has inadequate strength to fix the head while using accessory muscles to raise the thorax. As a result much accessory muscle effort is wasted, because those muscles work to move the head rather than the thorax. Audible sounds of respiratory distress can be heard during inspection of the head and neck. Expiratory grunting, which does not have a clearly defined mechanism, is thought to be an attempt to improve distribution of ventilation, enhance the ventilation:perfusion ratio, or increase functional residual capacity, a lung volume commonly used in times of increased respiratory demands.[26,27] Stridor is an inspiratory "crowing" sound commonly associated with obstruction of the extrathoracic portion of the trachea.

Evaluation of skin color is also part of the head and neck evaluation. Shortly after birth, normal neonates have pink skin, mucous membranes, and nailbeds. Cyanosis is a well-known bluish tinge to the skin, nailbeds, and mucous membranes secondary to some cardiopulmonary disorder. Cyanosis is often associated with severely reduced arterial oxygenation. Pallor, a general sign of distress caused by some cardiopulmonary or vascular abnormality, can be associated with respiratory distress and asphyxia. Plethora is a ruddy color that may be associated with polycythemia or neonatal hyperviscosity and may be related to some degree of respiratory distress.[28]

Unmoving Chest. This portion of the examination involves the shape and symmetry of the thorax and may include such items as rashes, scars, incisions, bruises, and obvious musculoskeletal deformities. The overall configuration of the neonatal thorax is one of greater roundness than in the older child or adult. The neonate will have an anteroposterior thoracic diameter approximately equal to the transverse diameter. In the adult, the anteroposterior diameter is only about one-half of the transverse diameter. This increase in the anteroposterior to transverse diameter, often called the *thoracic index,* results in the rounded thorax found in the neonate. In addition to this normal variation in thoracic configuration, congenital defects of the thorax may also be found. These include pectus excavatum, funnel chest, and pectus carinatum, pigeon breast. The therapist should also determine if scoliosis exists and attempt to ascertain whether the cause is skeletal, muscular, or neurologic. Muscular development should be examined, with particular emphasis upon symmetry.

Moving Chest. Respiratory rate should be the first item evaluated. The normal respiratory rate for a neonate is between 40 and 60 breaths per minute and is often variable, particularly during the first few days of life.[27] When the rate exceeds 60, tachypnea is said to exist, and when the rate falls to between

20 and 30, bradypnea is the case. Neonates commonly exhibit irregular breathing that includes differences in rate and depth and that makes it mandatory to count respirations for at least 60 seconds for a reliable reading. Periodic breathing is seen in premature and very young neonates. This periodic pattern is characterized by alternating periods of irregular rate and depth of breathing with periods of apnea, usually of less than 15 seconds duration. True apnea occurs with cessation of respiration for greater than 20 seconds, associated with bradycardia of less than 100 beats per minute and cyanosis.

Motion of the thorax should be evaluated for symmetry and synchrony. Symmetry is usually viewed by comparing the right to the left hemithorax for similar degree of motion. Synchrony is examined by comparing thoracic and abdominal movement. Thoracic expansion during inspiration is associated with abdominal protrusion as the diaphragm descends. Asynchronous movements between the thorax and abdomen often suggest respiratory distress and respiratory muscle weakness or fatigue. Retractions are also evaluated during this portion of inspection. Retractions, or indrawing of the thorax during inspiration, occur primarily in the sternal and intercostal areas. The indrawing is caused by the negative inspiratory pressure generated by the diaphragm, which can overcome the highly compliant thorax and cause a reduction, rather than expansion, in thoracic diameter during the inspiratory effort. An early study suggested a scoring system for retractions, but this system has not gained wide acceptance.[29] Bulging of the intercostal spaces and musculature may also occur, particularly when some pathology results in the generation of excessive expiratory pressures. Increasing severity of retractions usually indicates worsening pulmonary status, while decreasing severity suggests improvement.[30]

Coughing and Sneezing. Although coughing is critically important in the older child and adult, sneezing appears to be the main process by which the neonate clears the airways. The therapist may stimulate the nasal or oral pharynx in an attempt to elicit either a sneeze or a cough to determine which is functional for the infant.[13]

Auscultation

Auscultation, listening to the sounds generated in the thorax, although a sine qua non in pediatric and adult chest evaluation, may be less reliable and less valid for the neonate. The rapid respiratory rate, thinness of the thorax, and proximity of the thoracic surface to the lung tissue and airways that generate sounds often diminishes anatomic specificity of sounds from the neonatal thorax. Nonetheless, auscultation, with its limitations, is a major portion of the neonatal chest evaluation.

The stethoscope employed for neonatal examination is identical to the adult model in all aspects except size. Most models will have both a bell, which transmits all sounds, with particularly strong transmission of low-pitched sounds, and a diaphragm, which appears to favor transmission of high-pitched sounds.[31] Others have more fully described the techniques for auscultation by physical therapists.[13,32] Some authors suggest that, when possible, auscultation be performed during the long inspiratory phase of a neonate's cry.[31]

Breath Sounds.   Normal breath sounds are said to rustle. They reach maximum intensity during inspiration and diminish shortly after expiration begins. These sounds should be heard over the entire periphery of the lungs. Bronchial breath sounds are loud and harsh, heard throughout inspiration and expiration, and have been described as air passing through a hollow tube. Decreased breath sounds have qualities similar to normal breath sounds except that they are less intense, or more distant. Absent breath sounds describe a complete lack of sound from a lung area.

Abnormal or Adventitious Sounds.   Crackles are noncontinuous, nonmusical sounds that are superimposed over breath sounds. Crackles may be characterized by the portion of the respiratory cycle in which they are heard: early inspiratory or late expiratory. Inspiratory crackles are believed to represent the ''popping'' open of previously closed or collapsed airways, whereas expiratory crackles may represent fluid or secretions in the airways. Crackles are sometimes referred to as *rales*.

Wheezes are musical and continuous sounds. High-pitched wheezes have been compared with whistles and low-pitched wheezes with growling or snoring. Wheezes are often referred to as *rhonchi*. They are most commonly heard during expiration and almost universally considered a result of airways obstruction, either local or diffuse.

Extrapulmonary Sounds.   Rubs are sounds generated within the pleural or pericardial spaces. Rubs are thought to represent the rubbing together of inflamed surfaces of visceral and parietal pleura and pericardial membranes when these surfaces become inflamed. Pleural rubs, heard most distinctly during inspiration, are coarse and have been compared with leathery surfaces rubbing over one another.

Palpation of the Thorax

Palpation of the neonatal thorax, performed with the palmar surface of the distal fingers, provides only limited information to the therapist. The trachea can be palpated in an effort to determine whether the mediastinum is in midline or shifted to one side. A mediastinal shift could mean greater lung volume in the side *from which* the trachea is shifted or reduced volume in the hemithorax *toward which* the trachea is shifted. Palpation can also be used to identify vocal fremitus: the vibrations generated to the thorax due to phonation. Decreased fremitus may be caused by airways obstruction, pleural disease, or large lung cysts, each of which interferes with transmission of the vibratory wave to the surface of the thorax. Increased vocal fremitus occurs when transmission of the vibratory wave is enhanced, as occurs in lung consolidation (e.g., pneumonia). Other findings with palpation commonly include edema and subcutaneous emphysema. In the older child and adult, palpation is often employed for identifying chest pain or evaluating thoracic motion. These two items become more difficult to determine in neonates due to their inability to respond specifically to questioning about pain and their very limited thoracic motion and very rapid respiratory rate.

Percussion of the Thorax

Mediate, or indirect, percussion of the thorax of a neonate is considered inappropriate in many cases by some[12] and appropriate by others.[31] A characteristic sound is generated as the percussing finger strikes a finger of the opposite hand that is positioned in a rib interspace on the neonate's thorax. One of the reasons that some oppose percussion of the neonate is the tiny rib interspaces that cannot be strictly percussed without overlap onto the rib. As a result of the overlap, the sound generated probably becomes distorted and may be less meaningful. Five classic sounds have been described, ranging from the sounds denoting the most air-filled thorax to the least air-filled thorax: tympanic, hyperresonant, resonant, dull, and flat. These sounds have clear diagnostic implications to physicians, but in my opinion the therapist need only discern normal or resonant percussion notes from either increased resonance or decreased resonance. The normal note, which can only be appreciated after experience with many babies, is consistent with a normally air-filled thorax. The note with increased resonance suggests too much air in the thorax, while the note with decreased resonance suggests a thorax with too little air. I use the term *thorax* rather than *lung* because, with percussion alone, one cannot discern where the air is located (e.g., in the lung or in the pleural space).

CLINICAL APPLICATION OF FINDINGS FROM THE EVALUATION

A finite group of treatments can be applied to the pulmonary system of the neonate. These treatments have limited, but extremely important, goals. The underlying goals are not necessarily exclusive: (1) improve ventilation, (2) clear the airways of secretions or debris, and (3) reduce the work of breathing.

Each evaluation technique may provide information to suggest one or more treatment goals, and the therapist must integrate the information gleaned from each part of the evaluation to arrive at the proper goals. Portions of the evaluation should agree. For example, inspection of a neonate may indicate flaring of the alae nasi, expiratory grunting, tachypnea, and a cyanotic tinge to the mucous membranes. Mediate percussion may result in a dull note that indicates airless lung in a particular area. The accompanying auscultatory finding should be consistent, such as bronchial sounds, which indicates lung consolidation or lack of aeration in that area. Palpation may be expected to indicate increased vocal fremitus, also indicative of poor lung expansion in the area in question. These findings are all consistent with poor lung aeration and suggest treatment goals of improving ventilation to the airless lung. Had wheezes or crackles been heard in the area of abnormal findings in addition to bronchial sounds, airways clearance would have been an additional treatment goal.

This chapter has described the developmental background of the pulmonary system and the several anatomic and physiologic features of the system that make the neonate unique. Unlike published neuromuscular, motor, developmental, and other assessments, evaluation of the neonate's lungs remains an art and science largely based on the medical model. I have tried to offer a scheme of evaluation by which the physical therapist can gather information about the neonatal pulmonary system with which to prepare a rational treatment plan.

REFERENCES

1. Blessey R: The beneficial effects of aerobic exercise for patients with coronary artery disease. p. 187. In Irwin S, Tecklin JS (eds): Cardiopulmonary Physical Therapy. 2nd Ed. CV Mosby, St. Louis, 1990
2. Thurlbeck WM: Lung growth. p. 1. In: Pathology of the Lung. Thieme Medical Publishers, New York, 1988
3. Stahlman MT: Acute respiratory disorders of the newborn. p. 371. In Avery G (ed): Neonatology. JB Lippincott, Philadelphia, 1980
4. Avery ME: Hyaline membrane disease. Am Rev Respir Dis 111:657, 1975
5. Weibel ER: Morphometry of the Human Lung. Academic Press, New York, 1963
6. Dunnill MS: Quantitative observations on the anatomy of chronic non-specific lung disease. Med Thorac 22:261, 1965
7. Vidyasagar D: Clinical diagnosis of respiratory failure in infants and children. p. 2. In Gregory GA (ed): Respiratory Failure in the Child. Churchill Livingstone, New York, 1981
8. Kuhn C III: Normal anatomy and histology. p. 11. In Thurlbeck WM (ed): Pathology of the Lung. Thieme Medical Publishers, New York, 1988
9. Keens TG, Ianuzzo CO: Development of fatigue resistant fibers in human ventilatory muscles. Am Rev Respir Dis 119:139, 1979
10. Muller NL, Bryan AC: Chest wall mechanics and respiratory muscles in infants. Pediatr Clin North Am 26:503, 1979
11. Tecklin JS: Pulmonary disorders in infants and children and their physical therapy management. p. 144. In: Pediatric Physical Therapy. JB Lippincott, Philadelphia, 1989
12. DeCesare JA, Graybill CA: Physical therapy for the child with respiratory dysfunction. p. 418. In Irwin S, Tecklin JS (eds): Cardiopulmonary Physical Therapy. 2nd Ed. CV Mosby, St. Louis, 1990
13. Crane L: Physical therapy for the neonate with respiratory dysfunction. p. 389. In Irwin S, Tecklin JS (eds): Cardiopulmonary Physical Therapy. 2nd Ed. CV Mosby, St. Louis, 1990
14. Crone RK: Assisted ventilation in children. p. 20. In Gregory GA (ed): Respiratory Failure in the Child. Churchill Livingstone, New York, 1981
15. Pagliara AS, Karl IE, Haymond M, Kipnis DM: Hypoglycemia in infancy and childhood. J Pediatr 82:365, 1973
16. Brackbill Y, Douthitt TC, West H: Psycho-physiologic effects in the neonate of prone versus supine placement. J Pediatr 82:82, 1973

17. Martin RJ, Herrell N, Rubin D, Fanaroff A: Effects of supine and prone positions on arterial oxygen tension in the preterm infant. Pediatrics 63:528, 1979
18. Wagaman MJ, Shutack JG, Moomjian AS et al: Improved oxygenation and lung compliance with prone positioning of neonates. J Pediatr 94:787, 1979
19. Finer NN, Boyd J: Chest physiotherapy in the neonate: a controlled study. Pediatrics 61:282, 1978
20. Finer NN, Moriartey RR, Boyd J et al: Postextubation atelectasis: a retrospective review and a prospective controlled study. J Pediatr 94:110, 1979
21. Apgar V: Proposal for a new method of evaluation of newborn infants. Anesth Analg 32:260, 1953
22. Wennergen M, Krantz M, Hjalmarson O, Karlsson K: Low Apgar score as a risk factor for respiratory disturbances in the newborn infant. J Perinatal Med 15:153, 1987
23. Dubowitz LMS, Dubowitz V, Goldberg C: Clinical assessment of gestational age in the newborn infant. J Pediatr 77:1, 1970
24. Long JG, Philip AG, Lucey JF: Excessive handling as a cause of hypoxemia. Pediatrics 65:203, 1980
25. Yeh TF, Lilien LD, Leu ST, Pildes RS: Increased O_2 consumption and energy loss in premature infants following medical care procedures. Biol Neonate 46:157, 1984
26. Chrisman MK: Respiratory Nursing: Continuing Education Review. Medical Examination Publishing Co., New York, 1975
27. Polgar G: Practical pulmonary physiology. Pediatr Clin North Am 20:303, 1973
28. LeBlanc KB, Forestell FE: Assessment of the neonatal respiratory system. Clin Issues Crit Care Nurs 1:401, 1990
29. Silverman WA, Anderson DH: A controlled clinical trial of effects of water mist and obstructive respiratory signs. Pediatrics 17:1, 1956
30. Davis GM, Bureau MA: Pulmonary and chest wall mechanics in the control of respiration in the newborn. Clin Perinatol 14:551, 1987
31. Scarpelli E: Examination of the lung (physiologic and anatomic basis). p. 1. In Scarpelli EM, Auld PAM, Goldman HS (eds): Pulmonary Disease of the Fetus, Newborn, and Child. Lea & Febiger, Philadelphia, 1978
32. Humberstone N: Respiratory assessment and treatment. p. 287. In Irwin S, Tecklin JS (eds): Cardiopulmonary Physical Therapy. 2nd Ed. CV Mosby, St. Louis, 1990

7 | Oral–Motor Assessment

MaryBeth Mandich

Clinical oral–motor assessment in infancy as an objective evaluation presents several challenges to the therapist. First, structural and developmental variations are common in the anatomy of the face and oral cavity. Second, much of the oral–motor pattern is difficult to visualize clinically as it occurs. Finally, direct palpation of various structures as they are activated in the motor pattern is difficult if not impossible. For these reasons, oral–motor assessment of the infant demands a great deal more clinical judgment and interpolation of findings than do other types of assessment routinely performed by therapists.

A complete oral–motor assessment should include an assessment of facial and intraoral anatomy, a neurodevelopmental assessment of oral function, an evaluation of suck and swallow, an assessment of strength and endurance, and, finally, a behavioral assessment. Clinical assessment may be supplemented by radiographic imaging techniques. Specific structural and functional aberrations that compromise the integrity of the oral–motor pattern must be identified. The completion and correct interpretation of the comprehensive oral–motor assessment is essential to planning an effective intervention program.

ASSESSMENT OF ORAL AND INTRAORAL STRUCTURE

When evaluating the structural integrity of the feeding mechanism, several considerations must be taken into account. First, the structure of the infant's face and oral cavity is different from that of the adult. An understanding of normal developmental variations is essential to identification of deviations from normal structure. Second, several common structural abnormalities should be familiar to any therapist performing oral motor assessments. Finally, the therapist should be aware of available radiographic techniques that are helpful supplements to the clinical assessment in many cases.

Normal Developmental Anatomy of the Infant's Face and Mouth

The infant facial structure differs from that of the adult not only in size, but also in proportion. In general, the eyes are set relatively lower in the infant face than in that of the adult. This is because the upper third of the face grows most rapidly in fetal and early life, in accordance with the rapid growth of the frontal lobes of the brain. The maxillary and mandibular structures grow more slowly, not reaching maturity until late adolescence. The facial contour is further sculpted in later fetal life by a subcutaneous panniculus adiposis, most notably in the cheek. This buccal fat pad serves the function of preventing collapse of the cheeks during suckling.[1] The lips are short relative to their skeletal attachment, and each labial frenum is prominent compared with the length of the lip.[2] Tight seal of the lips is not seen at rest, and, even when activated, the labial seal on the nipple will characteristically allow some liquid to seep at the corners of the mouth.

The size of the oral cavity is smaller in the infant than in the adult; hence the tongue fills the mouth, touching the cheeks laterally. The infant tongue rests more anteriorly than in the adult; thus it tends to touch the lower lip at rest. Furthermore, the soft palate, tongue, and epiglottis are in approximation, resulting in nasal respiration. The larynx is higher in the infant than in the adult, and the pharynx is shorter. As postnatal development proceeds, the pharynx lengthens and enlarges as the larynx assumes a lower position. During the first 6 months, as postural control develops, the mandible and hyoid bones descend, producing a more mature relationship of these structures to the upper face.[3] As with all skeletal structures, the face and oral cavity respond during normal development to stresses placed on them by gravity, by repetitive pull of muscle action, and by the relative development of other structures. Motor use of the oral mechanism promotes generation of form.[2] A disruption in any functional aspect of the oral mechanism, including prolonged nonoral feeding, may have effects on structural development. These effects are evident in older children with neuromotor problems such as cerebral palsy. These children frequently demonstrate abnormalities in relative relationship and structure of oral and facial components, presumably due to interference with normative effects of gravity and muscle action on the development of facial and oral structures.[4]

Common Structural Problems Affecting Oral–Motor Patterns

By far the most common structural anomalies producing dysfunctional feeding in infancy are the clefts of lip and palate. Cleft lip occurs most frequently, with or without cleft palate. Cleft lip occurs when the mesenchymal masses of the medial nasal and maxillary prominence fail to merge. Cleft palate occurs when mesenchymal masses of the palatine processes fail to fuse. Both cleft lip and cleft palate are caused by multifactorial inheritance (e.g., a combination of genetic and environmental factors).[5] The infant with a cleft lip or combined cleft lip and palate has several obstacles to overcome in oral feeding.

First, a deficit exists in the ability to get strong labial closure on the nipple. Second, a cleft in the palate opens the intraoral cavity, thereby prohibiting or limiting the ability to express milk from the teat by pressure against the palate and also the ability to generate negative pressure within the oral cavity. Finally, cleft palate disrupts the patency of the separation between nasal and oral cavities, thereby permitting liquid to flow out through the nose.

Pierre-Robin syndrome is a congenital syndrome associated with cleft palate and micrognathia. In addition to mandibular hypoplasia, it is characterized by mandibular retrusion and deficient mobility. This syndrome illustrates the importance of intact developmental processes in all structures concurrently, as the micrognathia is believed to result in posterior displacement of the tongue and obstruction to full closure of palatine processes, thereby producing a bilateral cleft palate. Defects of the eye and ear are also associated.[5] Infants with the Pierre-Robin syndrome may benefit from feeding in the prone position, which permits the mandible to drop forward and down by the effect of gravity.[6]

Overdevelopment of the tongue (*macroglossia*) sometimes occurs. Relative macroglossia is most commonly seen in infants with Down syndrome,[1] in whom the mouth is frequently open and tongue protrusion is evident. The tongue does not perform normally in feeding patterns, as it tends to fill the mouth, thereby restricting movement.

Evaluation of Oral and Intra-Oral Structure

The evaluation of structures of the feeding apparatus may be done clinically through observation and palpation. The preliminary results may indicate a need for further radiographic examination.

Observation

Oral–motor assessment begins with observation. The infant's facial structure should be examined for obvious deformity or asymmetry. The activation of facial musculature can be noted as the infant is crying. During cry, the lips and mouth are opened wide. The soft palate is elevated and displaced downward. The tongue tip and lateral margins are elevated during the phonated expiratory phase, as they stand free of alveolar ridges, lips, and buccal surfaces.[2]

Palpation

Palpation of the facial and intraoral structures is done with a scrubbed or gloved hand. Sustained posterior displacement of the tongue and jaw indicate mandibular retraction. Patency of the palate must be assessed. Tonus in the soft palate may be determined by passive elevation of this structure. The normal tongue should actively oppose the palpating finger. The junction of mouth and pharynx should be palpated, because the pharynx is normally difficult to visualize.[7] The amount of information that can be obtained through observation and palpation is, however, limited. Clinicians fail to identify aspiration in about 40 percent of cases when clinical examination alone is used.[8]

Radiographic Examination

Radiographic examination is frequently necessary to obtain an assessment of intraoral and pharyngeal integrity. By far the most common radiographic technique for evaluation of structure and function in feeding is videofluoroscopy. The videofluoroscopic procedure known as the *modified barium swallow* will enable diagnosis of problems in the oral cavity and pharynx that impede swallowing. The criocopharyngeal and pharyngoesophageal juncture and cervical esophagus are examined, and motility problems in the oral cavity and pharynx can be identified. This differs from the barium swallow, which focuses on the pharynx and esophagus, with less attention to the oral cavity.[8]

The modified barium swallow involves a low-dose videofluoroscopic system delivering 30 to 40 mrad/min. A bolus water-soluble barium is administered orally with a syringe or via a nipple, depending on the infant's ability to suck. The fluoroscopy image is recorded on videotape, thereby eliminating the need for repetitive fluoroscopy. The videotape can be played back in slow motion to permit diagnostic evaluation.[9]

Zerilli et al.[10] reported a clinical and research protocol for videofluoroscopy in pediatric swallowing dysfunction. The protocol was used to compare sensitivity and clinical value of clinical versus fluoroscopic assessment of oral–motor dysfunction. The authors reviewed 33 videofluoroscopy studies performed at their facility. Prior to the videofluoroscopy, children were ranked in one of three categories of feeding recommendations. The children were ranked again following the videofluoroscopy procedure. Results indicated that 14 of the 33 children changed category following videofluorscopy, with five moving to a more restrictive category and nine to a less restrictive category. The authors concluded that videofluoroscopy, as compared with clinical oral–motor evaluation, could lead to a more definitive delineation of etiology and prognosis in pediatric swallowing dysfunction. They also reported that caregivers felt more comfortable in making clinical decisions following swallowing fluoroscopy.[10]

Although videofluoroscopy is the single most useful tool in evaluating structural and functional integrity of the oral–motor mechanism, other imaging techniques may be useful. Lateral radiographs of the nasopharynx can identify Pierre-Robin syndrome and choanal atresia. Computed tomography can be useful in some cases and involves less radiation exposure than x-ray radiography. Ultrasound is also being used more commonly to image the oral–motor apparatus.

The evaluation of structures associated with feeding provides a starting point for oral–motor assessment. Structural anomalies are frequently easiest to detect. Once structural integrity has been assessed, a basis for the function of the oral–motor mechanisms has been established.

ASSESSMENT OF ORAL–MOTOR FUNCTION

As in structural assessment, normal development of oral–motor function must be understood before assessment of the infant can occur. The neurodevelopmental processes underlying infant feeding, like most motor patterns, begin in the fetal period. With maturation, the early oral–motor patterns become less stereotypic as they come under increasing volitional control. The primary oral–motor activities associated with earliest feeding include rooting, gag, bite, and suck–swallow patterns. These innate patterns, characteristic of the normal term infant, have been described by Gesell[11] and later by Morris.[12]

The *rooting reaction* is normally present from week 28 of gestation and disappears between ages 2 and 4 months. It is stimulated by applying tactile stimulation or stroking at upper and lower lips and at the corners of the mouth. The normative response is head turning toward the stimulus, thereby seeking out food.[12] Rooting in a normal term infant is highly state dependent and is best observed before a scheduled feeding when the infant is hungry.

The *gag reflex* develops around 32 weeks of gestation and persists throughout life. The presence of an adequate gag reflex is considered to be a prerequisite for oral feeding in premature neonates.[13] Some authors, however, have suggested that the presence or absence of a gag reflex is not consistently correlated with aspiration.[10,14] The gag reflex is stimulated by touching the anterior of the tongue and moving back to the posterior half of the tongue and pharynx. A normal gag reflex is not elicited at the lips or anterior half of the tongue.[12]

The *bite reaction* is stimulated by touching the gums. The normal bite pattern is phasic and consists of a rhythmic bite and release. A sustained tonic bite reflex is never normal and is associated frequently with severe central nervous system damage, as in the asphyxiated infant. The phasic bite pattern is normally present at birth and disappears at 3 to 5 months.

The *suck–swallow pattern* develops in utero and persists essentially unchanged until about age 6 months, when it is replaced with a more volitional pattern that disassociates the suck and swallow. The stimulus for eliciting a suck–swallow is downward pressure on the lips, lower alveolar ridge, and tongue. The earlier response is a suckling pattern, which is a normal but primitive oral–motor pattern.

Normal Development of Oral–Motor Patterns

The assessment of oral–motor patterns in infants depends on an understanding of normal development of these patterns. In particular, the suck–swallow patterns undergo a maturational process that has been described in detail.[15,16] Sucking consists of two components, negative and positive. The negative component is suction created within the oral cavity. The positive component is expression, which consists of "stripping" the milk from the nipple by pressing it against the roof of the mouth. The neonatal or primitive suckling pattern has been determined to be much more strongly dependent on the expression component than on suction. Sameroff[15] reported that the suction component was tied to the expression component; however, expression occurred quite frequently in the absence of suction.

The Suckle Pattern

The suckle pattern is a stereotypic sequence of alternating motions. The nipple is first compressed between the upper gum and palate by the tongue. Tongue, lip, and mandible move as a unit, first down and forward, then up and back.[2] This activity expresses the liquid from the nipple. The liquid is then squirted back into the oropharynx by this rhythmic action. Swallow is linked with suck in the normal-term infant.[16] The tongue approximates the palate in a front-to-back sequence. The tongue makes sequential contact with the soft palate and then the pharyngeal wall. These structures form a closure behind the bolus, which passes into the pharynx. A peristalsis-like action is initiated by the pharyngeal constrictors and the functional sphincter at the pharyngealosophageal junction opens, allowing the bolus to pass into the esophagus. Concurrently, the hyoid bone moves anteriorly and up, the larynx elevates, and the laryngeal airway closes, with the epiglottis folding over the entrance to the laryngeal space.[7,17] Initially, swallow appears to be initiated by the suckle, but as the infant matures swallow will become independent of the preceding suckle pattern.

Suck and swallow in infants has been described in terms of the temporal characteristics of the pattern. Sucking patterns are characterized by bursts, defined as a group of sucks with less than 1 second between them, interspersed with pauses.[18] The temporal organization of suck and swallow patterns varies with the presence or absence of liquid in the nipple, as well as with maturity of the infant.[18,19] Non-nutritive sucking occurs when the nipple contains no liquid. The burst–pause pattern of non-nutritive sucking is characterized by shorter bursts of sucking than in the nutritive condition. Nutritive sucking has a lower overall rate of sucking and higher rate of swallowing compared with non-nutritive sucking. The lower rate of sucking in the nutritive condition may be related to the necessity to coordinate suck with respiration for swallow.[15]

The effect of maturational level on infant suck and swallow has been studied by several authors.[19,20] Suck and swallow behaviors are demonstrated early in fetal life.[21] Despite this fact, the demands of coordinating feeding with respiration prohibit most premature infants from achieving functional oral feeding before 32 to 34 weeks of gestation.[19] The premature infant, however, is often able to perform non-nutritive sucking on a nipple or pacifier while being gavage fed.[22–24] Dubignon et al.[19] studied the development of non-nutritive sucking in preterm infants and concluded that it is a form of automatic motor behavior that is relatively unaffected by experience. In comparing nutritive sucking in term and preterm infants, the latter group tends to have shorter suck bursts, preceded or followed by swallows. Term infants tend to have a higher suck rate and are able to swallow simultaneously.[20] Bosma[16] suggested that oral feeding competency is a pharynx-guided accomplishment. He observed that the pharyngeal swallow is functional prior to functional oral feeding. This may explain the frequently observed incidence of the preterm infant who sucks avidly in the non-nutritive mode but is unable to obtain functional nutritive sucking. Non-nutritive sucking and pharyngeal swallow may be maturationally driven, as isolated individual patterns, but the organization of nutritive sucking may only occur when its strong linkage with pharyngeal swallow is routinely practiced.[10]

Transition to Oral Feeding

The transition to oral feeding in preterm infants may be influenced by a number of factors. Medical complications, particularly those of a digestive, respiratory, cardiac, or neurologic nature, have been shown to correlate positively with length of transition to oral feeding.[25] The environmental experience of the preterm infant may adversely influence oral–motor competence. Aversive stimuli such as endotracheal and gavage tubes or tape on the face can lead to the onset of avoidance behaviors upon perioral or intraoral tactile stimulation.[26,27] Visual and auditory stimuli commonly present in the neonatal intensive care environment may overly stress the infant and result in difficulty with the infant's organization of feeding patterns.[26] Barrett and Miller[28] demonstrated a decreased sucking rate in term and preterm infants when patterned and unpatterned lights were flashed. Thus a number of maturational, physical, and environmental factors contribute to a poor transition to oral feeding in the preterm infant.

Beyond the neonatal period, significant changes occur in oral–motor function over the first year of life. As previously mentioned, the linkage between suck and swallow begins to become less strong, and the suckle pattern is replaced by a more mature sucking response. The mature suck differs from the immature suckling pattern in that the former has a greater negative pressure component. The mature suck is also characterized by increasing autonomy of tongue, lips, and mandible. The latter structure becomes a stable base from which the tongue can perform a wide variety of autonomous functions.[16]

Eating from a spoon is usually introduced at ages 4 to 6 months. Initially, the lips are not receptive to the presence of the spoon, and the infant attempts to use a suck-like pattern to withdraw the food from the spoon.[4] By approximately age 7 months, the upper lip becomes active in withdrawing the food from a spoon. Around the same time, the lower lip begins to draw inward after removal of the spoon.[29]

Drinking from a cup may be introduced in the latter half of the first year. Initially, the suckle-like pattern is also attempted in withdrawing liquid from a cup. Early sucks from a cup are poorly coordinated with swallow, and the infant will pull back after several sucks. Subsequently, around age 15 months, the child will be able to coordinate a longer sequence of sucks with intake of several ounces of liquid.[29]

Development of biting and chewing does not occur in strict continuity with suckle actions, although in primitive form they appear in phasic alteration not dissimilar to the cyclic actions of suckle.[16] When deciduous incisors erupt, protrusive mandibular movements occur and lateral movements follow rapidly.[4] The early chewing pattern, which is confined primarily to vertical movements of the jaw, is called *munching*. Munching appears sometime around age 8 months. Nearly concurrently, if food is placed to the side, a diagonal rotary movement of the jaw is seen. These diagonal jaw movements are related to increasing tongue lateralization. The mature circular rotary pattern of chewing, which transfers food across the midline, appears at 2 to 3 years of age.[29]

Assessment of Oral–Motor Patterns

The oral–motor patterns of suck–swallow, eating from a spoon, drinking from a cup, and biting and chewing compose a large portion of the oral–motor assessment in the first year of life. The assessment of structural integrity is the most obvious starting point for identification of feeding problems. Presence and absence of the early oral–motor reactions underlies the functional maturity of the oral–motor patterns. The patterns themselves must then be assessed for quality of movement and functional effectiveness.

The Suck–Swallow Pattern

To assess the suck–swallow pattern, both non-nutritive and nutritive conditions should be included. For non-nutritive sucking, the clinician can observe the infant in hand-to-mouth behavior or sucking on a pacifier. A better judgment of the qualitative aspects of non-nutritive sucking may be obtained by placing a nipple over the finger and inserting it into the infants mouth, with slight downward pressure on the tongue. Note the lowering and elevation of the mandible, as well as labial acceptance of the nipple. Palpate the tongue, which should cup and accept the nipple. Allow the infant to begin a suckle pattern. Assess the rhythmicity and the coordinated alternating forward–down and up–back movements of lip, tongue, and jaw. Upward pressure on the examiner's finger from the infant's tongue should also be palpated.

Nutritive sucking may then be assessed. Offer the nipple by stimulating the lower lip, looking for mouth opening. Note lip closure. A small amount of laxity permitting some seepage of liquid at the corners of the mouth is acceptable, but the lips should purse around the nipple. Note the rhythmicity of the sucking pattern and frequency of gasping, gagging, or choking. The presence of liquid seeping through the nose may indicate a palatal cleft.

The swallow pattern is not directly visible, but inference of adequate swallow is made when the sucking pattern is rhythmic and gasping or choking is infrequent. In addition, palpation of the hyoid bone movement should reveal the characteristic forward and upward movement, followed by downward and backward movement characteristic of a normal swallow. Logemann[8] described a palpation strategy in which the examiner's index finger is placed under the mandible, the middle finger at the hyoid, the third at the top of the thyroid cartilage, and the fourth at the bottom of the thyroid cartilage, thereby permitting an assessment of submandibular, hyoid, and laryngeal movement in the swallow. Of course, in the neonate, only two of the examiner's fingers will be needed to cover the same landmarks. If the examiner is concerned about the adequacy of the swallow after the clinical examination, a videofluoroscopy of the swallow is recommended.

Strength and endurance are important aspects of feeding, especially in the first few months. Infants with select problems such as heart conditions and Down syndrome will have a naturally weak suck and poor endurance. The nature of weak suck and disinterest in feeding is more subtle in other cases. To assess strength of suck, attempt to pull the nipple out of the mouth during nutritive suck in a hungry infant. The infant's seal on the nipple should tighten, and the head will come forward to resist withdrawal of the nipple. Endurance for feeding is an arbitrary judgment. Some authors have suggested that a bottle feeding session should be completed in as little as 15 minutes. When dealing with premature infants, up to 20 to 30 minutes is reasonable for a single feeding of a sufficient amount of formula for weight gain.[27] This is in accordance with suggested time allotments for breast feeding.[30] If more than 30 minutes are required for the infant to take a sufficient amount of formula, the probability is slim that the caregiver will be able to feed the infant within a reasonable schedule during a day. This may lead to frustration on the part of the caregiver and may play a role in the disproportionate representation of high-risk infants in populations of failure-to-thrive and abused children.[31]

Eating from a Spoon

In assessing the oral–motor patterns of the more mature infant, the following observations should be made. In eating from a spoon, the stability of the mandible should be noted. In children with neuromotor dysfunction, such as cerebral palsy, a tongue thrust may be present when the spoon enters the visual field. The lowering of the upper lip to the spoon is an important component of the mature pattern. The coordinated movement of the food back to the pharynx to initiate the swallow can be roughly estimated by intraoral transit time (i.e., the time it takes from removal of the bolus from the spoon until palpation of the swallow occurs).

Drinking from a Cup

In drinking from a cup, the stabilization of the mandible and activation of the upper lip are once again important. Note the ability to draw the liquid into the mouth through suck as opposed to tilting back of the head. The tongue should be noted to cup and groove. Ability to manage amount of liquid with the swallow is noted through absence of choking. Also, the number of sucks that can be taken and swallowed without stopping is an index of the coordination of this pattern.

Biting and Chewing

For assessing bite, first a soft cookie and later a harder cracker is presented. The ability of the upper incisors to obtain a functional bite against the stable mandible and lower incisors is noted. The chewing pattern is observed for vertical, diagonal, and rotary components. Tongue lateralization may be inferred from diagonal or rotary movement.[29] To assess tongue lateralization better, a small piece of banana or cereal may be placed in the mouth laterally near the molars.

Assessment of Sensory and Behavioral Components

The ultimate goals of any oral–motor intervention are safe feeding, functional feeding, and pleasurable feeding. The ability to attain these goals is inherently linked to the infant's overall behavioral state during feeding. The behavioral state itself is usually a reflection of the sensory experience of the infant within a single feeding session or over several sessions. Previously, infants who have difficulty making the transition to bottle feeding have been described as lackadaisical or aversive feeders.[27] The lackadaisical feeder is listless throughout the session. Oral hyposensitivity is noted through perioral touch and tongue walking, a technique of moving successively backward on the tongue with a finger or tongue blade. The lackadaisical feeder may be difficult to arouse for feeding and may fall asleep long before adequate nutrient intake has occurred.

On the other hand, the aversive feeder tends to be hypersensitive to perioral or intraoral touch. A hyperactive gag reflex may be noted. Behavioral manifestations include crying, arching, turning the head away from the nipple, and spitting or coughing. Both of these behavioral types can be related to organic conditions such as neurologic damage or heart disease. The extent to which abnormal experiences in the face, mouth, and pharynx influence these sensory and behavioral sequelae is unknown; however, prolonged absence or abnormality of oral sensory experience may play a role in producing these behavioral types. Since motion is intimately related to sensory experience, the importance of afferent satisfaction derived from the oral area should not be underestimated.[16]

Feeding behaviors can be noted and operationally defined for the purposes of evaluation as follows:

1. Alert and responsive; sucks vigorously, with rate decreasing over time until apparently satiated

2. Displays behaviors indicative of hunger (rooting, non-nutritive suck); on presentation of bottle, sucks briefly and seems satiated; may fall asleep and cannot be roused to continue feeding

3. No indication of hunger or interest in the bottle; disinterested, and may fall asleep

4. Bottle feeding aversive; infant squirms or withdraws; often breaks into insulated crying[27]

STANDARDIZED FEEDING ASSESSMENTS

The oral–motor assessment most commonly performed by therapists is subjective and qualitative, based on knowledge of normal development and common abnormalities. Some standardized assessments of oral–motor function, however, are available.

Pre-Speech Assessment Scale

By far the most extensive standardized assessment is the Pre-Speech Assessment Scale (PSAS).[29] This is a rating scale of pre-speech behaviors from birth through 2 years. Twenty-seven pre-speech performance areas are divided into six categories for evaluation: feeding behavior, sucking, swallowing, biting and chewing, respiration–phonation, and sound play. A double scaling system of scoring is employed. One scale ranging from −1 through −9 is used to score abnormal behaviors. Another scale, ranging from +1 to +24 months, is used to score normal developmental patterns from primitive to higher level mature patterns. A pre-speech assessment form permits an open-ended descriptive evaluation to be filled out by the therapist for each of the twenty-seven behaviors, plus some general postural motor patterns and behaviors relating to feeding and pre-speech. From the assessment form, a pre-speech assessment scale score is assigned. A summary of scores for repeated evaluation and a graph may subsequently be filled out.[29]

The PSAS in its entirety is lengthy and many choose to use only parts of the entire scale. It has not been used for clinical research and does not have established reliability values. Because it is by far the most specific and in-depth assessment available, research efforts directed toward establishing reliability and perhaps also toward streamlining the assessment would be valuable. As it currently exists, the PSAS presents valuable information for therapists wishing to develop expertise in oral–motor assessment.

Oral–Motor Feeding Rating Scale

A much shorter oral–motor assessment is the Oral–Motor Feeding Rating Scale.[32] The scale contains five sections: identifying information, oral–motor/feeding patterns, related areas of function, respiration–phonation (optional), and rating scale synopsis. It is recommended for use with children aged 1 to 3 years. With particular attention to Section II, oral–motor/feeding patterns, eight behaviors are evaluated and analyzed for lip and cheek movement, tongue movement, and jaw movement. A grading scale from zero to five is used. In Section III, related areas of function are scored as "normal," "inconsistent problem area," or "consistent problem area."[22] The Oral–Motor/Feeding Rating Scale is simple to administer, and scoring is easily read and interpreted. Reliability and validity information is not provided for this scale. It has potential value in clinical application for evaluation of patients and documentation of progress, pending further work to establish reliability.

Neonatal Oral–Motor Assessment Scale

A neonatal oral–motor assessment scale (NOMAS) has been devised to identify oral–motor problems in the neonate.[33] The NOMAS is designed to evaluate jaw and tongue movements in nutritive and non-nutritive sucking modes. The scoring scale was originally divided into normal and abnormal categories of feeding patterns. Twelve points were assigned in each characteristic category for tongue and jaw motion in nutritive and non-nutritive sucking, respectively. An optimal score was given, anything less indicating oral–motor difficulty.

The authors of the NOMAS reported on the correlation between NOMAS scores and certain polygraphic data (ratio of suction/expression pressures and duration of sucking bursts). The authors found that oral-motor performance was disorganized or dysfunctional in infants with intraventricular hemorrhage and asphyxia. They did not find that the polygraphic data distinguished the same infants who had abnormal NOMAS scores.[33]

The NOMAS was subsequently revised by Palmer to differentiate between normal, dysfunctional, and disorganized feeding patterns in neonates. The author proposed that differentiating between disorganization and dysfunction allows therapists to concentrate on children with dysfunctional patterns.[34] Case-Smith[35] used another revision of the NOMAS in a study of treatment efficacy in high-risk infants. Test–retest reliability for that study was reported to be 0.67 to 0.83 and inter-rater reliability was calculated as 0.93 to 0.97. Discriminative analysis revealed that the NOMAS accurately classified feeding capabilities in at-risk infants. The treatment efficacy component of this study was a single-subject design with replication on three subjects. Results showed that typical oral-motor interventions performed by occupational therapists could improve sucking in preterm neonates, as measured by the NOMAS.[35]

Case-Smith et al.[36] reported on the validity of the revised NOMAS scale. Results showed that the revised NOMAS scores accurately differentiated between efficient and nonefficient feeders in both nutritive and non-nutritive sucking conditions. Furthermore, several characteristics that were found to be associated with inefficient feeding were lack of rhythm, disorganization in jaw and tongue movements, and pauses of more than 6 seconds.[36]

Behavioral Assessment Scale of Oral Function in Feeding

The Behavioral Assessment Scale of Oral Functions in Feeding[37] provides an objective format for documenting skills and deficits as they relate to feeding. A columnar format is used for easy scoring and interpretation. The range of functions are given vertically, and six grades representing increasing levels of function are listed horizontally. This scale is most useful for infants older than 8 to 10 months and can be used for a wide age range of patients with feeding difficulty.[37] Reliability values for the Behavioral Assessment Scale of Oral Functions in Feeding have been reported for two samples of children with feeding problems. Inter-rater reliability and test–retest reliability values ranged from 0.68 to 0.84 with the intraclass correlation–generalizability theory approach. The authors concluded that this was marginally acceptable by current standards.[38]

Both the NOMAS and Behavioral Assessment Scale have potential utility, pending further research on reliability and validity, not only for clinical evaluation but also for research on oral–motor treatment efficacy. The former is useful only for neonates, while the latter is useful for older infants. The establishment and reported use of standardized oral–motor assessments such as those reviewed will enhance the therapist's objectivity and credibility in oral–motor evaluation and assessment of treatment effectiveness.

SUMMARY

Oral–motor assessment in infancy is complex and presents many challenges to the therapist. An understanding of normal development of structure and function of oral–motor mechanisms is essential. The development of improved imaging techniques assists the therapist in making determinations about safe and functional feeding patterns. The publication of standardized oral–motor assessments is helpful in providing clinical and research assessment tools. The oral–motor assessment as performed by most therapists in the clinic, however, is still based on an understanding of form and function, developmental and behavioral characteristics, as well as typical abnormalities of oral–motor function. Utilizing knowledge and experience in these areas, therapists can effectively assess infants with oral–motor dysfunction and plan treatment programs that will lead the infant toward achieving a feeding experience that is safe, functional, and pleasurable.

REFERENCES

1. Sperber GH: Craniofacial Embryology. 4th Ed. Wright Publishing, London, 1989
2. Bosma JF: Form and function in the infant's mouth and pharynx. p. 3. In Bosma J (ed): Third Symposium on Oral Sensation and Perception. Charles C. Thomas, Springfield, IL, 1972

3. Bosma J: Physiology of the mouth, pharynx and esophagus. p. 356. In Paparella M, Shumrick D (eds): Otolaryngology. Vol. 1. Basic Sciences and Related Disciplines. WB Saunders, Philadelphia, 1973

4. Tulley J: The development of the oral and facial musculature. p. 69. In Refrew C, Murphy K (eds): The Child Who Does Not Talk. Clinics in Developmental Medicine No. 13. Heinemann Medical Books, London, 1964

5. Moore KL: The branchial apparatus and the head and neck. p. 179. In: The Developing Human: Clinically Oriented Embryology. 3rd Ed. WB Saunders, Philadelphia, 1982

6. Takagi Y, Bosma JF: Disability of oral function in an infant associated with displacement of the tongue: therapy by feeding in the prone position. Acta Pediatr Scand 123(Suppl):62, 1960

7. Logan WJ, Bosma JF: Oral and pharyngeal dysphagia in infancy. Pediatr Clin North Am 14(1):67, 1967

8. Logemann JA: Evaluation of swallowing disorders. p. 89. In: Evaluation and Treatment of Swallowing Disorders. College-Hill Press, San Diego, 1983

9. Bowen A, Ledesme-Medina J, Fujioka M et al: Radiologic imaging in otorhinolaryngology. Pediatr Clin North Am 28(4):905, 1981

10. Zerilli KS, Stefans VA, DiPietro MA: Protocol for the use of videofluoroscopy in pediatric swallowing dysfunction. Am J Occup Ther 44(5):441, 1989

11. Gesell A: Morphologies of mouth and mouth behavior. *Am J Orthod* 28:367, 1942

12. Morris SE: Normal Acquisition of Oral Feeding Skills: Implications for Assessment and Treatment. Therapeutic Media, New York, 1982

13. Fanaroff AA, Klaus MH: Feeding and selected disorders of the gastrointestinal tract. p. 113. In Klaus M, Fanaroff A (eds): Care of the High Risk Neonate. 3rd Ed. WB Saunders, Philadelphia, 1986

14. Linden P, Siebens AA: Dysphagia: predicting laryngeal penetration. Arch Phys Med Rehab 64:281, 1983

15. Sameroff A: Reflexive and operant aspects of sucking behavior in infancy. p. 135. In Bosma J (ed): Fourth Symposium on Oral Sensation and Perception. Charles C. Thomas, Springfield, IL, 1973

16. Bosma J: Human infant oral function. p. 98. In Bosma J (ed): Symposium on Oral Sensation and Perception. Charles C. Thomas, Springfield, IL, 1967

17. Donner MW, Bosma JF, Robertson DI: Anatomy and physiology of the pharynx. Gastrointest Radiol 10:196, 1985

18. Dubignon J, Campbell D: Sucking in the newborn during a feed. J Exp Child Psychol 7:282, 1969

19. Dubignon JM, Campbell D, Partington MW: The development of non-nutritive sucking in premature infants. Biol Neonate 14:270, 1969

20. Gryboski JD: Suck and swallow in the premature infant. Pediatrics 43(1):96, 1969

21. Humphrey T: Reflex activity in the oral and facial area of the human fetus. p. 195. In Bosma J (ed): Second Symposium on Oral Sensation and Perception. Charles C. Thomas, Springfield, IL, 1970

22. Measel CP, Anderson GC: Non-nutritive sucking during tube feeding: effect on clinical course in premature infants. J Obstet Gynecol Neonatal Nurs 8(5):265, 1979

23. Bernbaum JC, Perura GR, Watkins JB, Peckham GJ: Non-nutritive sucking during gavage feeding enhances growth and maturation in premature infants. Pediatrics 71(1):41, 1983

24. Field T, Ignatoff E, Stringer S et al: Non-nutritive sucking during tube feedings: effects on preterm infants in an intensive care unit. Pediatrics 70:381, 1982

25. Bvazyk S: Factors associated with the transition to oral feeding in infants fed by nasogastric tubes. Am J Occup Ther 44(12):1070, 1990

26. Vandenberg KA: Nippling management of the sick neonate in the NICU: the disorganized feeder. Neonatal Network 9(1):198, 1990

27. Harris MB: Oral motor management of the high risk neonate. p. 231. In Sweeney J (ed): The High-Risk Neonate: Developmental Therapy Perspectives. Haworth Press, New York, 1986

28. Barrett TE, Miller LK: The organization of non-nutritive sucking in the premature infant. J Exp Child Psychol 16:472, 1973

29. Morris SE: Pre-Speech Assessment Scale. JA Preston Corp, Clifton, NJ, 1982

30. Warner MP: A Doctor Discusses Breast Feeding. Budlong Press, Chicago, 1975

31. Klein M. Stern L: Low birthweight and the battered child syndrome. Am J Dis Child 122:15, 1971

32. Jelm JM: Oral-Motor/Feeding Rating Scale. Therapy Skill Builders, Tucson, AZ, 1990

33. Braun MA, Palmer MM: A pilot study of oral-motor dysfunction in "at-risk" infants. Phys Occup Ther Pediatr 5(4):13, 1985/86

34. Palmer MM: Assessment of early sucking patterns in the high-risk infant: disorganization versus dysfunction. p. 161. In: Proceedings of Developmental Interventions in Neonatal Care, New Orleans, 1989. Contemporary Forums, Danville, CA

35. Case-Smith J: An efficacy study of occupational therapy with high risk neonates. Am J Occup Ther 42(8):499, 1988

36. Case-Smith J, Cooper D, Scala V: Feeding efficiency of premature neonates. Am J Occup Ther 43(4):245, 1989

37. Stratton M: Behavioral assessment scale of oral functions in feeding. Am J Occup Ther 35:719, 1981

38. Ottenbacher K, Dauck BS, Gruhn V et al: Reliability of the behavioral assessment scale of oral functions in feeding. Am J Occup Ther 39:436, 1985

8 | Theoretical Issues in Assessing Postural Control

Anne Shumway-Cook
Marjorie Woollacott

During the first 2 years of life, the child develops an incredible repertoire of skills, including crawling, independent walking and running, climbing, eye–hand coordination, and the manipulation of objects in a variety of ways. If one looks at each of these skills carefully, one can see that each contains a postural or balance component. This postural component underlies the primary movement and is essential to accomplishing the skill.

The development of postural control can limit the rate at which manipulatory and mobility skills are acquired during development. Amiel-Tison and Grenier[1] found that, when one stabilizes the head of a neonate, the normally chaotic movements of the arms commonly seen in newborn infants no longer occur. Instead behaviors typically seen in older, more mature infants emerge, such as coordinated hand and arm movements, inhibition of the grasp and Moro reflex, and better selective attention to the examiner and the task. This study suggests that the neonate's postural system is immature at birth, and this immaturity is a rate-limiting factor for the emergence of other behaviors such as coordinated arm and hand movements.

Similarly, delayed or abnormal development of the postural system potentially constrains the child's ability to develop independence in mobility skills.[2] Understanding the emergence of mobility and manipulatory skills in children therefore requires an understanding of the developing postural substrate for these skills. In addition, the capacity to assess effectively the development of these skills is tied to effective assessment of the systems contributing to the control of posture and balance.

The purpose of this chapter is to present concepts important to the assessment of postural control in children 0 to 24 months. We first define postural control and discuss two models for explaining it's development. We then discuss our conceptual framework for assessing postural control in infancy based on a systems model of motor control and present several examples of how these concepts can be applied to clinical practice.

DEFINING POSTURAL CONTROL

Postural control is defined here as the control of the body's position (posture) in space for the dual purposes of stability and orientation.[3] *Stability* is a term used interchangeably with *balance,* and is defined as the ability to maintain the center of body mass within stability limits largely determined by the base of support. Orientation is defined as maintaining a configuration or alignment of body segments with respect to one another that is appropriate to the movement or task. Most motor skills have an underlying postural substrate. For example, the emergence of locomotion requires the maturation of postural control, including the development of stability (the ability to control the center of mass relative to the support base of the feet), while maintaining a vertical orientation (the body aligned vertically with respect to gravity).

BEHAVIORAL INDICES OF POSTURAL DEVELOPMENT

The development of postural control is a continuous process, associated with a predictable sequence of motor behaviors. This sequence and timing of motor development has been well described by developmental researchers such as McGraw[4] and Gesell[5] and is depicted in Figure 8-1. During assessment individual behaviors within this sequence are often singled out as "motor milestones"; however, this can lead to the misconception that development of postural control follows a stage-like rather than a continuous progression. What is the basis for developing postural control? Currently two alternative models are cited to explain the neural correlates of emerging postural behavior.

TWO MODELS FOR UNDERSTANDING POSTURAL CONTROL

Reflex/Hierarchical Model

Traditionally, developmental theorists have attributed the development of motor skills primarily to central nervous system (CNS) maturation.[6-8] More specifically, the maturation of a series of hierarchically organized reflexes and reactions within the CNS forms the basis for the acquisition of postural stability and mobility skills. This approach to explaining motor development has been

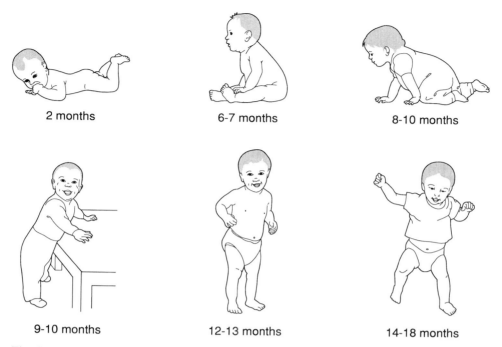

2 months

6-7 months

8-10 months

9-10 months

12-13 months

14-18 months

Fig. 8-1. Six motor milestones depicting critical behaviors within the motor development sequence.

referred to as a *reflex/hierarchical model* of motor control and development and is shown in Figure 8-2.[3,9]

Based on this model, motor behavior during infancy is seen to be dominated largely by primitive reflexes organized at the spinal cord level. As the child matures one can observe the emergence and subsequent disappearance of re-

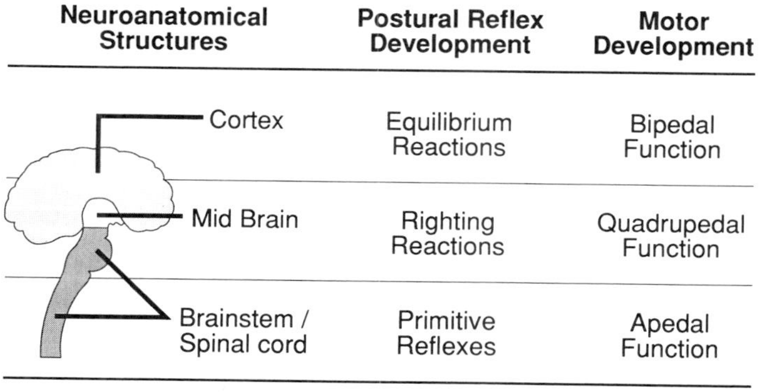

Neuroanatomical Structures	Postural Reflex Development	Motor Development
Cortex	Equilibrium Reactions	Bipedal Function
Mid Brain	Righting Reactions	Quadrupedal Function
Brainstem / Spinal cord	Primitive Reflexes	Apedal Function

Fig. 8-2. A reflex/hierarchical model of motor development. Development of motor function is attributed primarily to CNS maturation and the subsequent emergence of hierarchically organized postural reflexes.

flexes and reactions associated with ascending maturation within the CNS. For example, the tonic neck reflexes emerge with maturation of the brain stem, but disappear with the emergence of righting reactions organized hierarchically at the midbrain level of the CNS. Finally, with complete maturation of the cerebral cortex, the equilibrium reactions emerge, which are the basis for the child's ability to maintain balance during functional activities such as sitting, standing, and walking independently.[7]

As described by Palisano (Ch. 9) in detail, assessment of postural control using a reflex/hierarchical model focuses on both behavioral measures of motor milestones and postural reflexes and reactions.[7,10-16] This combination of measures is thought to provide the health care professional with an understanding of the functional abilities of the child and insight into the "level" of neurologic maturation that has occurred.

Systems Model

An alternative model for explaining motor control and development is the systems model.[2,9,17,18] In the systems model, the control of body posture for stability and orientation results from a complex interaction of neural and musculoskeletal systems referred to collectively as the *postural control system*.[18]

The development of postural control is seen as a continuous process involving the simultaneous development of multiple interacting systems. During development not all of the systems important to postural control develop at the same rate. Results from research examining the development of postural control from a systems perspective suggest that some of the rate-limiting systems and processes of postural control include (1) the development of the somatosensory, visual, and vestibular systems and central sensory processes that organize these multiple inputs for orientation; (2) changes in musculoskeletal components, including the development of muscle strength and changes in body morphology; (3) the development of neuromuscular synergies involving the head, trunk, and legs, which are used in maintaining stability; (4) the development of adaptive mechanisms that allow the child to modify sensory and motor processes for posture in response to changing tasks and environment; and (5) the development of anticipatory processes that allow the child to pretune sensory and motor processes for posture in anticipation of potentially destabilizing tasks.[18-26] These rate-limiting components are summarized in Figure 8-3.

We need to understand which systems and processes are rate limiting to the emergence of motor functions at various stages in development or, conversely, which push the system to a new level of function. This understanding of the relationship between critical rate-limiting components of postural control and the development of functional motor skills forms the basis for both assessment and treatment strategies in the pediatric patient.

The development of clinical assessment tools based on a systems model is just beginning. The authors are in the process of developing and testing a pediatric tool for assessing postural control in infancy using a systems model.

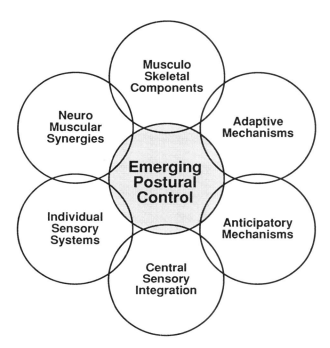

Fig. 8-3.   A systems model suggests the emergence of postural control results from the development of multiple interacting systems, each of which develop at different rates.

In the remainder of this chapter are described our conceptual framework and preliminary applications for assessment.

ASSESSING POSTURAL CONTROL— A SYSTEMS PERSPECTIVE

Our systems-based assessment of postural control requires the assessment of (1) sequences of functional motor behaviors representing postural development, traditionally referred to as *motor milestones;* and (2) the relative contribution of individual systems and processes important to achieving motor functions. In addition, during assessment, spontaneous movements and variability of performance of motor skills are evaluated as determinants of the child's capacity to explore and adapt to changing tasks and environments. In our systems-based assessment, the ability to explore and adapt is considered as important an index of normalcy as the acquisition of motor milestones.

Motor Milestones

In our approach to assessment of motor milestones we have divided motor behaviors related to postural control into four functional categories: (1) ability to sustain a posture, (2) ability to regain a posture, (3) ability to transition between postures, and (4) the ability to integrate posture into movement, specifically mobility and manipulatory and exploratory movements. These four categories of behaviors are then applied to motor development sequences involving the progressive control of head, trunk, and full body.

Figure 8-4 provides an example of how the four categories can be applied to examining functional behaviors related to stance posture control. The child's ability to maintain independent stance for varying intervals of time is examined. The child's ability to regain stance when perturbed in the sagittal and lateral planes is evaluated. The child's ability to assume the standing posture is assessed, including the type of movement pattern used. In addition, the ability to adapt movement patterns for assuming a stance position depending on changing initial constraints is determined. Finally, the child's ability to maintain an upright posture during ongoing movement is assessed. Shown in Figure 8-4 is postural control during gait; however, assessing the integration of posture into movement also includes determining the presence of anticipatory postural adjustments essential for maintaining stability prior to goal-directed reaching or manipulatory tasks.

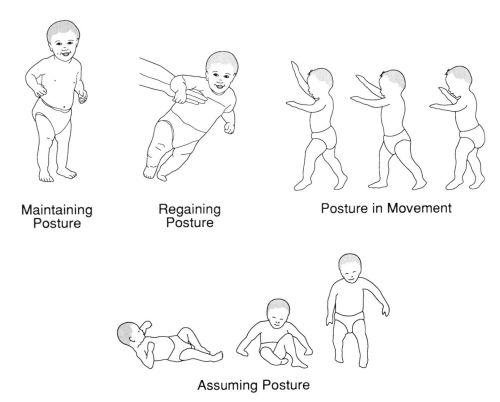

Maintaining   Regaining   Posture in Movement
Posture   Posture

Assuming Posture

Fig. 8-4. Four functional categories of postural control applied to understanding and assessing the control of upright stance.

Systems Analysis

In addition to the assessment of functional motor behaviors, we examine the major systems and processes underlying the acquisition of postural control.[27-29] These systems include the following.

Motor Systems

Both musculoskeletal components (i.e., range of motion, strength, and alignment of body segments) and neuromuscular components (i.e., the process of constructing neuromuscular synergies, allowing progressive control of body segments) comprise the motor systems.

Sensory Systems

Testing the efficacy of individual sensory systems themselves and the process of organizing sensory information for postural orientation is performed. In addition, perceptions essential to postural control are evaluated, specifically, the child's changing representation of stability limits.

Stability limits are defined as the area or domain in which the center of mass can be moved without changing the base of support.[27] Accurate perceptions regarding stability limits are an essential aspect of stability, since they often form the basis for movement strategies used to maintain balance.[29] For example, when a child cruises using furniture or toys for support, limits of stability incorporate support external to the child. When the child begins to stand and walk independent of external support, however, stability limits must be modified to reflect this loss of external support, as must movement strategies used for balance.

Adaptive and Anticipatory Mechanisms

Central processes that modify or pretune sensory and motor postural strategies to changing tasks and contexts are also studied. We believe a critical aspect underlying development of adaptive and anticipatory mechanisms is the child's role as an active explorer of the environment. With increasing experience the child learns to predict the postural requirements associated with various tasks and environments. The child minimizes instability by adjusting posture in anticipation of potentially destabilizing movements.

Unlike the reflex/hierarchical model, which places little emphasis on experience and learning, the systems model considers these as essential elements in the development of motor skills. Thus the child's capacity to explore and interact with a continuously changing environment is as essential to the emergence of

Table 8-1. Assessment of Head Control

Functional behaviors observed
  Ability to sustain head posture
    Supported vertical position
    Prone position
    Supine Position
  Ability to regain head posture
    Vertical - tip child from vertical
    Prone - tip child in prone
    Supine - tip child in supine
  Ability to maintain head posture during movement
    Primitive stepping
    Moving from supine to sit
    Spontaneous movements

Systems tested
  Motor
    Musculoskeletal constraints
      Range of motion, cervical region
      Strength, neck muscles
    Motor coordination, neuromuscular synergies involving neck and upper trunk
  Sensory
    Capacity of vision to regulate posture
    Capacity of vestibular and somatosensory inputs to regulate posture
  Adaptive/anticipation
    Active exploration
    Adapting behavior to externally controlled head position
    Anticipating postural adjustments of head to repeated tips

motor skills as a maturing nervous system. Table 8-1 provides a preliminary example of how the above concepts could be translated to evaluating head control in the child from ages 0 to 2 months.

We believe assessment based on these concepts will provide the therapist with insight as to (1) the child's level of function, (2) whether delayed or abnormal postural control is a contributing factor to decreased function, and (3) which systems and processes contributing to postural control are rate limiting to the emergence of stability and mobility functions. Most important, this information then forms the basis for intervention strategies designed to remediate delayed or abnormal postural control leading to improved function.

REFLEX TESTING IN A SYSTEMS-BASED ASSESSMENT

What is the role of reflex testing in a systems model of motor control and development? Inherent in a reflex-based model of motor development is the assumption that reflexes themselves are the rate-limiting constraints on normal motor development.[7,15] As a result, assessment focuses on evaluating the progression of reflexes throughout development. Therapeutic intervention centers on changing reflex activity in order to help the child progress to more mature motor behaviors.[15] What are the arguments for and against inclusion of reflex testing in a systems model of motor development?

One argument for performing reflex testing during infancy is based on research that suggests that the presence of abnormal reflexes early in development may predict long-term motor dysfunction. Several authors have suggested that the best predictor of long-term dysmobility in children with cerebral palsy is the persistence of primitive reflexes during infancy.[30,31] While the presence of primitive persisting reflexes may be predictive of dysfunction, the persistence of primitive reflexes is not necessarily the rate-limiting constraint on mobility. Directing therapy at the inhibition of primitive reflexes will not necessarily ensure the emergence of mobility skills.

Classic reflex testing during infant assessment may help to determine the integrity of specific neuronal circuitry. For example, testing deep tendon reflexes (DTRs) provides insight into the integrity of the stretch reflex circuit, while the doll's eye phenomenon allows one to examine otolith-ocular function.[32] The relationship of various reflex circuits to function and pathology, however, is in many cases not completely understood. For example, the presence of abnormal stretch reflexes as evidenced by abnormal DTRs, is not evidence that "spasticity" is the rate-limiting factor to function.[33,34]

Thus a growing number of developmental theorists are questioning the contribution of reflex testing in diagnosis, prognosis, and prescribing therapy for neurologically impaired children. Is reflex testing critical to the assessment of motor development? The answer to this question is not clear; however, assessment of reflex control during infancy should not preclude the evaluator from considering potentially more serious rate-limiting constraints on motor development.

SUMMARY

Assessment of postural control is an essential part of evaluating motor development in children. Postural control is the capacity to control the body's position in space so as to maintain balance and an appropriate orientation of the body with respect to the task. The development of postural control is a continuous process involving the development of multiple interacting systems within the body. Since these systems develop at different rates, each will affect the development of postural control and the emergence of functional motor skills differently throughout the course of development.

The primary focus of this chapter has been to consider clinical and theoretical implications of a systems-based model of motor control on understanding and assessing the development of postural control. The development of clinical methods based on a systems model of motor control is just beginning. As systems-based research provides an increased understanding of the factors that affect the development of postural control, new methods for assessing and treating postural disorders in infancy will emerge.

REFERENCES

1. Amiel-Tison C, Grenier A: Neurologic Evaluation of the Newborn and the Infant. Masson, New York, 1983
2. Thelen E, Ulrich B: Hidden skills. Monogr Soc Res Child Dev 56(1), 1991

3. Woollacott M, Shumway-Cook A: Changes in postural control across the lifespan—a systems perspective. Phys Ther 70:759, 1990

4. McGraw MB: From reflex to muscular control in the assumption of an erect posture and ambulation in the human infant. Child Dev 3:291, 1932

5. Gesell A: The ontogenesis of infant behavior. In Carmichael L (ed): Manual of Child Psychology. Wiley, New York, 1946

6. Easton T: On the normal use of reflexes. Am Scientist 60:591, 1972

7. Fiorentino MR: Reflex Testing Methods for Evaluating CNS Development. Charles C. Thomas, Springfield, IL, 1973

8. Twitchell TE: Attitudinal reflexes. In Davies E (ed): Growth and Development. American Physical Therapy Association, Washington, DC, 1975

9. Shumway-Cook A: Equilibrium deficits in children. In Woollacott M, Shumway-Cook A (eds): Development of Posture and Gait Across the Lifespan. University of South Carolina Press, Columbia, SC, 1989

10. Capute AJ, Wachtel RC, Palmer FB et al: A prospective study of three postural reactions. Dev Med Child Neurol 24:314, 1982

11. Chandler LS, Skillen MS, Swanson MW: Movement Assessment of Infants. A Manual. Rolling Bay Press, Rolling Bay, WA, 1980

12. Paine RS: Evolution of postural reflexes in normal infants. Neurology 14:1036, 1964

13. Milani-Comparetti A, Gidoni EA: Pattern analysis of motor development and its disorder. Dev Med Child Neurol 9:625, 1967

14. Haley S: Sequential analyses of postural reaction in nonhandicapped infants. Phys Ther 66:531, 1986

15. Bobath B, Bobath K: Motor Development in Different Types of Cerebral Palsy. Heinemann, London, 1976

16. Haley S: Postural reactions in infants with Down syndrome. Phys Ther 66:17, 1986

17. Bernstein N: Coordination and Regulation of Movements. Pergamon Press, New York, 1967

18. Woollacott MJ, Shumway-Cook A, Wiliams H: The development of posture and balance control in children. In Woollacott M, Shumway-Cook A (eds): Development of Posture and Locomotion Across the Lifespan. University of South Carolina Press, Columbia, SC, 1989

19. Shumway-Cook A, Woollacott M: The growth of stability: postural control from a developmental perspective. J Motor Behav 17:131, 1985

20. Bertenthal BI, Bai DL: Infants' sensitivity to optical flow for controlling posture. In Butler C, Jaffe K (eds): Visual-Vestibular Integration in Early Development: Technical and Clinical Perspectives. RESNA, Washington, DC, 1988

21. Harbourne RT, Guiliani CA, Mac Neela JC: Kinematic and electromygraphic analysis of the development of sitting posture in infants. Dev Med Child Neurol 29:31, 1987

22. Jouan F: Visual–proprioceptive control of posture in newborn infants. In Amblard B, Berthoz A, Clarac F (eds): Posture and Gait: Development, Adaptation and Modulation. Elsevier, Amsterdam, 1988

23. Lee DN, Aronson E: Visual–proprioceptive control of standing in human infants. Percept Psychophys 15:529, 1974

24. Prechtl HFR: Development of postural control in infancy. In von Euler C, Forssberg H, Lagercrantz H (eds): Neurobiology of Infant Behavior. Stockton Press, New York 1989

25. Woollacott M, Debu B, Mowatt M: Neuromuscular control of posture in the infant and child: is vision dominant? J Motor Behav 19:167, 1987

26. Woollacott M, Sveistrup H: Changes in the sequencing and timing of muscle response coordination associated with developmental transitions in balance abilities. Hum Movement Sci (in press)
27. McCollum G, Leen T: The form and exploration of mechanical stability limits in erect stance. J Motor Behav 21:225, 1989
28. Shumway-Cook A, McCollum G: Assessment and treatment of balance disorders in the neurologic patient. In Montgomery T, Connolly B (eds): Motor Control Theory and Practice. Chattanooga Corporation, Chattanooga, TN, 1990
29. Horak F, Shupert C, Mirka A: Components of postural dyscontrol in the elderly: a review. Neurobiol Aging 10:727, 1987
30. Effgen SK: Integration of the plantar grasp reflex as an indicator of ambulation potential in developmentally disabled infants. Phys Ther 62:433, 1982
31. Molnar GE, Fordon SU: Cerebral palsy: predictive value of selected signs for early prognostication of motor function. Arch Phys Med Rehabil 57:153, 1976
32. Eviatar L, Eviatar A: Neurovestibular examination of infants and children. Adv Oto-Rhino-Laryngol 23:169, 1978
33. Burke D: Reassessment of muscle spindle contribution to muscle tone in normal and spastic man. In Feldman RG, Young RR, Koella WP (eds): Spasticity: Disordered Motor Control. Year Book Medical Publishers, Chicago, 1980
34. Katz R, Rymer Z: Spastic hypertonia: mechanisms and measurement. Arch Phys Med Rehabil 70:144, 1989

9 | Neuromotor and Developmental Assessment

Robert J. Palisano

Physical therapists traditionally have included neuromotor and motor development in their assessment of infants. In the neuromotor area, physical therapists have placed the greatest emphasis on assessment of muscle tone, primitive reflexes, and righting, equilibrium, and protective reactions. This practice reflects the importance of abnormal neuromotor findings for diagnosis and the emphasis these areas of neuromotor function have received in treatment, particularly neurodevelopmental treatment (NDT).[1] Physical therapists also stress the importance of documenting motor development, including the quality of movement or how a movement is performed. Although assessment of motor development has been a common practice of physical therapists, a survey by Lewko[2] in 1976 indicated that health professionals including physical therapists used a multitude of different motor assessments and that the vast majority of tests were not rigorously constructed or standardized. Campbell[3] has attributed this practice to inadequate preparation of physical therapists in principles of measurement and technical measurement skills at the entry level of education.

In recent years, greater emphasis on early diagnosis and intervention, the practice of developmental follow-up of infants who as newborns were admitted to neonatal intensive care units, and passage of PL 99-457, the Education of the Handicapped Act Amendment of 1986, have all contributed to an expanded role for physical therapists in the neuromotor and developmental assessment of infants. Greater involvement of physical therapists in interdisciplinary teams, a proliferation of new standardized assessment tools, and an increase in the number of published articles on developmental assessment in journals and books commonly read by physical therapists suggest a trend toward increased use of standardized motor development scales. In contrast, current concepts of motor development and motor control and a greater focus on functional outcomes in treatment have created controversy regarding the significance of traditional methods of neuromotor assessment. This is especially true when the purpose of testing is to evaluate the effects of treatment.

Neuromotor and motor development assessments can be classified as either norm referenced or criterion referenced. Norm-referenced scales are designed to compare an infant's performance with the performance of a representative sample of infants of the same age. Criterion-referenced scales are designed to compare an infant's performance with external criteria such as development of specific postures and movements without regard to the performance of other infants of the same age. *Standardization* refers to the process of establishing uniform testing procedures. Standardization is often synonymous with *norm-referenced assessments* but is also a desirable feature of criterion-referenced assessments. A standardized assessment includes or specifies the necessary material or equipment. The manual should indicate the qualifications needed to administer the test, provide clear instructions for administering and scoring each item, and include guidelines for determining and interpreting results. In this chapter, the types and purposes of neuromotor and developmental assessments and issues relevant to assessment of infants are discussed, and selected assessments currently used by physical therapists are critiqued. The focus of the chapter is on providing information pertinent to selection, application, and interpretation of the results of standardized neuromotor and developmental assessments.

NEUROMOTOR ASSESSMENT

This section presents research on the value of neuromotor assessment for early diagnosis. Rationale and methods of assessing muscle tone, primitive reflexes, and automatic reactions are discussed in reference to current concepts of motor development and control, treatment planning, and evaluation of the effects of treatment. The section will conclude with a review of the Movement Assessment of Infants, the Milani-Comparetti Motor Examination, and the Primitive Reflex Profile, three standardized neuromotor assessments used by physical therapists.

Implications for Early Diagnosis

Abnormalities of muscle tone, primitive reflexes, and automatic reactions have implications for early diagnosis of infants with disorders in motor development. Neuromotor assessment therefore is part of the physician's neurologic examination as well as the physical therapist's assessment. Support for the diagnostic value of neuromotor findings is provided by Ellenberg and Nelson.[4] The investigators examined retrospectively the relative value of neurologic signs at age 4 months in predicting cerebral palsy at age 7 years. The subjects were approximately 32,000 infants born between 1959 and 1966 who were part of a National Collaborative Perinatal Project. Infants demonstrating abnormal muscle tone at 4 months of age were 19 to 74 times more likely to have cerebral palsy at 7 years. The presence of hypertonia was more predictive of later cerebral palsy than was hypotonia. Furthermore, hypertonia in the neck or trunk was more predictive than hypertonus of the limbs. Twenty percent of infants with hypertonia of the neck extensors or trunk were later diagnosed as having cerebral palsy.

Noteworthy in the study by Ellenberg and Nelson[4] are the findings that the predictive value of an abnormal neurologic examination increased when accompanied by delayed developmental milestones and that low-risk neurologic status at 4 months did not preclude a later diagnosis of cerebral palsy. For infants who failed at least one of the six developmental milestones that were assessed, the risk for cerebral palsy increased with increased number of abnormal neurologic findings. All infants with neck or trunk hypertonia who were diagnosed as having cerebral palsy failed at least one developmental milestone, and most had other signs of central nervous system (CNS) dysfunction, including abnormal head circumference. In contrast, infants who passed all of the milestones were unlikely to have cerebral palsy even if they had abnormal neurologic findings. Although the incidence of cerebral palsy was low among children classified low risk, 44 percent of children diagnosed as having cerebral palsy were from the low-risk group.

The diagnostic value of neuromotor findings may be increased for items that require only minimal handling of the infant. Support for this position is provided in a retrospective study by Harris[5] in which a sample of 154 high-risk infants were administered the Movement Assessment of Infants (MAI) at age 4 months. The MAI scores of 36 infants who were diagnosed between ages 3 and 8 years as having cerebral palsy were compared with the scores of 118 infants who did not have cerebral palsy upon follow-up examination. Eleven of the 17 items that were found to be highly significant predictors of cerebral palsy ($p < 0.001$) did not involve handling the infant. Muscle extensibility (resistance to quick stretch) was the only passive muscle tone item, and the tonic labyrinthine reflex in both prone and supine were the only primitive reflexes that were highly significant predictors.

Although abnormal neuromotor findings increase the risk of a disorder in motor development, the ability to make an early diagnosis is complicated by the variable outcomes of infants who demonstrate abnormal neuromotor findings during the first year. Several researchers have reported that the incidence of abnormal findings in preterm infants decreases during the first year.[6-9] The pattern of early motor development referred to as *transient dystonia of prematurity* illustrates this point. Transient dystonia occurs most often in preterm infants with birth weights of less than 1,500 g. Characteristic findings at ages 5 to 8 months are extensor hypertonia of the legs, retention of primitive reflexes, brisk deep tendon reflexes, and asymmetries, which all have been reported to resolve by 12 to 18 months.[6] Amiel-Tison[10] states that between 5 and 8 months there is no reliable method to distinguish infants with transient abnormal neurologic findings from those who will eventually be diagnosed as having spastic diplegia. Drillien and associates[6] concluded that, during the first year, the neuromotor status of preterm infants can be classified as normal, abnormal, or transient abnormal.

Coolman and associates[7] reported that, in addition to the three categories described by Drillien et al., preterm infants also demonstrate a pattern of persistent neuromotor abnormalities that are not as severe as those associated with cerebral palsy. The investigators performed a retrospective chart review of 219 infants who were in the University of Washington Hospital's neonatal intensive care nursery and attended all follow-up appointments during the first 2 years. The degree of neuromotor abnormality in each examination was rated as none, mild, moderate, or severe based on criteria that were operationally defined. During the first year, mild abnormalities were identified in 50 percent of the infants, moderate abnormalities were identified in 7 percent, and severe abnormalities in 20 percent. At age 2 years, 23 percent of the infants were classified as always normal, 43 percent as having transient neuromotor abnormalities, 21 percent as having persistent neuromotor abnormalities, and 13 percent as having cerebral palsy. The group of infants classified at age 2 years as having persistent neuromotor abnormalities included 25 percent of infants rated as having mild abnormalities during the first year, 50 percent rated as having moderate abnormalities, and 33 percent rated as having severe abnormalities.

Research supports the value of early neuromotor assessment to identify infants at risk for disorders in motor development. The ability to make an early diagnosis, however, is complicated by the variable developmental outcomes of preterm infants with neuromotor abnormalities during the first year. There is evidence to suggest that assessment items that require less handling of the infant are better predictors of cerebral palsy. This implies that physical therapists should not limit neuromotor assessment to elicited responses but should also assess muscle tone, primitive reflexes, righting, and equilibrium reactions within the context of posture and movement. Physical therapists who evaluate muscle tone and primitive reflexes to determine the effects of therapy should be aware that change may reflect transient abnormalities and not the direct effects of treatment.

Assessment of Muscle Tone

The French pediatric neurologists Andre-Thomas and Saint-Anne Dargassies were influential in formulating methods of clinical assessment of muscle tone. The neurologic examination of the infant developed by Andre-Thomas and colleagues[11] is based on the assessment of muscle tone, which they classified into active and passive components. Saint-Anne Dargassies[12] defined passive muscle tone as the viscoelastic properties of the muscle and all the spinal and supraspinal neurologic influences on the muscle at rest. This definition is consistent with the concept that muscle and muscle connective tissue have elastic or spring-like properties and that the intrinsic stiffness of muscle contributes to muscle tone.[13] Passive muscle tone is assessed by the capacity of the muscle to lengthen and by the resistance to passive movement. Although not clearly defined by Andre-Thomas and colleagues,[11] they assessed active tone by observation of recoil of a muscle that had been passively stretched, posture and spontaneous movement, and by the strength of elicited reflexes and automatic responses.

Hypertonia and hypotonia are clinically defined respectively as an increased or decreased resistance to quick stretch. Muscle spasticity is characterized by hypertonia, hyperactive deep tendon reflexes, and clonus.[14] Although the clinical definition of muscle tone is accepted, the causes of CNS muscle tone disorders are not fully understood. Clinical findings for muscle tone may reflect a number of primary and secondary pathologic processes, including abnormal supraspinal and spinal level inhibition, change in muscle fiber properties, and change in muscle length.[15] Furthermore, the relationship between muscle tone at rest and during active movement is unclear.

The most frequent method used by physical therapists to assess muscle tone involves eliciting a quick stretch to a muscle group through passive limb movement. The therapist makes a judgment of whether the resistance encountered is normal, hypotonic, or hypertonic. To qualify abnormal muscle tone, the therapist may further describe hypotonia or hypertonia as mild, moderate, or severe. Other methods of clinical assessment of muscle tone that require instrumentation such as a hand-held dynamometer or an isokinetic dynamometer are not feasible for assessment of young infants.

In a recent study, inter-rater reliability of muscle tone assessment was examined by having six physical therapists use their preferred method to assess children with abnormal muscle tone.[16] The therapists were provided a scoring form with ratings for normal muscle tone and mild, moderate, and severe hypo- or hypertonia. Definitions of each rating and instructions for scoring were not provided. Agreement was 55.6 percent for overall tone, 40.7 to 51.9 percent by body part, and 61.1 percent for clinical impression. Not surprisingly, poor inter-rater reliability was attributed to the lack of a standardized procedure. Variability in positioning of the child, the therapist's hand placement, the rate of limb displacement, the number of trials, and the child's behavior state are factors that may have adversely affected reliability.

Reliability of muscle tone assessment is an issue even when standardized protocols are used. Harris et al.[17] examined both inter-rater and intrarater reliability of the muscle tone section of the MAI. The muscle tone section contains 10 items. Three items involve handling the infant to assess passive tone, three items involve observation of posture in supine and prone, two items involve counting asymmetries and distribution variations observed when testing the first six items, and two items ask for the therapist's clinical impression. Items are scored on a six-point scale, and criteria for each rating are described. Eleven physical therapists and occupational therapists were trained with the MAI and then, working in pairs, tested 53 preterm infants at age 4 months, 29 of whom were retested within 7 days. Using the Pearson correlation coefficient, an intrarater reliability of 0.87 and an inter-rater reliability of 0.57 were reported. The results indicate that each therapist was consistent in rating infant muscle tone, but reliability between therapists was poor.

Assessment of Primitive Reflexes and Automatic Movements

Assessment of primitive reflexes has been traditionally performed by physical therapists within the context of a hierarchical view of brain development. In hierarchical theory, primitive reflexes are considered to be mediated by the spinal cord and brain stem, righting reactions by the midbrain, and equilibrium reactions and voluntary movement by the cerebral cortex.[18] As part of normal development, as each level of the CNS matures, lower levels of motor control are inhibited. At birth, spinal cord and brain stem levels are considered the most mature, and hence primitive reflexes characterize neonatal motor behavior. As midbrain and cortical levels of motor control mature, automatic reactions emerge and primitive reflexes are inhibited. Consequently by about 4 months primitive reflexes no longer characterize posture and movement. The term *integration of primitive reflexes* has traditionally been used to describe this process.

In this theoretical context, the inhibition normally exerted by midbrain and cortical centers of motor control is considered to be disrupted following a CNS lesion. Primitive reflexes therefore are not inhibited by higher levels of the CNS and often persist in a stereotyped manner that is not typical of normal development. Bobath[19] has proposed that persistence of abnormal primitive reflexes prevents the normal development of automatic righting and equilibrium reactions, which are requisites for voluntary movement. A focus of neurodevelopmental treatment therefore is to use positioning and handling techniques in treatment to inhibit abnormal primitive reflexes and facilitate righting and equilibrium reactions.

The work of Fiorentino[18] is a classic illustration of how physical therapists applied hierarchical theory to assess primitive reflexes and automatic reactions. Fiorentino categorized primitive reflexes, righting, and equilibrium reactions according to the level of the CNS presumed to mediate them. For each reflex, the test position and stimulus are described and guidelines are provided for determining a positive or negative response. Fiorentino stated that results are valuable in determining the maturational level of the CNS and identifying abnormal reflexes for the purpose of treatment planning. In the 1970s reflex assessments based on similar methods of testing were published by physical therapists.[20,21]

A little over a decade ago, Milani-Comparetti[22] proposed that the concept of primitive reflexes as stereotyped responses produced by sensory inputs was too limited a perspective. Using real-time ultrasound, he observed the movements of over 10,000 fetuses. Based on his observations, Milani-Comparetti proposed that primitive reflexes are actually innate primary movement patterns that the fetus is capable of initiating in the absence of a sensory stimulus. Furthermore, he hypothesized that primary motor patterns have functional significance. For example, Milani-Comparetti considered the positive support reflex a propulsive pattern that the fetus uses to push off the uterine wall to assist in the birth process.

Research by Zelazo et al.[23] and Thelen et al.[24] on early stepping supports the concept that primitive reflexes are innate patterns of movement that are modified through the interaction of a number of systems. Zelazo and associates reported that infants who were provided regular practice in stepping during the first year did not demonstrate a dormant period during which stepping was not observed. To the contrary, practice actually increased the frequency of stepping. Zelazo[25] proposed that the stepping reflex is not inhibited but rather through experience and neuromaturation the control of stepping undergoes transition from reflexive to cognitive control.

Thelen and associates[24] proposed that biomechanical factors account for the decrease in stepping movements that occurs between birth and age 4 weeks. Using kinematic and electromyographic (EMG) analysis, they reported that newborn supine kicking and stepping were similar and characterized by movement of the hip, knee, and ankle in synchrony. At 1 month, infants with the greatest weight gain took the fewest number of steps; however, supine kicking was not affected. To examine why the frequency of leg movement decreased in standing, small weights were attached to the infants' legs and a decrease in the number of steps was observed. When the infants' legs were submerged in water, however, the number of steps increased. The investigators concluded that the relative increase in leg mass that occurs between birth and 4 weeks constrains stepping movements. Thelen[26] also examined developmental changes in leg movements during the first year and suggested that the transition from newborn stepping to independent walking involves individuation of joint movement and subsequent organization of more complex movement, a process that involves the interaction of CNS maturation and biomechanical changes that occur as a result of physical growth.

The concepts and the research summarized in the previous three paragraphs are not all encompassing or presented in detail. The intent in presenting this information is to illustrate that, as knowledge of motor development has increased, theory has evolved. Systems theories of motor development and motor control have recently have generated considerable interest among physical therapists[27] (see also Chs. 1, 4, 8, 10, and 12). In systems theory, the CNS is viewed as an information-processing system capable of both feedback and feedforward controls. Motor control is distributed among the anatomic levels of the CNS in a heterarchical manner. Each level of motor control is relatively autonomous and control is distributed among each level based on the task and prior experience.[28] Dynamic systems theory[29,30] is based on the concepts of the Russian physiologist Bernstein[31] and on the application of principles of nonequilibrium phenomena in physics (dynamics) to human movement. Motor development is conceptualized as task and context oriented and arising from the interaction of multiple subsystems, such as neuromotor, musculoskeletal, cognitive, perceptual, social, and environmental. Current theories of motor development and motor control have heightened the controversy as to whether passive muscle tone and elicited primitive reflexes and automatic reactions are related to functional movement and responsive to change through physical therapy. As assumptions regarding the cause and significance of neuromotor findings are challenged by current theories, physical therapists have questioned the value of traditional assessment practices (see Ch. 8) and have suggested that greater emphasis be placed on assessment of self-initiated functional movement (see Ch. 10).[32-34]

CRITIQUES OF NEUROMOTOR ASSESSMENTS

Movement Assessment of Infants*

Brief Description of the Test

The MAI[35] was developed by physical therapists to address the need for a standardized neuromotor assessment to assist in early identification of infants with neuromotor dysfunction. In addition to use in high-risk infant follow-up clinics, the MAI can be used to monitor the effects of physical therapy on infants and children whose motor development is below a 12-month level. The MAI is also appropriate for use in research. The test can be administered by physical therapists, occupational therapists, physicians, nurses, psychologists, and others with a specialized knowledge of and experience in infant development. The test includes a manual and scoring sheets. A list of the test materials needed is included in the manual.

The MAI is criterion referenced and consists of 65 items divided among four sections muscle tone, primitive reflexes, automatic reactions, and volitional movement. Fifty-two items are administered, and the remaining 13 items are scored based on the examiner's impression or by counting asymmetries and distribution variations for the items that are administered. In the muscle tone section, antigravity postures, resistance to passive stretch, and muscle consistency are assessed. Items in the primitive reflexes section examine the relative presence or absence of reflexes observed in early infancy. The automatic reactions section includes items for righting, equilibrium, and protective reactions. The volitional movement section includes gross motor and fine motor behaviors and items that screen hearing and vision. Directions for administering and scoring each item are contained in the manual. Items for the muscle tone section are scored on a six-point numerical rating scale, while items for the remaining

---

* The authors of this assesment are Lynette S. Chandler, Mary Skillen, and Marcia W. Swanson. It was published in 1980 by the authors, P.O. Box 4631, Rolling Bay, WA 98061.

three sections are scored on four-point scales. Emphasis is placed on the quality of movement.

Scoring is based on the total number of risk points, a high score indicating poor performance. Interpretation of the 4-month profile is based on the performance of 35 high-risk infants who were administered the MAI at age 4 months, then re-examined at 1 year. All 8 of the infants diagnosed as having cerebral palsy as opposed to only 4 of 27 infants without cerebral palsy had 4-month risk scores of 8 or higher. The authors caution that the 4-month profile is preliminary and should not be the sole basis for any clinical decisions. Recently, an 8-month profile was developed, but the manual does not provide information on how risk points were determined or on interpretation of results. Research is in progress to establish a 6-month profile.

Technical Evaluation

Research on reliability and validity was conducted after publication of the manual. A summary of reliability and validity studies has been published.[36] As described earlier, Harris et al.[17] investigated inter-rater and intrarater reliability for both total risk scores and section risk scores. Inter-rater reliability for total risk scores was 0.72. Inter-rater reliability for section risk scores was 0.57 for muscle tone, 0.51 for primitive reflexes, 0.78 for automatic reactions, and 0.65 for volitional movement. The magnitude of the correlations indicates fair inter-rater reliability for total risk scores and poor to fair inter-rater reliability for section risk scores. Intrarater reliability for total risk scores was 0.76. Intrarater reliability for section risk scores was 0.87 for muscle tone, 0.62 for primitive reflexes, 0.70 for automatic movements, and 0.16 for volitional movements. The magnitude of the correlations indicates fair intrarater reliability for total risk scores and poor to good intrarater reliability for section risk scores.

Haley et al.[37] examined the item reliability of the MAI using the scores of the subjects included in the study by Harris et al.[17] Inter-rater reliability was excellent for only 2 percent of the items and fair to good for 58 percent of the items. Intrarater reliability was excellent for 10 percent of the items and fair to good for 42 percent of the items. The authors suggested that factors that enhance the clinical value of the MAI such as ability to handle the infant, the rating scale, and documentation of asymmetry may have contributed to poor reliability for many items. The amount of handling required to administer the MAI and differences in technique among examiners are potential sources of scoring error. Similarly, although a four-point rating scale is advantageous for assessing quality of movement, examiners are required to make more subtle distinctions, including the presence of asymmetry, than a scale in which items are scored as pass–fail.

Schneider et al.[38] examined the construct that the MAI is able to differentiate infants at risk for cerebral palsy from normal infants. Fifty healthy 4-month-old infants were administered the MAI. Seventy percent had total risk scores ranging from 0 to 7, 28 percent had total risk scores ranging from 8 to 13, and one subject had a total risk score greater than 13. Follow-up of the 15 infants with total risk scores of 8 or higher indicated that none had motor problems at 18 to 24 months. The investigators concluded that the MAI 4-month profile does not accurately reflect or predict neuromotor development of normal infants.

The major focus of research has been the ability of the 4-month score to identify infants who will eventually be diagnosed as having cerebral palsy, a measure of predictive validity. Harris[39] compared the ability of 4-month MAI risk scores and Bayley Motor Scores to identify infants who at ages 3 to 8 years were diagnosed as having cerebral palsy. Of 152 infants assessed, 34 were later diagnosed as having cerebral palsy. The MAI correctly identified 73.5 percent of children with cerebral palsy (sensitivity) and 62.7 percent of children who did not have cerebral palsy (specificity). The Bayley Motor Scale identified 35.3 percent of the children with cerebral palsy and 94.9 percent of children without cerebral palsy. Harris suggested that the broader spectrum of neuromotor behaviors and ability to measure quality of movement accounted for the finding that the MAI was more accurate than the Bayley Motor Scale in identifying infants with cerebral palsy. In contrast, the resolution of abnormal neuromotor signs that are not assessed on the Bayley Motor Scale may have contributed to the finding that the Bayley was more accurate in identifying infants without cerebral palsy. Harris recommended using the MAI in conjunction with a norm-referenced motor scale such as the Bayley for developmental follow-up of high-risk infants and performing repeated assessments during the first year.

Paban and Piper[40] included 4-month MAI scores in their prospective study of 1-year predictors of neurologic status and developmental outcome for 26 high-risk infants. Using a total risk score of 8 or greater, six of nine infants were correctly identified as suspect or abnormal (67 percent sensitivity), while only 6 of 17 were correctly identified as normal (35 percent specificity). The moderately good sensitivity but poor specificity concurs with the results reported by Harris.[39]

Although the MAI is intended to monitor progress in physical therapy, this has not been a focus of research with one exception. Lydic et al.[41] compared the ability of the MAI and the revised experimental edition of the Peabody Developmental Gross Motor Scale to measure change for a 6-week period in 10 infants with Down syndrome. Peabody total raw scores were used to allow for direct comparison to MAI risk points. The mean change score of -2.1 was significant for the MAI, while the mean change score of 7.3 for the Peabody Scale was not. The authors suggested that the MAI may be preferable for measuring change over short periods of time in infants with Down syndrome.

Qualitative Evaluation

The MAI can be administered in 45 to 60 minutes, depending on the experience of the examiner and on the behavior of the infant. The materials needed include a bell, rattle, ring, ball, cubes, and pellets. For clinical use, the authors recommend that the examiner should have knowledge of infant development, experience in handling infants, familiarity with the manual, and practice using the test. Formal training is recommended for use in research. The areas of neuromotor development assessed and emphasis on quality of movement are appealing to physical therapists. The administration time, however, may preclude routine use in high-risk infant follow-up clinics, especially if a norm-referenced assessment is also administered. Although the sensitivity of the MAI in predicting cerebral palsy compares favorably with other neuromotor assessments, the high rate of false positives is of concern. Caution must be exercised in interpreting the MAI, and test scores should not be the sole basis for decision making.

Summary Evaluation

The concept and content of the MAI make it a useful neuromotor assessment. The standardized administration and scoring procedures provide physical therapists a method of systematic assessment. Research suggests that the MAI has potential as a diagnostic tool; however, further test construction to improve reliability and validity is needed. The lack of information on interpretation of scores, particularly for infants who are not 4 months of age, and the high rate of false positives preclude the ability to diagnose cerebral palsy on the basis of MAI score. The time needed to administer the MAI is a limitation for use in high-risk infant follow-up clinics.

Milani-Comparetti Motor Development Screening Test[†]

Brief Description of the Test

The Milani-Comparetti Motor Development Screening Test (M-C) was first published in 1967.[42] Milani-Comparetti, an Italian pediatric neurologist, and his colleague Gidoni were interested in the inter-relationships between motor function and underlying primitive reflexes and automatic movements. The test is based on the construct that integration of primitive reflexes is necessary for full expression of automatic reactions and that the development of automatic reactions is necessary for antigravity control of posture and movement. The construct for the examination met with favor among physical therapists, and in 1977 the test was published with standardized directions for administration and scoring.[43]

The revised edition[44] is normed for ages 1 to 16 months. All of the original

---

[†] The authors: of this test are A. Milani-Comparetti and E. A. Gidoni. It was published in 1987 (revised edition; Wayne Stuberg, project director) by Meyer Children's Rehabilitation Institute, University of Nebraska Medical Center, 444 South 44th Street, Omaha, NE 68131-3795.

items are retained; however, the order and position for testing some items were modified. The test consists of 27 items scored "present" or "absent." Items address primitive reflexes; righting, tilting, and protective reactions; and spontaneous posture and movement through attainment of independent walking. The title of the manual indicates that the test is a screening tool; however, no summary score or cut-off scores are suggested to differentiate between infants with normal and infants with delayed development. The test includes a manual and scoring sheets. The only equipment needed is a firm cushion for testing tilting reactions. On the original scoring sheet items are grouped by category. In the revised edition, items are listed on the scoring sheet by order of testing to minimize position changes.

Technical Evaluation

The revised edition of the M-C[44] was standardized and normed on 312 infants who resided in the Omaha, NE, area. Infants born more than 2 weeks preterm and infants with medical problems and developmental delays were excluded. Infants were screened using the Denver Developmental Screening Test. Testing was done by four pediatric physical therapists. Items are placed at the age when they were passed by 85 percent of the infants in the normative sample.

Evidence of inter-rater and intrarater reliability is provided in the manual and in a subsequent article.[45] Inter-rater reliability was examined by having three physical therapists score 60 assessments from videotape. Agreement between the primary observer and each therapist ranged from 90 to 93 percent. Inter-rater reliability for individual items ranged from 79 to 98 percent. Intrarater reliability was examined by testing 43 infants twice within a 1-week interval. Mean agreements were 93 percent for all items and 80 to 100 percent for individual items. The validity of the revised edition has not been determined.

Qualitative Evaluation

The M-C can be administered in 10 to 15 minutes. The procedure and criteria for scoring each item are described in the manual. Figures that depict each response are provided. Physical therapists are familiar with the items, and instructions are clear. Criteria for scoring items incorporate quality of movement. No formal method of presenting results is published; rather, the therapist compiles a summary profile.

Summary Evaluation

The construct of the M-C is appealing to physical therapists who subscribe to traditional methods of neuromotor assessment. Administration time is suitable for use in high-risk infant follow-up clinics or as part of a comprehensive developmental assessment. Although the revised edition is standardized and normed on a local sample, the lack of a total score and specific guidelines for interpretation of results are major limitations. Until the validity of the M-C is determined, discretion must be used in interpreting results. The lack of cut-off scores prevents use of the M-C as a formal screening tool.

Primitive Reflex Profile‡

Brief Description of the Test

The Primitive Reflex Profile (PRP)[46] is a standardized assessment of seven primitive reflexes scored on a five-point ordinal scale. The PRP was constructed to provide a method of quantifying primitive reflexes. After the manual was published, a profile of the scores of normal infants for each reflex was developed. The authors chose to examine primitive reflexes because they are present at birth, and hence delay in integration may serve as the earliest indication of motor dysfunction including cerebral palsy. Reflexes were selected based on clinical observations of persistance of primitive reflexes in children with cerebral palsy. No equipment is needed to administer the PRP.

The reflexes included in the PRP are the asymmetrical tonic neck reflex, symmetrical tonic neck reflex, tonic labyrinthine reflex (tested supine and prone), derotational righting (both body on body and head on body), positive support reflex, Moro reflex, and Galant reflex. The five-point scoring scale is defined as follows: 0, the response is absent; +1, the response is transient and only elicited by passive movement; +2, the response is elicited by voluntary movement; +3, the response is exaggerated or sustained beyond what is seen in normal infants; and +4, the response is obligatory. The manual includes instructions for administering and scoring each item. Consistency on three of five trials is required for a particular score. Guidelines are not provided for interpretation of the total score.

Technical Evaluation

Profiles of mean scores for each reflex were obtained by administering the PRP longitudinally to 381 healthy full-term infants. Each infant was assessed in the newborn nursery and at each well baby visit through ages 24 months. Composite bar graphs and graphs of the mean scores have been published.[47]

---

‡ The authors of this assessment are Arnold J. Capute, Pasquale J. Accardo, Eileen P.G. Vining, James E. Rubenstein, and Susan Harryman. It was published in 1978 in *Monographs in Developmental Pediatrics* Vol. 1, by University Park Press, 233 East Redwood Street, Baltimore, MD 21202.

None of the infants received scores of +4 on the reflexes expected to decline in the first year.

Inter-rater reliability was examined by having four researchers examine four children with cerebral palsy and four full-term newborn infants. When reliability was determined for exact agreement, reliability coefficients for each item ranged from 0.50 to 0.88 for the children with cerebral palsy and from 0.50 to 1.00 for the newborn infants. Intrarater reliability for the children with cerebral palsy ranged from 0.44 to 0.88.

The construct that decreased reflex activity is related to the emergence of rolling and sitting was supported in a study of 177 normal infants.[48] The ability of the PRP to discriminate functional levels of ambulation in children with cerebral palsy was investigated in 53 subjects and 18 months to 21 years.[49] The mean PRP score was 3.79 (range, 1 to 5) for subjects classified as independent ambulators, 6.08 for subjects classified as intermediate ambulators (range, 4 to 9), and 7.80 for nonambulators (range, 6 to 11). The results indicate that the PRP was able to discriminate ambulation status. The authors suggest that when used prospectively with children having cerebral palsy, the PRP might be of value in monitoring progress and decision making. The validity of the PRP in early diagnosis has not been reported.

Qualitative Evaluation

Qualifications for administration of the PRP are not discussed in the manual. The authors suggest that primary health care providers use the PRP for screening motor dysfunction. Criteria for assigning scores include both measurable criteria such as angles and time and descriptors that are not defined, such as "mild," "marked," and "exaggerated." Behavioral state is not strictly controlled. The authors maintain that younger infants should be in states 3, 4, or 5 as defined by Prechtl. Habituation to repeated trials is not discussed.

Summary Evaluation

The PRP is standardized, and reflexes are scored on a five-point scale, distinct strengths compared with most reflex assessments. The PRP is short, which allows time for other developmental assessments. The validity of using the PRP for early diagnosis or to monitor change in neurologic status of children with a diagnosis of cerebral palsy has not been determined.

NORM-REFERENCED DEVELOPMENTAL ASSESSMENTS

Norm-referenced developmental scales are used to compare the development of an infant who is being assessed to the development of infants of the same age. A *norm* is defined as the normal or average performance of the population of interest.[50] Norm-referenced assessments are designed to identify infants with significant developmental delay and therefore are administered as part of a diagnostic assessment. Norm-referenced assessments are also used for the purpose of classification. *Classification* refers to the process of determining whether an infant meets eligibility criteria for a particular service such as early intervention. States that receive funding for early intervention under PL 99-457 are required to establish guidelines for determining eligibility for service. The law requires professionals from at least two disciplines to administer a multido-main assessment that includes motor development. Determination of degree of developmental delay or other criteria that will be used to determine eligibility is left to the discretion of each state. Developmental screening tests that are typically norm-referenced are presented in a separate section.

Norm-referenced developmental scales are based on the construct that normal development is characterized by a predictable rate and orderly sequence. Older infants demonstrate abilities that are not seen in younger infants and hence are expected to receive higher scores on norm-referenced scales. The representative sample, also called the *normative sample,* should reflect the characteristics of infants in the United States, although norms are often estab-lished by testing infants from a smaller geographic area. In addition to age and geographic representation, factors considered in selecting a normative sample include gender, race, family socioeconomic status, and rural–urban residency. The raw scores obtained from the infants in the normative sample are trans-formed into one or more units of measure, including age-equivalents, percen-tiles, and standard scores. Standard scores include developmental quotients, z-scores, and T-scores. An important feature of standard scores is that variance of scores about the mean is also determined and typically presented as the standard deviation. The manual for a norm-referenced assessment contains tables that enable the test user to convert the raw score to a norm or standard score and thereby compare the performance of the infant with the performance of the normative sample.

When assessing development for the purpose of diagnosis or classification, the primary concern is not whether an infant achieves the mean score but rather whether the score falls within the variability demonstrated by the infants in the normative sample. For standard scores, the variability of the normative sample is expressed by the standard deviation of the mean score. By convention, a standard deviation of -1.0 or -1.5 is used as a cut-off score between normal and delayed development. This corresponds to the 16th and 6th percentiles, respectively, indicating that the infant scored higher than only 16 or 6 percent of infants in the normative sample. A standard score equal to or below the cut-off score is considered to represent a delay in development.

In the chapter introduction, the perspective was provided that, although physical therapists have traditionally assessed motor development, they have not relied on norm-referenced scales. The lack of entry-level training in measure-ment is one explanation for this practice. Physical therapists also have asserted that the use of norm-referenced assessments is inappropriate for children with moderate to severe motor dysfunction. Therapists contend that the focus of treatment is not to increase the rate of development but to assist the infant to develop and improve the efficiency of postures and movements that represent areas of greatest need. In particular, therapists have questioned the practice of using norm-referenced motor scales to evaluate the effects of physical therapy.[51,52] Rosenbaum and colleagues[53] support this perspective and state that norm-referenced motor assessments should not be used to evaluate the effects of intervention until they are validated as responsive to changes made by children with motor dysfunction.

The objection to the use of norm-referenced scales to evaluate the effects of treatment in children with moderate to severe motor dysfunction is justifiable but should not preclude the use of norm-referenced scales as part of a diagnostic assessment, for classification, or to monitor development of infants. The results of norm-referenced scales provide an indication of developmental status and therefore compliment the neuromotor assessment of high-risk infants. Abnormal neuromotor findings during the first year may be transient or persistent and have a variable influence on development. Recommendations for an infant with abnormal neuromotor findings who attains a score on a norm-referenced developmental scale that is within 1 SD of the mean are likely to differ from those for an infant who displays abnormal neuromotor findings and a norm-referenced scale score that is -3.0 SD below the mean.

Pertinent to the assessment of preterm infants is the issue of basing the results of norm-referenced scales on chronologic age (CA), as is done for the full-term infant, or making adjustments to account for the infant's gestational age at birth. Gesell and Amatruda[54] consider development of the preterm infant a function of conceptual age, with maturation of the CNS the most important determinant of development in infancy. They recommend that for the first 2 to 3 years of life development should be based on the preterm infant's adjusted age (AA) (also referred to as *corrected age*) to account for differences in gestational age at birth. For example, an infant born at 27 weeks of gestation (3 months preterm) and assessed at 12 months CA would have an AA of 9 months.

To examine the effect of gestational age on motor development and to determine the appropriateness of making age adjustments when assessing motor development of preterm infants, Palisano[55] administered the Peabody Developmental Motor Scales (PDMS) to 23 preterm and 21 full-term infants at 12, 15, and 18 months CA. The preterm infants were born between 29 and 32 weeks of gestation and met preestablished criteria that classified them at lowrisk for a disorder in motor development. Neither the preterm nor the full-term infants had major medical, neurologic, or orthopedic problems during the first year. The preterm and full-term groups were comparable in gender, race, and family socioeconomic status. The PDMS developmental motor quotient is based on variable and wide age ranges that were not discrete enough for the purpose of this study. Therefore, in this study, motor developmental quotients were calculated by dividing the normed age equivalent score by either CA or AA.

When quotients were based on CA, the mean gross motor and fine motor developmental quotients for the full-term group were significantly higher than those of the preterm group of all three test ages, indicating that the full-term infants had higher levels of motor development. When the quotients of the preterm infants were based on AA, however, the motor quotients of the two groups did not differ significantly. The results support the concept that the motor development of healthy preterm and full-term infants differ primarily as a function of gestational age and the practice of making age adjustments when administering norm-referenced motor assessments to preterm infants. These results also suggest that factors in addition to gestational age at birth are affecting the motor development of preterm infants if test scores based on AA remain below age expectations.

The norm-referenced developmental scales selected for critique are the Bayley Scales of Infant Development, the Gesell Developmental Schedules, the PDMS, and the Battelle Developmental Inventory. These scales meet criteria for a well-constructed test, are used by professionals from a number of disciplines including physical therapy, and are prominent in research on developmental outcome of infants with various biological and environmental risk factors. Emphasis will be placed on assessment of motor development.

Bayley Scales of Infant Development[§]

Brief Description of the Test

The Bayley Scales of Infant Development (BSID)[56] consist of norm-referenced Mental and Motor Scales and a descriptive Infant Behavior Record. The Mental and Motor Scales were constructed to provide a standardized measure of infant development during the first 30 months. The scales are designed for both clinical and research use. At the time the BSID were published, no nationally normed infant developmental scales were available. The test kit includes a manual, scoring forms, and materials needed for testing. Directions are provided for construction of stairs and a balance beam. Bayley was sensitive to the fact that assessment of infants requires special methods and procedures. In developing items, an effort was made to create situations that would capture interest and to use materials and toys that would enhance participation.

The Mental Scale is used to assess early cognitive and language abilities, including perception, object permanence, memory, learning, problem solving, vocalizations, verbal communication, and early evidence of the ability to form generalizations and classifications, a basis for abstract thinking. The Mental Scale consists of 163 items that are scored pass–fail. Items are ordered by the age at which the item was passed by 50 percent of the normative sample. Similar items are grouped by situational codes, but there are no formal subscales. Kohen-Raz[57] performed a scalogram analysis and, based on the results, grouped

---

[§] The author of this assessment is Nancy Bayley. It was published in 1969 by The Psychological Corporation, 555 Academic Court, San Antonio, TX 78204-9990.

items into five subscales: eye–hand, manipulation, object–relations, imitation–comprehension, vocalization–social contact–active vocabularly.

The Bayley Motor Scale is used to measure control and coordination of the body for posture, locomotion, and fine motor manipulation. The Motor Scale consists of 81 items, 69 of which measure gross motor behavior. No fine motor items appear after the 8.9-month level. A format similar to that of the Mental Scale is followed for placement of items, scoring, and situational codes.

Guidelines are provided in the manual for determining the lowest and highest items that need to be administered (basal and ceiling levels). The number of items passed is summed, and the total raw score is used to determine the standard score. The manual contains tables that are divided into 1-month age levels and used to convert the total raw score to a standard score. The standard score for the Mental Scale is the Mental Development Index (MDI), and the standard score for the Motor Scale is the Psychomotor Development Index (PDI). For each scale the mean is 100 and the standard deviation is 16. A difference of 20 points between the two scales is considered significant. Scores may also be presented as an age equivalent.

A revised edition of the BSID is presently being constructed. The revised scales will be expanded but retain a similar format. Plans are to norm the revised edition on a national sample of infants and preschool children from birth to age 42 months.

Technical Evaluation

The BSID were standardized and normed on a national sample of 1,262 infants, aged 2 through 30 months, whose characteristics and demographics reflected the 1960 U. S. Census of Population. Infants who were born more than 1 month preterm or who demonstrated developmental disorders were excluded from the sample.

Werner and Bayley[58] examined reliability for the 1958–60 version of the Mental and Motor Scales. Inter-rater reliability was examined in 90 infants aged 8 months. The mean agreement for individual items was 89.4 percent for the Mental Scale and 93.4 percent for the Motor Scale. To determine intrarater reliability, 28 infants were retested 1 week later. The mean agreement for individual items was 76.4 percent for the Mental Scale and 75.3 percent for the Motor Scale.

Evidence of concurrent validity of the Bayley Mental Scale and the Stanford-Binet Intelligence Scale is provided in the test manual. Correlations were determined between the scores of 120 children aged 24, 27, and 30 months who passed all six tests at the 2-year level on the Stanford-Binet. A correlation coefficient of 0.57 was obtained between scores on the two tests. In view of the restricted range of scores, Bayley concluded that the results support the concurrent validity of the Mental Scale.

Support for the need to renorm the BSID is provided by Campbell et al.[59] As part of a study on the effectiveness of a regionalized perinatal care program in rural North Carolina, a population-based sample of 305 12-month-old infants were administered the BSID. The mean MDI was 111, and the mean PDI was 110. The authors raised the concern that developmental outcomes of 12-month-old high-risk infants whose scores are in the low average range may be overestimated using the BSID and recommended renorming.

Coryell et al.[60] analyzed longitudinal data relative to the stability of the Bayley Motor Scale and concluded that a single score may not reflect an infant's true abilities. Subjects were 15 low-risk and 8 high-risk infants who were administered the Bayley Motor Scale at 2, 3, 4, 8, and 12 months. Based on test scores at 24 to 36 months, infants were classified as having normal or non-normal outcomes. For the normal outcome group, subjects did not change ranks over the different test ages, and mean scores were not significantly different. Subjects in the non-normal outcome groups also did not change ranks over the different test ages; however, mean scores varied significantly from test to test. For the majority of individual infants in both groups, scores were not stable during the first 12 months. In particular, 4-month scores were inflated. The high 4-month scores are of particular interest in light of the findings by Harris[39] that 4-month Bayley Motor scores were not as accurate as 4-month MAI scores in identifying infants who later were diagnosed as having cerebral palsy. Coryell and associates[60] concluded that an infant's score on the Bayley Motor Scale at one age cannot be used to predict his or her score at another age. The conclusion that Bayley Motor scores during the first year are not predictive of development at later ages is supported by the results of Crowe et al.[61]

Qualitative Evaluation

The BSID can be administered in about 45 minutes; the Motor Scale usually requires no more than 20 minutes. Instructions for administration and scoring items are generally clear. Test materials are attractive to infants and are durable. Physical therapists are familiar with the items on the Motor Scale. Administration of the Mental Scale would be more difficult and is not appropriate for routine administration by physical therapists. No specific examiner certification requirements are published; however, the publisher does appraise the professional qualifications of individuals who seek to purchase the BSID.

BSID scores do not delineate cognitive and fine motor development or gross motor and fine motor development. Many of the items on the Mental Scale require fine motor manipulation of pellets, cubes, pegs, formboard pieces, and a crayon. Consequently, the Mental Scale may not provide a valid indication of cognitive development for an infant with limited fine motor control. The Motor Scale contains only a few items for each age level and omits stages in the motor development sequence. For example, it contains no items for running and kicking, and a single item incorporates all methods of prewalking progression. Quality of movement is not emphasized.

Summary Evaluation

The BSID meet the criteria of a well-constructed test and are the prominent norm-referenced assessment used by psychologists and in research on normal development and developmental outcome of high-risk infants. The BSID are recommended for the purpose of discriminating between infants with and without delayed development, although caution should be exerted when interpreting scores in the low average range and scores of infants aged 4 months and younger. A limitation of the BSID is the lack of formal subscales to delineate different areas of development. The large number of items on the Mental Scale that require manipulation of objects is a concern for infants with fine motor dysfunction. The time needed to administer the Motor Scale makes it suitable for use in high-risk infant follow-up clinics. Although the Motor Scale has been used to evaluate the effects of physical therapy in infants with cerebral palsy,[62,62] no evidence exists to suggest that it is responsive to change in infants with motor dysfunction.

Revised Gesell and Amatruda Developmental and Neurologic Examination ‖

Brief Description of the Test

The Gesell Developmental Schedules are based on the work of Arnold Gesell, a pioneer in the study of child development in the United States. The original Gesell Schedules were standardized in 1929.[64] The revised edition[65] was standardized and normed between 1975 and 1977 on infants and preschool children 4 weeks to 36 months of age. The test includes a manual, scoring forms, and test materials. The Gesell Schedules were constructed for use by pediatricians in the developmental diagnosis of young children. They are based on the concept that maturation of the CNS is the primary factor that determines the rate and sequence of early development. Behavior in several areas is assessed in order to make inferences about the integrity and functional maturity of the child's nervous system.

The revised Gesell Schedules consist of 489 items divided into five domains of behavior: adaptive, gross motor, fine motor, language, and personal–social. The adaptive domain consists of 145 items that are concerned with organization of stimuli, perception, and problem solving. The authors consider this domain as a forerunner of later intelligence. The gross motor domain consists of 98

‖ The authors of this assessment are Hilda Knobloch, Frances Stevens, and Anthony F. Malone. It was published in 1987 as a test kit with the *Manual of Developmental Diagnosis: the Administration and Interpretation of the Revised Gesell and Amatruda Developmental and Neurologic Examination*. They are available from Gesell Developmental Materials, Inc., P.O. Box 272391, Houston, TX 77277-2391.

items that include postural reactions, head control, sitting, creeping, standing, walking, running, and jumping. The fine motor domain consists of 56 items designed to assess use of the hands and fingers to reach, grasp, and manipulate objects. The language domain consists of 109 items for examining facial expressions, gestures, vocalizations, words, sentences, and comprehension. The personal–social domain consists of 81 items intended to assess "the child's personal reactions to the social culture in which he lives." This domain includes items for eating, dressing, playing, cooperating, and responding socially.

Directions for administration and scoring are provided in the manual. On the scoring form, items that represent temporary behavior patterns are distinguised from those for permanent behavior patterns, as are items that may be scored from parent report. The scoring code is as follows. A "+" sign is used to indicate that the child displays the behavior consistently, and "+/−" or "±" indicates that the behavior is observed but inconsistently. Guidelines for making this distinction are not provided. A "++" sign is used for earlier items in a sequence when a child has displayed a more advanced pattern. "N" indicates a temporary pattern that has been replaced by a more mature behavior. A "−" sign indicates a failure. The examiner may also use the letter "A" to note a behavior that is present but abnormal in quality (guidelines are not provided), the letter "D" if a child has a disability that prevents the item from being administered (e.g., hearing loss), and the letter "R" for an item that is refused.

Technical Development

The Gesell Schedules were standardized and normed on 927 infants in the Albany, NY, area. Infants were selected to match the demographics of families residing in that area. All infants were born full-term and demonstrated no congenital anomalies or developmental delays. Children were tested 4 weeks apart between 4 and 56 weeks and 3 months apart between 15 and 36 months. Initially over 1,000 items were evaluated. The 489 items selected were placed at the age passed by 50 percent of the normative sample.

Age equivalent scores for each domain are determined by deciding the point where the aggregate of + scores change to − scores. Examples are provided in the manual, but the procedure involves judgment on the part of the examiner. The Developmental Quotient (DQ) for each domain is determined by dividing the age equivalent (referred to as the *maturity age*) by the child's CA and multiplying this ratio by 100. The authors of the revised edition suggest that in infancy a DQ below 85 is a cause for concern. The DQ is not a true standard score. The mean DQ and standard deviation of the normative sample are not provided for each test age; therefore interpretation of a DQ of 85 is based on the authors' recommendations and not on the performance of the normative sample.

Inter-rater reliability was examined for individual items on a sample of 48 infants between ages 16 and 21 months. The overall percentage of agreement was 94 percent, ranging from 88 percent for the fine motor domain to 97 percent for the language domain. Support is also provided for inter-rater reliability in determining DQs. DQs for 184 children were independently calculated by two examiners. Pearson correlation coefficients were determined by domain for nine test ages and ranged from 0.84 to 0.99.

Schneider and Brannen[66] reported evidence of concurrent validity of the revised Gesell Schedules and the BSID. Twenty children with Down syndrome, aged 6 through 36 months, were administered both assessments. Scores for each assessment were represented by developmental lag expressed in months. No significant difference was found between mean mental lag on the Gesell (adaptive and language domains) and Bayley Mental Scale. A significant difference in mean motor lag was found between the Gesell (gross motor and fine motor domains) and Bayley Motor Scale. When only the gross motor domain of the Gesell was used to calculate motor lag, however, the two scales did not differ. The authors suggest that the lack of fine motor items on the Bayley Motor Scale may have skewed the comparison between the two tests. The results suggest that the two tests may be used interchangeably. The authors stated that the Gesell may be preferred in a clinical setting because it is less rigorous and takes less time to administer, but they recommended use of the BSID for research.

Qualitative Evaluation

No formal training is required to administer the Gesell Schedules. The assessment can be administered in 30 minutes. The test user may initially have difficulty locating items in the manual. Test materials are attractive and durable. Items are representative of developmental milestones and fairly easy to administer. Items included in the motor section are familiar to physical therapists. Some emphasis is placed on quality of movement; however, broad descriptions such as "good control" are used. Separate adaptive and fine motor domains are helpful in differentiating fine motor from perception-cognitive delays. The number of items included at each age level is variable and ranges from 2 to 10 for the gross motor domain and from 1 to 5 for the fine motor domain. Differentiating between a score of + and +/- or ± and determining DQs are problematic for infants whose scores are greatly scattered.

Summary Evaluation

The Gesell Schedules include five domains of development, which is a strength when used as part of an interdisciplinary or transdisciplinary assessment. Compared with the BSID, the Gesell Schedules place greater emphasis on developmental sequences, which is advantageous for program planning. The scoring system is not precise, and, although the test is normed, standard scores are not available. The ability to determine separate gross motor and fine motor age equivalents is an advantage over the Bayley Scales.

Peabody Developmental Motor Scales[¶]

Brief Description of the Test

The PDMS[67] consist of separate Gross Motor and Fine Motor Scales standardized and normed for the ages birth through 83 months. The test includes a manual, scoring booklets, some of the necessary fine motor materials, and activity cards which correspond to test items. The authors whose backgrounds are in education and physical education developed the PDMS to (1) identify children with delayed or aberrant motor development, (2) allow for comparison of gross motor and fine motor development, (3) enable development to be assessed across time or in response to intervention, (4) be appropriate for use with children having motor handicaps, and (5) serve as a curriculum-based assessment when used with accompanying activity cards.

The Gross Motor Scale consists of 170 items divided into 17 age levels with 10 items at each age level. The Fine Motor Scale consists of 112 items with 6 or 8 items divided among 16 age levels. Each scale is divided into skill categories, not actual subscales, which in the authors' opinion represent the clustering of items that place similar demands on the child. The Gross Motor Scale consists of five skill categories: reflexes, balance, non-locomotion, locomotion, and receipt and propulsion of objects. The Fine Motor Scale is divided into four skill categories: grasping, hand use, eye-hand coordination, and manual dexterity. Directions for administration and scoring of each item are contained in the manual. Items are scored on a three-point scale (0, 1, and 2), with a score of 1 indicating that the behavior is emerging but that the criterion for successful performance is not fully met. Specific criteria for a score of 1 are not provided for each item.

Technical Evaluation

The PDMS were normed on 617 children using a stratified sampling procedure. Twenty states were selected to represent the four major U.S. Census Bureau regions. Within each state, test sites were selected that represented the rural–urban and socioeconomic status of the region. The sample consisted of 85 percent white and 15 percent nonwhite (black and Hispanic) children. The number of children tested at each age level ranged from 27 to 55. Between 27 and 33 children were tested at each age level up to 18 to 23 months.

Using the tables provided in the manual, Gross Motor and Fine Motor Scale total raw scores can be converted into an age equivalent, percentile, or one of three standardized scores: developmental motor quotient (DMQ), Z-score, and T-score. The mean DMQ is 100 and the standard deviation is 15.

[¶] The authors of this assessment are M. Rebecca Folio and Rebecca R. Fewell. It was published in 1983 by DLM Teaching Resources, One DLM Park, Allen, TX 75002.

Raw scores have also been normalized into scaled scores that are recommended to measure change in children who are not expected to make a large amount of progress. Scores for each skill category may be transformed into a percentile, DMQ, Z-score, or T-score.

Inter-rater reliability for total scores was examined in 36 children, and correlations of 0.97 for the Gross Motor Scale and 0.94 for the Fine Motor Scale were obtained. Intrarater reliability for total scores was determined for 38 children who were readministered the PDMS within 1 week of initial testing. Correlations of 0.95 for the Gross Motor Scale and 0.80 for the Fine Motor Scale were obtained.

Test items were adapted from the Revised Experimental Edition of the PDMS, other motor assessments, and research. Content validity is supported by adherence to Harrow's hierarchical sequence of motor development.[68] The authors' provide evidence of construct validity by demonstrating that scores improved as a function of age (except for the 54- to 59-month level of the Gross Motor Scale) and that scores of 104 children with identified motor problems were significantly lower than those obtained by the normative sample except for the 0- to 5-month age level. Based on this finding, caution is recommended in interpreting the scores of infants under age 6 months. Concurrent validity was examined with the BSID on a sample of 43 infants. Moderate correlations of 0.37 and 0.36 were reported between the Bayley Motor Scale and the Peabody Gross Motor and Fine Motor Scales, respectively. Correlations of -0.03 and 0.78 were reported between the Bayley Mental Scale and the Peabody Gross Motor Scale and Fine Motor Scale, respectively. The absence of a relationship between Peabody Gross Motor Scale and Bayley Mental Scores was not unexpected, whereas the high correlation between scores on the Peabody Fine Motor Scale and the Bayley Mental Scale probably reflects the similar nature of many items on the two scales.

Palisano[69] examined concurrent and predictive validities of the PDMS and the Bayley Motor Scale by administering both assessments to 44 preterm and full-term infants at ages 12, 15, and 18 months. Correlation analysis of age equivalent scores indicated that Bayley Motor Scores had a high correlation with Peabody Gross Motor Scores ($r = 0.78$ to 0.96) and unacceptable correlation with Peabody Fine Motor Scores ($r = 0.20$ to 0.57). When results were reported using standard scores, mean Bayley quotients for the full-term infants was significantly higher than the Peabody Gross Motor quotients. Prediction of motor development at 18 months was limited ($r = 0.25$ to 0.60) with the exception of Peabody Fine Motor scores for preterm infants ($r = 0.75$). The results support the concurrent validity of Peabody Gross Motor and Bayley Motor age equivalent scores but not predictive validity of the PDMS.

Phillips et al.[70] examined whether infants with different types of cerebral palsy would be distinguished by test performances on the Peabody Gross Motor Scale. Forty infants, aged 6 to 24 months, were administered the PDMS. No differences in scaled scores were found when age was used at a covariate. Differences in skill category Z-scores were found for all but the locomotor skill category. The authors suggested that skill category scores may provide information on differences in motor ability among infants with different types of cerebral palsy.

Campbell et al.[71] examined the concurrent validities of the gross motor portions of the PDMS, BSID, and Gesell Schedules. Subjects were 32 infants with cerebral palsy and 12 normal infants. The sample ranged in age from 7 to 26 months. Testing was performed using a checklist that combined items from all three assessments. The mean age equivalents for the normal infants on the PDMS, BSID, and the Gesell were 12.5, 13.4, and 14.1 months, respectively. Mean scores for the infants with cerebral palsy were 5.3, 6.9, and 6.8 months, respectively. Statistical analysis indicated that Gesell scores were significantly higher than Bayley scores and that Bayley scores were significantly higher than Peabody scores. The normal infants' mean age equivalent for the PDMS was exactly equal to their mean chronological age. On the basis of this result, the investigators concluded that the Peabody Gross Motor Scale was the most accurate of the three assessments.

Qualitative Evaluation

Each scale can be administered separately in 20 to 30 minutes; total test time is 40 to 60 minutes. No special qualifications are required to administer the PDMS. The authors recommend establishing inter-rater reliability with an experienced tester prior to formal testing. Hinderer et al.[72] have published an extensive critique of the PDMS. Their focus is on the upper age levels; however, most comments are germane to the whole scale and concur with my experience using the PDMS to assess infants.[73]

The normal motor developmental sequence is addressed in more depth than other norm-referenced assessments. The ability to obtain scores for each skill category is another strength of the PDMS. The inability of the examiner to demonstrate some items and the limited number of trials permitted may confound the ability to distinguish primary motor problems from behavioral, cognitive, and language causes of motor failure. Testing equipment is also an area of concern. Some of the materials provided are not durable, and specifications for some of the materials that are not included are not precise.

Items from each skill category are not equally distributed at each age level and, depending on a child's area of strength or weakness, may skew the total score. Items are ordered from least to most difficult within each age level, and therefore all items are not discriminatory of the age level in which they are passed. Therapists therefore must be careful in interpreting the scores of infants who cannot be tested with the standardized procedure. The lack of specific criteria for a score of 1 poses a problem in establishing reliability, comparing a child's scores to test norms, and comparing findings among clinical centers. For skills in which items are sequenced at two or more age levels such as grasp of a cube and supported walking, I have recommended that a child should demonstrate ability that is above the criteria for a score of 2 on the first item to receive a score of 1 for the next item in the sequence.

Although the PDMS is intended for use in assessing infants with motor problems, emphasis is not placed on quality of movement or differentiation of normal and atypical movement. General guidelines are provided for modifying testing procedures for children with handicapping conditions. Modifications are not incorporated into the standardized administration and scoring procedures, however, as the normative sample did not include children with identified motor delays or disorders. The normative sample included a relatively small number of infants for each age level. Consequently, standardized scores should be interpreted carefully. Furthermore, the 3-month age range for the 12- through 14-month and the 15- through 17-month age levels and the 6-month range beginning at the 18- through 23-month age level may not permit determination of a standard score for preterm infants based on the adjusted age.

Summary Evaluation

The PDMS provides the most in-depth assessment of motor development and despite some limitations is recommended over the Bayley Motor Scale and the Gesell Gross Motor and Fine Motor domains for use by physical therapists. The greater number of items, three-point scoring scale, ability to obtain separate scores for the Gross Motor and Fine Motor Scales and for skill categories within each scale are desirable features. The PDMS also can be used to assess motor development through age 6 years. The Bayley Motor Scale takes less time to administer than the PDMS and therefore might be preferred for use in high-risk infant follow-up clinics. An advantage of the BSID and the Gesell is the ability to compare motor development with development in other areas. This is helpful in determining an infant's areas of strength and need.

Battelle Developmental Inventory¶

Brief Description of the Test

The Battelle Developmental Inventory[74] (BDI) was developed under a contract from Special Education Services, United States Department of Education. The BDI was constructed for use by educators, speech pathologists, psychologists, and adaptive physical education specialists in infant, preschool, and primary educational programs to develop individualized education plans. The BDI is standardized and normed for children aged 1 month through 9 years. The BDI consists of 341 items grouped into five domains: personal–social, adaptive, motor, communication, and cognitive. The BDI is unique among norm-referenced assessments in the inclusion of adaptations of items for chil-

---

¶ The authors of this assessment are Jean Newborg, John R. Stock, and Linda Wnek. It was published in 1984 by DLM Teaching Resources, One DLM Park, Allen, TX 75002.

dren with visual, hearing, motor, and emotional handicaps. The BDI consists of scoring forms, an examiner's manual, and six separate test books, one for each domain and one for the screening test. The BDI screening test is presented in the section "Developmental Screening." A list of materials needed by age levels is given at the beginning of each test book.

The final stages of test construction and the national standardization were completed by the same corporation that published the PDMS. Determination of basal and ceiling age levels, the three-point scoring scale, and the types of scores obtained are similar to the PDMS. The number of domains and the wide age range of the test restricts the number of items at each age level. Items are grouped by age levels of either 6 or 12 months. The first three age levels are 0 to 5, 6 to 11, and 12 to 17 months. The motor domain, which includes the subdomains muscle control, body coordination, locomotion, fine muscle, and perceptual motor, contains only 30 items through the 12 to 17 month age level. There are no items for rolling, creeping, or cruising, and consequently the BDI is not inclusive of the motor development sequence.

Technical Evaluation

Content was determined by a panel of professionals who analyzed items for inclusion on the BDI. The procedures used to standardize and norm the BDI are similar to those used for the PDMS. The normative sample consisted of a national sample of 800 children aged 1 to 95 months. Norms for the first three age levels are based in the performance of 148 infants. Tables are provided in the manual for converting raw scores to age equivalents and standard scores.

Inter-rater and intrarater reliabilities for the BDI were determined on 148 and 183 children, respectively. Correlation coefficients for each item and for each domain by age level ranged from 0.71 to 1.00. Several studies are reported in the examiner's manual to support validity. Evidence of construct validity is suggested as a result of high correlations between scores for each domain and for items within each domain for children with normal development. The authors also report that with few exceptions older children received higher scores in each domain, and children in the normative sample received higher scores than a clinical sample of 160 children. Concurrent validity was examined by simultaneously administering the BDI and five other assessments, including the Stanford-Binet and Wechsler Intelligence Scale for Children, to between 10 and 37 children. Correlations for total scores ranged from 0.41 to 0.94, which the authors conclude provides support for concurrent validity. In a recent study, a correlation of 0.73 was reported between the total scores on the Developmental Edition of the Pediatric Evaluation of Disability inventory and the BDI.[75]

Qualitative Evaluation

The BDI can be administered in 1 hour or less. All assessments are designed to be administered by professionals from a number of disciplines, and formal training is not required. The role of the physical therapist in administration of the BDI within an educational setting is not discussed. Physical therapists are familiar with items in the motor domain and should find them easy to administer. The limited number of items restricts the value of the BDI for infants who receive physical therapy.

Summary Evaluation

The BDI has the fewest items for the first 2 years of development than the other norm-referenced scales reviewed in this section and is not suitable for treatment planning and evaluation of the effects of physical therapy. Standard scores for infants are based on a small normative sample and provided for 6-month age levels. The BDI therefore is not recommended for use as part of a diagnostic assessment. The most appropriate use of the BDI is for classification. The ability to obtain standard scores and the inclusion of multiple domains are desirable features of an assessment used to determine eligibility for early intervention and levels of function for multiple domains of development.

DEVELOPMENTAL SCREENING

The purpose of developmental screening is to identify infants who exhibit or who are at risk for a delay or disorder on one or more areas of development. The American Academy of Pediatrics[76] has stated that a role of the primary care pediatrician is to screen infants and preschool aged children for potential developmental problems. Physical therapists have become involved in developmental screening through participation in high-risk infant follow-up clinics and by the passage of PL 99-457. The rationale for developmental screening is that early identification and subsequent intervention will either prevent or minimize long-term disability. A well-care clinic may institute a developmental screening program to identify infants who are likely candidates for early intervention with the long-term goal of preventing mental retardation and learning disabilities attributable to environmental factors. A goal of neonatal intensive care nursery follow-up clinics is to identify among infants with biologic risk factors those with developmental delays or disabilities and recommend services to prevent or minimize long-term disability and secondary problems. PL 99-457 mandates that states establish a comprehensive child find system to identify infants from birth through age 2 years who experience developmental delays or who are at high risk for developmental delays in one or more areas. The domains listed in PL 99-457 are cognitive, physical (which includes motor development), language, self-help, and psychosocial.

Several characteristics are typical of a good developmental screening tool.[77] The test should be short (15 to 20 minutes), inexpensive, able to be administered by paraprofessionals, and acceptable to families and infants. These characteristics are intended to make it cost effective to screen large numbers of infants. A good developmental screening tool is also standardized, normed, and has acceptable reliability and validity. Glascoe[78] recommends inclusion of multiple sources of information (observation, direct elicitation, and parent report) to account for variability in infant performance. Results of screening tests are used to classify an infant's development into one of three categories: normal; suspect or questionable; or abnormal. Cut-off scores are intended to discriminate between low average and delayed development. Therefore a developmental screening test should not be used to determine an age equivalent or developmental quotient. Infants whose development is classified as suspect should be rescreened in a short period of time, whereas infants whose development is classified as abnormal should receive a more comprehensive assessment (diagnostic assessment). If the results of the diagnostic assessment confirm the presence of a delay or disorder in development, recommendations should be made for the appropriate services. In regard to PL 99-457, infants who upon screening have developmental delays are provided a more comprehensive assessment to determine eligibility for early intervention and develop the Individual Family Service Plan.

Determining the Accuracy of a Developmental Screening Test

The accuracy or validity of a developmental screening test is determined by concurrently administering the screening test and a reputable diagnostic assessment to a representative sample of infants. The results on the screening test are compared with the results of the diagnostic assessment using a four-cell classification table, which is presented in Table 9-1. The cells' "correct referrals" and "correct nonreferrals" represent agreement between the results of the screening test and the diagnostic assessment (infants who either were classified as normal or suspect/abnormal on both tests). The cells' "over-referrals" and "under-referrals" represent disagreement between the two tests in classifying infants as either normal or suspect/abnormal.

The percentage of infants classified as abnormal on both the screening test and diagnostic assessment indicate the sensitivity of the screening test. *Sensitivity* is a measure of how well a screening test identifies infants with delays. The percentage of infants classified as normal on both the screening test and diagnostic assessment indicates the specificity of the screening test. *Specificity* is a measure of how well a screening test identifies infants without delays. The percentage of infants classified as suspect/abnormal on the screening test but normal on the diagnostic assessment indicates the rate of over-

Table 9-1. Classification Table for Determining Validity of Developmental Screening Tests

Classification by Screening	Classification by Diagnostic Assessment	
	Abnormal	Normal
Abnormal (Positive)	Correct referrals	Over-referrals
Normal (Negative)	Under-referrals	Correct nonreferrals

referral. Over-referrals are also called *false positives,* since infants were incorrectly identified as having delayed development. The percentage of infants classified as normal on the screening test but abnormal on the diagnostic assessment indicates the rate of under-referral. Under-referrals are also called *false negatives,* because the screening test failed to identify infants with developmental delays.

In determining the cut-off scores for a screening test, the goal is to attain high sensitivity and specificity and a low rate of over-referral and under-referral. Glascoe[78] suggests that sensitivity should be a minimum of 80 percent and specificity 90 percent. The acceptable rate of over-referral is arbitrary but should be low enough so that the time gained by screening is not lost by having to perform comprehensive assessments on a large number of infants who receive scores within the normal range. Incorrect classification of infants as suspect/abnormal may also cause anxiety among families. A low rate of under-referral is particularly important. In general, an under-referral rate of 5 percent or less is acceptable. The validity of a screening test with a high rate of under-referral is questionable.

The Denver Developmental Screening Test[79] (DDST) is the most prominent developmental screening test used in the United States. A critique of the Denver II, the recently published revision and restandardization of the DDST, is presented in this section. Other developmental screening tests that have been published during the past decade include the Kansas Infant Development Screen[80] (KIDS) and screening versions of the Gesell Developmental Schedules[65] and the BDI.[74] The Chandler Movement Assessment of Infants Screening Test[81] and the Infant Motor Screen[82] are two recently constructed neuromotor screening tests. Each of these screening tools will be briefly summarized.

The Revised Developmental Screening Inventory (RDSI) consists of selected items from the Revised Gesell and Amatruda Developmental and Neurologic Examination and is published in Chapter 7 of the Gesell manual.[65] Based on guidelines provided in that manual, the RDSI is scored "normal," "questionable," or "abnormal." Validity was examined by administering the RDSI and the complete Gesell Developmental Schedules to 125 infants, some of whom had identified developmental disabilities. The authors report that sensitivity was 100 percent and specificity was 95 percent. The rate of over-referral was 5.1 percent. The Battelle Developmental Inventory Screening Test (BDIST) is a subset of items from the BDI,[74] which has been adopted for use under PL 99-457 by Utah, California, New Hampshire, Maine, and Montana.[78] Correlations between the 10 BDIST scores and the comparable BDI scores of 164 children were all above 0.90. The KIDS[80] was developed to provide a simple and efficient screening tool that could be incorporated into well-infant clinic visits in a variety of settings. The KIDS consists of 80 items that normally develop between birth and 24 months of age. Evidence of validity includes a high correlation between CA and developmental age on the KIDS for normal infants and a high correlation between developmental age on the KIDS and developmental age on a curriculum-based assessment for infants with developmental delays. Information on sensitivity and specificity are not reported for either the BDIST or the KIDS.

The Chandler Movement Assessment of Infants Screening Test (CMAI-ST)[81] was constructed to screen infants for movement disorders along a continuum from normal to delayed motor milestones to abnormal movement patterns. The four sections of the MAI are retained. Based on research on reliability and validity of the MAI, the number of items was reduced from 65 to 37, and a three-point scoring scale was adopted. The majority of items are scored from observation of spontaneous movement. Administration time is 10 to 15 minutes. Norms are being established on normal infants 2 to 12 months old. For each item, risk points are determined based on the age that either 85 percent or 90 percent of the normative sample passed the scoring criteria. Interpretations of the total risk score, reliability, and validity await the final stages of test construction. The CMAI-ST is a promising screening tool that appears well suited for use in high-risk infant follow-up clinics.

The Infant Motor Screen (IMS)[82] was adapted in part from the M-C and from the MAI to improve early detection of neuromotor problems, including cerebral palsy. The IMS consists of 25 items that assess the quality of movement between 4 and 16 months of age. Items are scored on a three-point scale, and results are presented as normal, questionable, or abnormal. Validity was examined by testing 111 infants at 4 months and 58 infants at 8 months on the IMS and either the Gesell Developmental Schedules or the RDSI.[83] A sensitivity of 93 percent and a specificity of 89 percent were reported at 4 months, and a sensitivity of 100 percent and a specificity of 96 percent were reported at 8 months.

Denver II**

Brief Description of the Test

The Denver II[84] is the revised and restandardized edition of the DDST,[79] which was originally standardized in 1967. The DDST was constructed for use by professionals and paraprofessionals to detect potential developmental problems in children from birth to age 6 years. The DDST was developed prior to the passage of the Education for All Handicapped Children Act (PL 94-142) and the widespread availability of publicly funded early-intervention programs. The DDST therefore was primarily designed to identify children with delays in multiple domains who were at risk for mental retardation. In a review of five subsequent studies on predictive validity, Greer et al.[85] concluded that for children over age 3 years those with an abnormal DDST

** The authors of this assessment are W.K. Frankenburg, J. Dodds, P. Archer, B. Bresnick, P. Maschka, N. Edelman, and H. Shapiro. It was published in 1990 by Denver Developmental Materials, Inc., P.O. Box 6919, Denver, CO 80206-0919.

were likely to have a poor school outcome but that many children with school-related problems who might benefit from early intervention were not identified by the DDST. The lack of test sensitivity in predicting school performance and concerns regarding the need for additional language items, the appropriateness of 1967 norms in 1990, the specific test item characteristics, and the appropriateness of the test for various subgroups were instrumental in the authors' decision to revise the DDST.

The Denver II retains the structure of the DDST, in which items are divided into four domains: personal–social, fine motor adaptive, language, and gross motor. Items were expanded from 105 to 125, and five "test behavior" items were added. The test behavior items are completed after administration of the test to assist the examiner to assess subjectively the child's overall behavior. The Denver II consists of a screening manual, scoring forms, and a kit of test materials that includes a red yarn pom-pom, small bell, rattle, raisins, a small bottle, 1 inch cubes, a tennis ball, red pencil, small doll, and a cup. The examiner only needs to supply paper for drawing. A separate technical manual includes details of the revision and standardization and a chapter on training.

The Denver II can be administered in less than 20 minutes. Some items may be passed by report. Items are arranged by domain and age level on a single-page scoring form. Each item is represented by a bar that spans the ages at which 25, 50, 75, and 90 percent of the standardization sample passed that item. In each domain, the examiner administers every item that intersects a line depicting the child's age and at least three items nearest to and totally to the left of the age line. Items are scored "pass," "fail," "no opportunity," or "refusal." A "fail" is scored when a child is unable to perform an item to the left of the age line, indicating that at least 90 percent of children of the same age in the normative sample passed the item. Based on guidelines that are provided, results are interpreted as "normal," "abnormal," "questionable," or "untestable." Children who receive an "abnormal" score should be referred for a diagnostic assessment; children whose performance is "questionable" should be rescreened in 3 months.

To reduce the amount of time necessary for routine developmental screening, a prescreening developmental questionnaire (PDQ) was developed for the DDST.[86] The PDQ consists of 97 items adapted from the DDST and is designed to be answered by parents in 5 minutes while waiting for their child's well-care appointment. Ten questions are answered based on the child's age. Children who pass six or fewer items receive a "suspect" score and should be administered the full DDST. A new PDQ is being developed for the Denver II. Until the new PDQ is available, children who are suspect on the PDQ may be screened using either the Denver II or the DDST.

Technical Evaluation

A pool of 326 potential items was created prior to restandardizion of the DDST. Normative data were collected by 17 screeners on a sample of 2,096 children. The children selected were divided into 10 age groups ranging from

0 to 2 months to 57 to 78 months. Only full-term children without obvious developmental problems were included in the sample. The children resided in the Denver metropolitan area and in several urban, semirural, and rural regions in the state of Colorado. A quota sample design was used that controlled for maternal education, residence, and ethnicity within age groups. Each item was administered at least 440 times. Selection of the 125 items that comprise the Denver II was based on statistical analysis and several qualitative factors, including the examiners' impressions about ease of administration and scoring, interest value for the child, and practicality.

Reliability was examined by administering the Denver II to 38 children from 10 age groups. Four trained examiners independently scored each child's performance. Seven to 10 days later, each child was readministered the Denver II. Mean inter-rater reliability was 0.99, and mean intrarater reliability was 0.90. The authors' suggest that the wide acceptance of the DDST is evidence of the content validity of the Denver II. Information on sensitivity, specificity, and the rates of over-referral and under-referral is not available.

Qualitative Evaluation

Like the DDST, directions for administering and scoring the Denver II are clear. The Denver II is relatively short, easy to administer, requires no special equipment, and is acceptable to both children and parents. Procedures for administration, scoring, and interpretation are similar to those for the DDST. Physical therapists who are familiar with the DDST will have no difficulty learning the Denver II. A training videotape, which includes a proficiency examination, is available from the publisher.

The decision to revise and renorm the DDST was timely, given the current emphasis on identification of infants with mild developmental problems and preschool children at risk for problems in school performance. The criteria for the abnormal and questionable are less stringent, which should increase the number of children who receive these two classifications. For the DDST, a child must demonstrate delays in two or more domains for an "abnormal" score and two delays in one domain for a "questionable" score. On the Denver II, in contrast, a child with two delays in only one domain receives an "abnormal" score, and a child with one delay in one domain receives a "questionable" score.

Summary Evaluation

The DDST is widely used in the United States and meets criteria for a well-constructed developmental screening tool. The revision and restandardization should increase test sensitivity; however, the validity of the Denver II has not been established. Physical therapists working in early intervention who are involved in child find programs or in the intake process are most likely to administer the Denver II. The Denver II can also be administered to monitor the development of infants who attend a high-risk infant follow-up clinic or a medical clinic in which a physical therapist is a member of the team. The Denver II is primarily intended for routine use in pediatric well care clinics and in pediatricians' offices to identify infants who, on the basis of an "abnormal" score, should be referred for a diagnostic assessment. For infants who receive an "abnormal" score in the gross motor domain, a referral may be made for a physical therapy assessment.

CRITERION-REFERENCED ASSESSMENTS

Criterion-referenced scales are designed to compare the performance of the infant with external criteria or standards for a particular domain. The items on a criterion-referenced assessment represent the sequential stages, the hierarchy involved in the development, or the mastery of the domain of interest. The infant's score reflects the extent of achievement within the content domain without regard to the performance of other infants of the same age. Curriculum-based assessments and client-centered measures of change are two special types of criterion-referenced scales. Curriculum-based assessments are designed for use in planning and measuring instructional objectives. Behavioral objectives and goal attainment scaling are client-centered measures of change in which criteria for success are specified for the individual infant.

A primary need of physical therapists is for reliable and valid assessments for treatment planning and evaluation of the effects of treatment. Although criterion-referenced assessments are intended for these purposes, few have been constructed specific to the needs of physical therapists. Consequently, assessments based on the rate and sequence of normal motor development are the predominate type of standardized motor assessment used by physical therapists. The responsiveness of motor scales based on normal development is a concern for infants with moderate to severe motor dysfunction. Guyatt et al.[87] define responsiveness as the ability of a test to measure clinically important changes over time. Responsiveness is a special form of validity that is necessary for a test that is used to evaluate the effects of treatment.[53] The limited information on the ability of standardized motor assessments to measure change in children receiving physical therapy partly reflects the fact that the majority of assessments used by physical therapists are constructed by professionals from other disciplines. Furthermore, children who receive physical therapy are heterogeneous in terms of age, diagnosis, and degree of involvement. The Gross Motor Function Measure, whose authors include physiotherapists, and the Erhardt Developmental Prehension Assessment, whose author is an occupational therapist, are two criterion-referenced assessments constructed for use in treatment planning and evaluation of the effects of treatment.

Gross Motor Function Measure††

Brief Description of the Test

The Gross Motor Function Measure[88] (GMFM) was recently constructed by a group of physiotherapists, physicians, and a biostatistician at McMaster University in Ontario, Canada. The GMFM was designed to evaluate change in gross motor function of children with cerebral palsy, to describe a child's current level of function, and to assist in treatment planning. The GMFM is intended for use in both clinical and research settings. The test consists of a manual and scoring forms. The manual lists the necessary equipment, which is common to physical therapy clinics.

The GMFM consists of 88 items divided among five domains: lying and rolling; sitting; crawling and kneeling; standing; and walking, running, and jumping. Items were selected to represent motor functions typically performed by children without motor problems by age 5 years. The focus is not only on what a child can do but also on the quality of performance. This is accomplished by use of a four-point rating scale. A score of 0 indicates that the child does not initiate the movement, a score of 1 indicates that the child initiates but completes less than 10 percent of the movement, a score of 2 indicates that the child partially completes the movement, and a score of 3 indicates that the child successfully completes the movement. Specific criteria are provided for scoring each item.

Standardized instructions for administration of the GMFM are included in the manual. A demonstration and three trials are allowed for each item. No specific instructions are required, and verbal encouragement may be provided. The therapist can physically assist the child to assume the starting position but cannot assist the child to perform the item. The authors recommend administering the GMFM with the child in bare feet and without assistive gait devices. The therapist may choose to target one or more domains that reflect the goals of treatment. For each dimension, the total score is expressed as a percentage of the maximum score for that dimension.

Technical Evaluation

Items were selected through a group process that involved the authors and physical therapists from sites used to pilot the GMFM. Six therapists from three centers participated in the reliability studies. The subjects were 12 children who

---

†† The authors of this assessment are Dianne Russell, Peter Rosenbaum, Carolyn Gowland, Susan Hardy, Mary Lane, Nancy Plews, Heather McGavin, David Cadman, and Sheila Jarvis. It was published in 1990 by Gross Motor Measures Group, c/o Dianne Russell, Building 74, Room 29, Station 9, Hamilton, ON, Canada L8N 3Z5.

were selected to represent a spectrum of ages and motor disabilities. Intraclass correlation coefficients of 0.92 or higher for both inter-rater and intrarater reliability were reported for each domain and for the total score. The one exception was inter-rater realiability for the lying and rolling domain, for which the correlation was 0.87.

Responsiveness of the GMFM is supported based on several methods of analysis. The procedures used by the authors are of interest, since the responsiveness of motor assessments has not been routinely examined. The sample included 86 children with cerebral palsy, 25 children with acute head injury, and 34 children without motor delays who ranged in age from less than 3 years to adolescence. Subjects were administered the GMFM and then retested 6 months later. In the absence of an accepted external standard of motor change for children with motor dysfunction, concurrent validity was examined three ways. Change scores on the GMFM were correlated with the ratings of independent physical therapists who viewed videotapes of the initial and follow-up test for 28 children. Each child's parent and physical therapist also completed a questionnaire that rated change. The correlation between GMFM change scores and the videotape scores was 0.82. Correlations between GMFM change scores and questionnaire ratings was 0.54 for the parent and 0.65 for the therapist.

Further analysis indicated that children rated by both a parent and the therapist as having made no change did not make significant change on the GMFM, whereas children rated as having made change did make significant change on the GMFM. Change was also examined for each group. Children with acute head injury had higher change scores than children with cerebral palsy. For children without delays, those who were under age 3 years made greater gains than those who were older, confirming that the GMFM is weighted toward motor functions that develop during the first 3 years.

Qualitative Evaluation

The GMFM can be administered in 45 to 60 minutes, depending on whether the child is able to walk. The test was constructed for use by physical therapists; however, qualifications for testing have not been determined. The authors plan to offer workshops for therapists interested in using the GMFM. Instructions for administration are clear, although the distinction between use of arms to stabilize oneself versus an external support is not explicit. The criteria for assigning scores are based on distinct differences in patterns of movement, time, and number of steps. GMFM items are of clinical importance, which is a strength for treatment planning. Rolling, cruising, and transitional movements are scored separately for the right and left. Sixty-eight items are below the level of independent walking, and all movement transitions are included. The GMFM includes items for both floor sitting and bench sitting, which is unique compared with norm-referenced scales. The focus is on transition onto and off of a large and small bench; however, only one item is included to rate balance in bench sitting. Items can be repeated with the child wearing an orthosis or using an assistive device, although progression from orthosis to no orthosis and from ambulation with assistive devices to no assistive device has not been formally incorporated into the scoring procedure.

Summary Evaluation

The GMFM was designed to evaluate change in children with motor dysfunction and hopefully will serve as a model for additional tests designed to measure change in clinical populations. As research on reliability and validity is performed, recommendations will undoubtedly be made for further development. The GMFM appears to be more suited for children over age 2 years with moderate to severe motor dysfunction but who can follow simple directions or demonstrations. Administration to infants under 1 year would provide a baseline to evaluate change and should assist in treatment planning.

Erhardt Developmental Prehension Assessment‡‡

Brief Description of the Test

The Erhardt Developmental Prehension Assessment[89] (EDPA) was constructed by an occupational therapist to describe the essential components of prehension that develop between birth and 15 months. The EDPA is intended for use in the assessment and treatment planning of children with fine motor dysfunction. The test consists of a manual and scoring forms that can be reproduced. The materials needed are specified and include rattles, cubes, pellets, and a pencil. The EDPA was constructed based on developmental theory, clinical observation, and other developmental tests. The manual is published as part of a book[89] that also includes a model of prehension used to develop the EDPA and three in-depth case studies.

The EDPA is divided into three sections: primary involuntary arm–hand patterns, primary voluntary movements, and pre-writing skills. Sections are divided by skill clusters. Six skill clusters are in section 1, nine in section 2, and two in section 3. The arms at rest during play in supine and in prone; the asymetrical tonic neck reflex; and the grasping, placing, and avoiding responses are the skill clusters for section 1. The arms on approach in supine, prone, and sitting; grasp of the dowel, cube, and pellet; manipulation; and release of the dowel and pellet are the skill clusters for section 2. Pencil grasp and drawings are the skill clusters for section 3. For each skill cluster, items are arranged by

‡‡ The author of this assessment is Rhoda P. Erhardt. It was published in 1982 as (the manual is part of the book) *Developmental Hand Dysfunction: Theory–Assessment–Treatment* by RAMSCO Publishing Company, P.O. Box N, Laurel, MD 20707.

developmental level and contain one or more pattern components that describe the quality of movement. More than 300 pattern components are included throughout the assessment. Each hand is scored separately. The EDPA is not standardized.

Pattern components are scores using a four-symbol ordinal scale (++, +, +/– or ±, –). The same four symbols are used to score each item. A score of ++ indicates that all pattern components have been replaced by more mature patterns, + indicates that all pattern components are present, +/– or ± indicates that some pattern components are present, and – indicates that no pattern components are present. Detailed instructions for scoring pattern components are not provided, nor are specific guidelines for interpretation of the results. The case studies are used to provide examples for goal setting, treatment planning, and measurement of progress.

Technical Evaluation

Studies on reliability and validity of the EDPA are not reported in the manual. Inter-rater reliability is reported for an earlier shorter version of the EDPA. Sixteen occupational therapists scored from videotape the performance of four children with cerebral palsy. Agreement with the test author ranged from 71.6 to 95.5 percent. Tomacelli and Palisano[90] examined construct and concurrent validity with the Peabody Developmental Fine Motor Scale. Both assessments were administered to 32 healthy infants less than 12 months of age. Operationally defined age equivalents for the right and left hands on the EDPA were compared to the normed age equivalents on the PDMS. Correlations between scores on the two tests were 0.95 (EDPA right hand) and 0.94 (EDPA left hand), supporting construct validity of the EDPA. Despite clear differences in content between the two assessments, the high correlations suggest that for healthy infants achievement of requisite posture, patterns of reaching, and automatic grasp (assessed by EDPA) are related to achievement of voluntary grasp and manipulation (assessed by PDMS). Mean EDPA scores for both the right and left hands were significantly higher than the mean PDMS score. The significant difference in mean age equivalents does not support concurrent validity and reflects the fact that the EDPA is not normed and does not provide a method of obtaining a total score.

Qualitative Evaluation

The time needed to administer the EDPA varies from 30 to 60 minutes, depending on the child and on the experience of the examiner. Physical therapists who are not familiar with components of reach, grasp, and release are likely to experience difficulty, particularly since instructions for administration of each item are not provided.

Summary Evaluation

The EDPA is a criterion-referenced assessment that is potentially responsive to change in the prehension of infants with fine motor dysfunction. The EDPA has several strengths for assessment and treatment planning of infants with identified fine motor dysfunction, including administration of items to both the right and left, emphasis on quality of movement, and incorporation of posture, reach, grasp, and manipulation within a single test. The lack of standardization, guidelines for interpretation of scores, and information on reliability and validity are areas of weakness.

Curriculum-Based Developmental Assessments

Curriculum-based assessments are a type of criterion-referenced assessment designed to measure student achievement specific to the content that is taught in the school curriculum. The purpose of assessing a student's mastery of the school curriculum is to determine instructional needs. Proponents of curriculum-based assessments argue that national norm-referenced tests are not specific to a school's curriculum and therefore, have limited value for instructional planning. Curriculum-based assessments are especially suited for special education settings in which students receive an individualized education plan. The passage of PL 94-142 in 1975 created an unprecedented need for eductional curricula for students under the age of 6 years with special needs. A number of instructional curricula and companion assessments have been published during the past 15 years in response to this need.

Bailey et al.[91] performed an informative analysis of published curricula and curriculum-based assessments intended for use in early intervention programs. Fifteen commercially available curricula published prior to 1983 were reviewed. Each curriculum was examined for (1) theoretical perspective, (2) teaching and learning strategies utilized, and (3) methods of assessing development. Bailey and associates identified three perspectives that have influenced content of curricula for infants with special needs. One perspective is that development of infants with special needs can be defined by the successive mastery of normal developmental milestones. A second perspective is that cognitive and language development are best understood within the theoretical framework of sensorimotor development described by Jean Piaget. A third perspective is that development of infants with special needs should emphasize acquisition of functional skills that have a high probability of improving independence. Content of all 15 of the curricula reviewed were based on normal development. Eight of the curricula reviewed were exclusively based on normal development, four also included components based on Piaget's theory of development, and three also included functional components. The vast majority of curricula did not present evidence to support feasibility and effectiveness. Methods of instruction were variable. Four curricula used an experiential model of teaching that emphasizes providing the infant a variety of opportunities to interact with the environment.

Six curricula used a behavioral model in which the teacher or therapist assumes a more directive and active role. These curricula placed greater emphasis on task analysis and instructional strategies. Five curricula used a combination of experiential and behavioral models.

All of the curricula addressed multiple domains of development, including motor development. Assessments varied in the number of items included in the birth to 24-month age levels. The number of items for each assessment ranged from 49 to 507, with a mean of 270. Explicit instructions for administering and scoring items were not provided in all of the assessments, and none were completely standardized. Although results are frequently presented using age levels, none of the assessments are normed. Information on reliability and validity was presented for only one assessment.

Curriculum-based assessments are designed for administration by an interdisciplinary or transdisciplinary team. Ideally, each team member participates in administration of the assessment. Based on the results, the team and family develop goals for the infant. The curriculum provides instructional activities for each goal. A concern of physical therapists is that, although curriculum-based assessments are intended to reflect goals of intervention for infants with delays or disorders in motor development, items primarily reflect normal motor milestones and do not emphasize the quality of movement. Methods of instruction often differ from treatment approaches advocated by many physical therapists, including NDT and sensory integration. Instructional activities generally do not consider the cause of an infant's motor delay and may not be appropriate for all infants. Furthermore, the focus of instructional activities tends to be on specific training of developmental milestones, with little attention given to motor behaviors that may be a prerequisite for successful emergence of a posture or movement.

The three curriculum-based assessments selected for discussion are critiqued collectively to enhance comparison and contrast. The assessments are (1) Early Developmental Profile (Volume 2 of Developmental Programming for Infants and Young Children)[§§]; (2) Hawaii Early Learning Profile[|||]; and (3) The Carolina Curriculum for Infants and Toddlers With Special Needs.[¶¶]

Brief Description of the Tests

The Early Intervention Developmental Profile (EIDP),[92] the Hawaii Early Learning Profile (HELP),[93] and the Carolina Curriculum for Infants and Toddlers With Special Needs (CCITSN)[94] are all used in early intervention programs

---

§§ The authors are Sally J. Rodgers, Carol M. Donovon, Diane B. D'Eugenio, Sara L. Brown, Eleanor Whiteside Lynch, Martha S. Moersch, and D. Sue Schafer. The revised edition was published in 1981 by The University of Michigan Press, P.O. Box 1104, Ann Arbor, MI 48106.

||| The authors are Setsu Furuno, Katherine A. O'Reilly, Carol M. Hosaka, Takayo T. Inatsuka, Toney L. Allman, and Barbara Zeislot. The revised edition was published in 1985 by VORT Corporation, P.O. Box 60132, Palo Alto, CA 94306.

¶¶ The authors are Nancy Johnson-Martin, Kenneth G. Jens, Susan M. Attermeier, and Bonnie J. Hacker. The second edition was published in 1991 by Paul H. Brookes Publishing Company, P.O. Box 10624, Baltimore, MD 21285.

throughout the United States. Each of the assessments has a physical therapist as an author and consists of a manual, scoring booklets or charts, and instructional activities for each assessment item. Test materials are not provided but are common to early intervention programs. The EIDP and HELP tests are designed to assess infants and children who function below the 36-month age level, while the CCITSN assesses children below the 24-month level of development. The EIDP and HELP each consists of six domains: cognition, language, social–emotional, self-care, fine motor, and gross motor. The EIDP has 299 items, and the HELP has 650. The CCITSN consists of five domains (cognition, communication, social adaptation, fine motor skills, and gross motor skills) that are divided into 26 curriculum or teaching sequences. Within each curriculum sequence, items are arranged according to skill progression. None of the assessments require specific training to administer.

The HELP test is based on the normal development sequence, while the EIDP and CCITSN are based on normal development and Piaget's theory of early cognitive development. The CCITSN is unique in placing emphasis on adaptive functional skills. The gross motor domain for the EIDP differs from the other assessments by including items on integration of primitive reflexes and development of automatic reactions. The EIDP also has the most explicit instructions for administration and scoring while procedures for administering the HELP are not standardized. Items on the EIDP, HELP, and CCITSN are scored pass–fail. Based on the examiner's judgment, an infant's performance on an item may also be scored as partially successful. The EIDP and CCITSN provide guidelines for establishing basal and ceiling levels. For the CCITSN a child must successfully perform an item for three of five trials to reach the teaching criterion.

Technical Evaluation

Items on the EIDP, HELP, and CCITSN were adapted from other developmental assessments and child development literature. Authors of the HELP and CCITSN report having field-tested the curriculum and assessment, but details are provided only for the CCITSN. The EIDP provides methods for estimating age equivalents and DQs. Scores, however, are not norm-referenced. Estimates of age levels are provided for each item on the HELP and for developmental sequences on the CCITSN.

Inter-rater reliability was examined for the EIDP by having nine raters score 100 items from videotape. Agreement between the tester and nine observers ranged from 80 to 97 percent with a mean of 89 percent. Inter-rater reliability of 96.9 percent agreement is reported for the first edition of the CCITSN based on two examiners having simultaneously scored the performance of 88 children. Information on reliability is not reported in the HELP manual.

Concurrent validity of the EIDP was examined in 14 children by correlation of the infants' scores on each domain of the EIDP with their scores on five other assessments, including the BSID. The majority of correlations were above 0.80 and ranged from 0.33 to 0.96. Two studies have been conducted to examine the concurrent validity and responsiveness of the EIDP gross motor domain and the Peabody Gross Motor Scale in infants receiving early intervention.[95,96] Haley et al.[95] compared the EIDP and Peabody by administering both assessments to 71 infants with motor delays. High correlations were found that support concurrent validity of the EIDP. Using an effect size statistic, the investigators reported that the Peabody Gross Motor Scale detected a greater amount of change over a 6-month period. Jones and Palisano[96] administered the EIDP and PDMS to 21 infants with motor delays three times over a 6-month period and reported that mean EIDP and Peabody age-equivalent scores increased significantly at 3 months and 6 months and the mean gain scores between the two assessments did not differ significantly. In both studies, the majority of infants had a diagnosis of nonspecific developmental delay, but both studies included infants with Down syndrome and cerebral palsy. Although the question of which gross motor scale is more responsive to change is unresolved, the results suggest that the EIDP is able to detect change over a 6-month period in infants with motor delays.

The ability to measure change has also been reported for the first edition of the CCITSN, the Carolina Curriculum for Handicapped Infants and Infants at Risk (CCHI).[97] As part of field testing, 92 children were retested on the CCHI at 3- and 6-month intervals. Children who were mildly or moderately handicapped made the most progress. The results suggest that 3 months was too short an interval to measure change for children with severe and profound handicaps. Validity for the HELP has not been reported.

Qualitative Evaluation

The EIDP can be administered in 1 hour or less. Time to administer the HELP and CCITSN is not addressed in the manuals. All assessments are designed to be administered by professionals from a number of disciplines, and formal training is not required. Since all three assessments are at least partially based on normal development, they contain many similar items. When administering the EIDP, HELP, and CCITSN the examiner is encouraged to record relevant information on how items were administered for uniformity upon retesting. The CCITSN format most effectively integrates assessment and instruction, particularly for infants with moderate to severe developmental disorders. Instructional activities for the CCITSN are the most process oriented, providing suggestions for incorporating activities into daily care and modifications for infants with motor, visual, or hearing impairments. Physical therapists should find most instructional strategies compatible with their discipline-specific approaches. Activities for each EIDP and HELP items are more general and not as integrated.

Summary Evaluation

From a technical standpoint, the CCITSN best meets the criteria of a well-constructed curriculum-based assessment. The CCITSN assessment format is most conducive to instructional programming and provides a direct measure of the effectiveness of intervention. Greater evidence of reliability and validity is published for the EIDP, than for the CCITSN and HELP. Perhaps because of this and the most specific guidelines for scoring, the EIDP has been used in program evaluations, including a comparison of progress in early intervention made by infants with different diagnoses.[98,99]

Individual Criterion-Referenced Measures

The behavioral objective and goal attainment scaling are unique types of criterion-referenced scales in that both the behaviors of interest and the criteria for success are based on the goals of the individual client. For infants receiving physical therapy, goals are established by the physical therapist in collaboration with the family and often other professionals providing early intervention services. Compared with norm-referenced assessments, individual criterion-referenced measures offer several advantages for evaluation of infants receiving physical therapy. Goals can be written that will measure the direct effects of the physical therapy. Criteria for success can represent important progress that is smaller than the change needed to pass items on a norm-referenced scale. Emphasis can also be placed on the quality of movement. The reliance on the clinical judgment of the person(s) who determine criteria for success is a potential limitation in that the infant's potential may be over- or underestimated.

Physical therapists in pediatric practice are familiar with the behavioral objective. The enactment of PL 94-142 mandated that children receiving special education receive an individualized education plan (IEP) that includes annual goals and short-term objectives. Physical therapists working in educational settings use the behavioral objective format to write IEP goals in the motor and self-care domains. The behavioral objective also provides physical therapists employed in pediatric acute care and rehabilitation hospitals a method to document objectively short-term treatment goals.

A behavioral objective has five components.[100] First, the learner or the person for whom the objective is being written is identified. Second, the target behavior is identified (the behavior must be observable, repeatable, and have a definite beginning and end). Third, the conditions are stated under which the behavior will be measured (examples of conditions are the setting, instructions, verbal or sensory cues, physical assistance, assistive devices, and adaptive equipment). Fourth, criteria for success are stated in measurable terms. (Time and distance are well suited for objective measurement of posture and movement. Observable anatomic relationships such as walking using a heel–toe progression and maintaining a prone posture with weight on forearms and elbows vertically in line with the shoulder are examples of criteria used to measure quality of movement. Criteria for success may also be expressed as the percentage of correct responses and rate of performance [frequency of a behavior within a specified time span].) Fifth, a time frame is stated for achievement of the objective. Examples of behavioral objectives are presented in Table 9-2.

Table 9-2. Comparison of Behavioral Objectives and Goal Attainment Scaling

Goal for 10-month-old infant for a 6-month period
  Behavioral Objective Format
    During freeplay, Anthony will creep reciprocally 10 feet
  Goal Attainment Scaling Format
    During freeplay, Anthony will
      −2 = Assume and maintain quadruped for 5 seconds
      −1 = Creep 3 feet using any pattern
       0 = Creep reciprocally 10 feet
      +1 = Creep reciprocally 20 feet
      +2 = +1 and creep up two steps using arms/legs
Goal for 18-month-old infant for a 6-month period
  Behavioral Objective Format
    When a toy is placed on a waist high surface, Jenna will pull to stand through half-kneeling
  Goal Attainment Scaling Format
    When a toy is placed on a waist high surface, Jenna will
      −2 = Pull partway to standing using primarily her arms
      −1 = Pull to stand with partial leg movement through half-kneeling
       0 = Pull to stand through half-kneeling
      +1 = 0 and lower herself from standing to floor sitting in any manner
      +2 = 0 and lower herself from standing to floor sitting with controlled trunk and leg
            movements

A study by Harris[63] on the effects of NDT on motor performance of infants with Down syndrome provides evidence to support the use of behavioral objectives to evaluate the short-term effects of treatment. The experimental group of infants received NDT three times a week for a 9-week period in addition to the weekly early intervention received by the control group. The groups did not differ significantly on gain scores for the BSID and the experimental edition of the PDMS. Infants in the NDT group, however, achieved a significantly higher number of individualized behavioral objectives. Harris attributed the discrepancy between the outcome measures to the fact that the behavioral objectives were direct measures of the goals of NDT.

Goal attainment scaling (GAS)[101] was originally designed to evaluate mental health services but recently has been applied to evaluation of children with developmental disabilities,[102] including infants receiving physical therapy as part of early intervention services.[103,104] Like the behavioral objective, goal attainment scaling requires selection of goals that are observable and repeatable, specification of the conditions under which performance is measured, statement of criteria for success in measurable terms, and a time frame for achievement of the goal. A unique feature of GAS is the inclusion of not only the expected outcome for each goal but also two possible levels of attainment that are less favorable and two possible levels that are more favorable than the expected outcome. By convention, scores of −2 and −1 represent the two less favorable levels of attainment, a score of 0 represents the expected level of attainment, and scores of +1 and +2 represent the two levels of attainment that exceed expectations. The infant's initial level of attainment is typically represented by a score of −2. For infants who might lose function, the initial level of attainment can be represented by a score of −1. A comparison of behavior objective and GAS formats is presented in Table 9-2.

The ability to compute a single change score for multiple goals and to weight each goal are other useful features of GAS. GAS may be used to evaluate achievement of goals for multiple areas of development or a single area such as motor development. The simplest method of expressing the change score is to subtract the sum of the follow-up scores from the sum of the initial scores. Kiresuk and Sherman[101] have derived a formula for determining a standard score that reflects the composite change score for multiple scores. The standard score is expressed as a T-score with a mean equal to 50 and a standard deviation of 10. Weights are based on the relative importance of each goal. For example, a physical therapist may select three goals for an infant and assign weights of 3, 2, and 1. The goal assigned a weight of 3 would receive the most emphasis in treatment and the goal assigned a weight of 1 the least emphasis. When determining the change score for weighted goals, the score for each goal (-2 to $+2$) is multiplied by the weight. Clark and Caudrey[105] have proposed a method to compute the T-score by assigning weights to each goal according to both importance and difficulty. Their recommendation addresses the conflict that arises when the most important goal for a child is also the most difficult. The reader is referred to Ottenbacher and Cusick[106] for a description of GAS and suggestions for clinical applications in rehabilitation.

The concurrent validity of GAS and the PDMS has been examined.[103,104] Heavlin and associates[107] proposed that the unique properties of GAS should result in low to moderate concurrent validity with norm-referenced scales. Stephens and Haley[103] selected for 54 infants with motor delays either one or two goals that were related to achievement of gross and fine motor milestones. Change was measured for a 6-month period. An innovative method was used to adjust GAS change scores to account for rate of development. Correlations of 0.35 and 0.14 were reported between GAS change scores for two goals and change in scaled score on the PDMS, indicating low concurrent validity. Palisano et al.[104] re-examined concurrent validity using the GAS T-score and the PDMS age equivalent. The subjects were the 54 included in the study by Stephens and Haley[103] plus 11 additional subjects. Two goals were selected for each infant and included not only goals that measured achievement of a motor milestone but also goals that reflected improved quality of movement, function, and range of motion. The correlation between GAS T-scores for gross motor goals and Peabody Gross Motor Scale age-equivalent change scores was 0.44. The correlation between GAS T-Scores for fine motor goals and Peabody Fine Motor Scale age-equivalent change scores was 0.18. The findings support those of Stephens and Haley[103] and suggest that differences exist in the aspects of motor performance that are measured by GAS and the PDMS.

The ability of GAS to measure change in motor development for infants receiving physical therapy has also been investigated. In the study by Stephens and Haley, [103] the sensitivity of GAS was compared with that of the PDMS. Large effect sizes were found, indicating that the infants made changes on both measures. Effect sizes for the PDMS were smaller than for the unadjusted GAS but larger than the effect sizes for the adjusted GAS. The ability of GAS to measure change was investigated further in 65 infants receiving physical therapy, occupational therapy, or both as part of an early intervention program.[104] The infants ranged from 3 to 30 months. Fifteen infants were diagnosed as having Down syndrome, 8 cerebral palsy, 4 myelomeningocele, and 1 autism. The remaining infants demonstrated delayed motor development. The therapist for each infant selected two motor goals for a 6-month period. Goals were put into GAS format, with a score of −2 representing the infants' initial level of attainment. Testing was performed by independent examiners. The mean GAS T-score was 55.4, which was significantly higher than the expected mean of 50, indicating that the change made by the infants' exceeded the therapist's expectations. Only one infant did not demonstrate change on both goals, while 13 attained scores of +2 for both goals.

In a third study, Palisano[108] compared the ability of GAS and behavioral objectives to measure change in individualized gross motor goals. The subjects were 21 infants who were receiving physical therapy as part of early intervention. The subjects ranged from 4 to 24 months of age and represented a heterogeneous group. Two gross motor goals were developed for a 3-month period, and then two new goals were developed for a second 3-month period. Goals were put into both behavioral objective and GAS formats. The criteria for passing the behavioral objective were equivalent to a score of 0 for GAS, and a score of −2 represented the infants' level of attainment at the start of the study. An independent examiner put all goals into GAS and behavioral objective format, and a second independent examiner performed the testing. The infants passed 83 percent of their behavioral objectives. The mean GAS T-score was 53.0 for the first 3 months and 60.3 for the second 3 months. The mean for the second 3 months was significantly higher than the expected mean of 50. Of the 17 behavioral objectives that were failed, the corresponding GAS documented progress toward the expected outcome for 2 (12 percent) of the goals. In contrast, of the 67 behavioral objectives passed, the corresponding GAS score documented progress that exceeded the expected outcome for 49 (73 percent) of the goals. The results indicate that both GAS and behavioral objectives measured change in infants receiving physical therapy. GAS, however, measured change that exceeded criteria for passing the behavioral objectives, suggesting that GAS is the more responsive measure.

The properties of behavioral objectives and GAS are well suited for measurement of qualitative change and small but clinically important improvement in the motor development of infants receiving physical therapy. Compared with norm-referenced scales, an advantage of individualized measures of change is the ability to account for the potential impact of relevant child, family, and program factors when selecting goals and expected outcomes. The validity of individualized measures of change, however, is dependent on the physical therapist making accurate judgments regarding an infant's potential for change and the impact of intervention. Research suggests that both behavioral objectives and GAS are able to measure change in infants receiving physical therapy and that GAS is the more responsive measure. Research also suggests that differences exist between client-centered measures of change and norm-referenced scales, and hence potential benefits may result from using both to obtain a comprehensive evaluation of change in infants with motor delays. In the studies reviewed, the PDMS provided a global measure of change in motor development while GAS measured change in postures and movement that were directly related to the goals of intervention.

SUMMARY

The role of physical therapists in the management of infants with delays or disorders in motor development has expanded to include participation in high-risk infant follow-up clinics, interdisciplinary diagnostic assessments, and inter-disciplinary and transdisciplinary assessments performed by early intervention teams. Physical therapists are also increasingly aware of the need to document objectively the effects of physical therapy. Documentation is becoming particularly important to physical therapists who contract their services or work in private practice. As practice moves toward greater autonomy, the use of standardized neuromotor and developmental assessments is necessary both to complement and to substantiate the pediatric physical therapist's clinical impressions.

Infants referred to physical therapy are a diverse group, and therefore neuromotor and developmental assessments are selected on an individual basis. Test selection is complicated by the limited number of assessments that have been developed specifically for infants with motor dysfunction, the large number of assessments that require further test construction, and the lack of research on the ability of assessments to measure changes made by infants with motor dysfunction. Furthermore, as theoretical assumptions regarding the significance of findings for passive muscle tone and elicited primitive reflexes and automatic reactions are questioned, physical therapists are challenged to reconsider traditional neuromotor assessment practices. Factors to consider when selecting an assessment include the purpose of testing, the infant's age, diagnosis, degree of motor involvement, and goals of physical therapy. Norm-referenced assessments are most appropriate when the purpose is to determine whether an infant has a motor delay or to determine eligibility for early intervention. Criterion-referenced assessments offer advantages for treatment planning and evaluation of the effects of physical therapy. For many infants, use of both a norm-referenced and a criterion-referenced assessment is recommended. The norm-referenced motor assessment enables the physical therapist to document the infant's level of development and to monitor general progress, while the criterion-referenced assessment serves as a measure of the direct effects of physical therapy. Careful selection and interpretation of neuromotor and developmental assessments are integral to the decision-making process and provision of quality physical therapy to infants with delays or disorders in motor development.

REFERENCES

1. Bobath B: The very early treatment of cerebral palsy. Dev Med Child Neurol 9:37, 1967
2. Lewko JH: Current practices in evaluating motor behavior of disabled children. Am J Occup Ther 30:413, 1976
3. Campbell SK: Measurement and technical skills—neglected aspects of research education. Phys Ther 61:523, 1981
4. Ellenberg JH, Nelson KB: Early recognition of infants at high risk for cerebral palsy: examination at age four months. Dev Med Child Neurol 23:705, 1981
5. Harris SR: Early neuromotor predictors of cerebral palsy in low-birth-weight infants. Dev Med Child Neurol 29:508, 1987
6. Drillien CM, Thomson AFM, Buroyne K: Low-birth-weight children at early school age: a longitudinal study. Dev Med Child Neurol 22:26, 1980
7. Coolman RB, Bennett FC, Sells CJ et al: Neuromotor development of graduates of the neonatal intensive care unit: patterns encountered in the first two years of life. J Dev Behav Pediatr 6:327, 1985
8. Nelson KB, Ellenberg JH: Children who "outgrew" cerebral palsy. Pediatrics 69:529, 1982
9. Georgieff MK, Bernbaum JC: Abnormal shoulder girdle muscle tone in premature infants during their first 18 months of life. Pediatrics 77:664, 1986
10. Amiel-Tison C: A method of neurologic evaluation within the first year of life. Curr Probl Pediatr 7:1, 1976
11. Andre-Thomas, Chesni Y, Saint-Anne Dargassies S: The Neurological Examination of the Infant. Little Club Clinics in Developmental Medicine, No. 1. National Spastics Society, London, 1960
12. Saint-Anne Dargassies S: Neurological Development in the Full-Term and Premature Neonate. Excerpta Medica, New York, 1977
13. Katz RT, Rymer WZ: Spastic hypertonia: mechanisms and measurement. Arch Phys Med Rehabil 70:144, 1989
14. Chapman CE, Wiesendanger M: The physiological and anatomical basis of spasticity: a review. Physiother Can 34:125, 1982
15. Craik RL: Abnormalities of motor behavior. p 155. In Lister MJ (ed): Contemporary Management of Motor Control Problems: Proceedings of the II STEP Conference. The Foundation for Physical Therapy, Alexandria, VA, 1991
16. Kathrein JE: Interrater reliability in the assessment of muscle tone of infants and children. Phys Occup Ther Pediatr 10(1):27, 1990
17. Harris SR, Haley SM, Tada WL et al: Reliability of observational measures of the Movement Assessment of Infants. Phys Ther 64:471, 1984
18. Fiorentino MR: Reflex Testing Methods for Evaluation of CNS Development. Charles C Thomas, Springfield, IL, 1965
19. Bobath B: Abnormal Postural Reflex Activity Caused by Brain Lesions. 3rd Ed. Aspen Systems Corp, Rockville, MD, 1985
20. Hoskins T, Squires J: Developmental assessment: a test for gross motor and reflex development. Phys Ther 53:117, 1973
21. Wilson J: A developmental reflex test. p. 335. In Vulpe S: The Vulpe Assessment Battery. National Institute on Mental Retardation, Toronto, Ontario, Canada, 1977
22. Milani-Comparetti A: Pattern analysis of normal and abnormal development: the fetus, the newborn, the child. p. 1. In Slaton DS (ed): Development of Movement

in Infancy. University of North Carolina at Chapel Hill, Division of Physical Therapy, Chapel Hill, NC, 1980

23. Zelazo PR, Zelazo NA, Kolb S: "Walking" in the newborn. Science 176:314, 1972
24. Thelen E, Fisher DM, Ridley-Johnson R: The relationship between physical growth and a newborn reflex. Inf Behav Dev 7:479, 1984
25. Zelazo PR: From reflexive to instrumental behavior. p. 87. In Lipsitt L (ed): Developmental Psychobiology: the Significance of Infancy. Lawrence Erlbaum Associates, Inc., Hillside, NJ, 1976
26. Thelen E: Developmental origins of motor coordination: leg movements in human infants. Dev Psychobiol 18:1, 1985
27. Horak FB: Assumptions underlying motor control for neurologic rehabilitation. p. 11. In Lister MJ (ed): Contemporary Management of Motor Control Problems: Proceedings of the II STEP Conference. The Foundation for Physical Therapy, Alexandria, VA, 1991
28. Brooks VB: Motor control. Phys Ther 63:664, 1983
29. Thelen E, Kelso JAS, Fogel A: Self-organizing systems and infant motor development. Dev Rev 7:39, 1987
30. Heriza C: Motor development: traditional and contemporary theories. p. 99. In Lister MJ (ed): Contemporary Management of Motor Control Problems: Proceedings of the II STEP Conference. The Foundation for Physical Therapy, Alexandria, VA, 1991
31. Bernstein N: The Coordination and Regulation of Movement. Pergamon Press, Ltd., London, England, 1967
32. Craik RL: Recovery processes: maximizing function. p. 155. In Lister MJ (ed): Comtemporary Management of Motor Control Problems: Proceedings of the II STEP Conference. The Foundation for Physical Therapy, Alexandria, VA, 1991
33. Keshner EA: How theoretical framework biases evaluation and treatment. p. 37. In Lister MJ (ed): Contemporary Management of Motor Control Problems: Proceedings of the II STEP Conference. The Foundation for Physical Therapy, Alexandria, VA, 1991
34. Fetters L: Measurement and treatment in cerebral palsy: an argument for a new approach. Phys Ther 71:244, 1991
35. Chandler LS, Skillen M, Swanson MW: Movement Assessment of Infants: a Manual. Authors, Rolling Bay, WA, 1980
36. Palisano RJ: Review of research on reliability and validity of the Movement Assessment of Infants. Pediatr Phys Ther 1:167, 1989
37. Haley SM, Harris SR, Tada WL et al: Item reliability of the Movement Assessment of Infants. Phys Occup Ther Pediatr 6(1):21, 1986
38. Schneider JW, Lee W, Chasnoff IJ: Field testing of the Movement Assessment of Infants. Phys Ther 68:321, 1988
39. Harris SR: Early detection of cerebral palsy: sensitivity and specificity of two motor assessment tools. J Perinatol 7(1):11, 1987
40. Paban M, Piper MC: Early predictors of one year neurodevelopment outcome for at risk infants. Phys Occup Ther Pediatr 7(3):17, 1987
41. Lydic JS, Short MA, Nelson DL: Comparison of two scales for assessing motor development in infants with Down's syndrome. Occup Ther J Res 3:213, 1983
42. Milani-Comparetti A, Gidoni EA: Routine developmental examination in normal and retarded children. Dev Med Child Neurol 9:631,1967
43. Trembath J: The Milani-Comparetti Motor Development Screening Test. Meyer Children's Rehabilitation Institute, Omaha, NE, 1977

44. Stuberg W: Milani-Comparetti Motor Development Screening Test. Rev. Ed. Meyer Children's Rehabilitation Institute, University of Nebraska Medical Center, Omaha, NE, 1987
45. Stuberg WA, White PJ, Miedaner JA, Dehne PR: Item reliability of the Milani-Comparetti Motor Development Screening Test. Phys Ther 69:328, 1989
46. Capute AJ, Accardo PJ, Vining EPG et al: Primitive Reflex Profile. Monographs in Developmental Pediatrics, Vol. 1. University Park Press, Baltimore, MD, 1978
47. Capute AJ, Palmer FB, Shapiro BK et al: Primitive Reflex Profile: a quantitation of primitive reflexes in infancy. Dev Med Child Neurol 26:375, 1984
48. Capute AJ, Shapiro BK, Accardo PJ et al: Motor functions: associated reflex profiles. Dev Med Child Neurol 24:662, 1982
49. Capute AJ, Accardo PJ, Vining EPG et al: Primitive Reflex Profile, Phys Ther 58:1061, 1978
50. Anastasi A: Psychological Testing. 5th Ed. Macmillan, New York, 1982
51. Mettler JL: Commentary. Phys Occup Ther Pediatr 9(2):1, 1989
52. Palisano RJ: Research on the effectiveness of neurodevelopmental treatment. Pediatr Phys Ther 3:143, 1991
53. Rosenbaum PL, Russell DJ, Cadman DT et al: Issues in measuring change in motor function in children with cerebral palsy: a special communication. Phys Ther 70:125, 1990
54. Gesell A, Amatruda CS: Developmental Diagnosis. Paul B Haeber, New York, 1947
55. Palisano RJ: Use of chronological and adjusted age to compare motor development of healthy preterm and fullterm infants. Dev Med Child Neurol 28:180, 1988
56. Bayley N: Bayley Scales of Infant Development. The Psychological Corporation, San Antonio, TX, 1969
57. Kohen-Raz R: Scalogram analysis of some developmental sequences of infant behavior as measured by the Bayley Infant Scale of Mental Development. Genet Psychol Monogr 76:3, 1967
58. Werner EE, Bayley N: The reliability of Bayley's revised scale of mental and motor development during the first year of life. Child Dev 37:39, 1966
59. Campbell SK, Siegel E, Parr CA, Ramey CT: Evidence for the need to renorm the Bayley Scales of Infant Development based on the performance of a population-based sample of 12-month-old infants. TECSE 6(2):83, 1986
60. Coryell J, Provost B, Wilhelm IJ, Campbell SK: Stability of Bayley Motor Scale scores in the first year of life. Phys Ther 69:834, 1989
61. Crowe TK, Deitz JC, Bennett FC: The relationship between the Bayley Scales of Infant Development and preschool gross motor and cognitive performance. Am J Occup Ther 41:374, 1987
62. Palmer FB, Shapiro BK, Wachtel RC et al: The effects of physical therapy on cerebral palsy: a controlled trial in infants with spastic diplegia. N Engl J Med 318:803, 1988
63. Harris SR: Effects of neurodevelopmental therapy on motor performance of infants with Down's syndrome. Dev Med Child Neurol 23:477, 1981
64. Gesell A, Amatruda C: Developmental Diagnosis. Paul B Haeber, New York, 1941
65. Knobloch H, Stevens F, Malone AF: Manual of Developmental Diagnosis: the Administration and Interpretation of the Revised Gesell and Amatruda Developmental and Neurologic Examination. Gesell Developmental Materials, Houston, TX, 1987
66. Schneider JW, Brannen EA: A comparison of two developmental evaluation tools used to assess children with Down's syndrome. Phys Occup Ther Pediatr 4(4):19, 1984

67. Folio RM, Fewell RR: Peabody Developmental Motor Scales and Activity Cards. DLM Teaching Resources, Allen, TX, 1983
68. Harrow AJ: A Taxonomy of the Psychomotor Domain. D. McKay Co., New York, 1972
69. Palisano RJ: Concurrent and predictive validities of the Bayley Motor Scale and the Peabody Developmental Motor Scales. Phys Ther 66:1714, 1986
70. Phillips WE, Campbell SK, Slaton DS, Wilhelm IJ: The relationship between differences in Peabody Developmental Motor Scale performance and cerebral palsy type, abstracted. Totline 14(1):20, 1988
71. Campbell SK, Wilhelm IJ, Phillips W, Slaton DS: Comparative performance of infants on three tests of gross motor development, abstracted. Phys Ther 68:818, 1988
72. Hinderer KA, Richardson PK, Atwater SW: Clinical implications of the Peabody Developmental Motor Scales: a constructive review. Phys Occup Ther Pediatr 9(2):81, 1989
73. Palisano RJ: Commentary. Phys Occup Ther Pediatr 9(2):81, 1989
74. Newborg J, Stock JR, Wnek L: Battelle Developmental Inventory. DLM Teaching Resources, Allen, TX, 1984
75. Feldman AB, Haley SM, Coryell J: Concurrent and construct validity of the Pediatric Evaluation of Disability Inventory. Phys Ther 70:602, 1990
76. Frankenburg WF, Fandal AW, Kamper MB: Developmental screening. p. 15. In Frankenburg WF et al (eds): Pediatric Developmental Diagnosis. Stratton, New York, 1981
77. Stangler SR, Huber CJ, Routh DK: Guidelines for screening test assessment. p. 34. In: Screening Growth and Development of Preschool Children: a Guide for Test Selection. McGraw-Hill, New York, 1980
78. Glascoe FP: Developmental screening: rationale, methods, and application. Inf Young Child 4(1):1, 1991
79. Frankenburg WK, Dodds JB, Fandal AW et al: Denver Developmental Screening Test. University of Colorado Medical Center, Denver, CO, 1975
80. Holmes GE, Hassanein RS: The KIDS chart. Am J Dis Child 136:997, 1982
81. Chandler LS: Screening for movement dysfunction. Phys Occup Ther Pediatr 6(3):171, 1986
82. Nickel RE: The Manual for the Infant Motor Screen. The Oregon Health Sciences University, Portland, OR, 1987
83. Nickel RE, Renken CA, Gallenstein JS: The Infant Motor Screen. Dev Med Child Neurol 31:35, 1989
84. Frankenburg WK, Dodds J, Archer P et al: Denver II. Denver Developmental Materials, Denver, CO, 1990
85. Greer S, Bauchner H, Zuckerman B: The Denver Developmental Screening Test: how good is its predictive validity? Dev Med Child Neurol 31:774, 1989
86. Frankenburg WK, van Doorninck WJ, Liddell TN, Dick NP: The Denver Pre-screening Developmental Questionnaire (PDQ). Pediatrics 57:744, 1976
87. Guyatt GH, Walter SD, Norman G: Measuring change over time: assessing the usefulness of evaluative instruments. J Chronic Dis 40:171, 1987
88. Russell D, Rosenbaum P, Gowland C et al: Gross Motor Function Measure. Gross Motor Measures Group, Hamilton, Ontario, Canada, 1990
89. Erhardt RP: Erhardt Developmental Prehension Assessment. RAMSCO, Laurel, MD, 1982
90. Tomacelli DL, Palisano RJ: Concurrent and construct validity of the Erhardt Developmental Prehension Assessment and the Peabody Developmental Fine Motor Scale. Pediatr Phys Ther 2:15, 1990

91. Bailey DB, Jens KG, Johnson N: Curricula for handicapped infants. In Garwood SG, Fewell RR (eds): Educating Handicapped Infants. Aspen, Rockville, MD, 1983
92. Rodgers SJ, Donovon CM, D'Eugenio DB et al: Early intervention Developmental Profile (Vol. 2 of Developmental Programming for Infants and Young Children). The University of Michigan Press, Ann Arbor, MI, 1981
93. Furono S, O'Reilly KA, Hosaka CM et al: Hawaii Early Learning Profile. VORT, Palo Alto, CA, 1985
94. Johnson-Martin N, Jens KG, Attermeier SM, Hacker BJ: The Carolina Curriculum for Infants and Toddlers With Special Needs. Paul H Brookes, Baltimore, MD, 1991
95. Haley SM, Robins SD, Jank PM, Coryell J: Concurrent validity and differential sensitivity of three developmental motor scales, abstracted. Phys Ther 68:818, 1988
96. Jones SL, Palisano RJ: Comparison of the PDMS and EIDP as measures of change in gross motor development in children 4 to 36 months with motor delays, abstracted. Pediatr Phys Ther 3:210, 1991
97. Johnson-Martin N, Jens KG, Attermeier SM: The Carolina Curriculum for Handicapped Infants and Infants at Risk. Paul H Brookes, Baltimore, MD, 1986
98. Holmes GE, Britain LA, Simpson RL, Hassanein RS: Developmental progress in five groups of disabled children attending an early intervention program. Phys Occup Ther Pediatr 7(1):3, 1987
99. Schafer DS, Spalding JB, Bell AP: Potential predictors of child progress as measured by the Early Intervention Developmental Profile. J Div Early Child 11:106, 1987
100. O'Neill DL, Harris SR: Developing goals and objectives for handicapped children. Phys Ther 62:295, 1982
101. Kiresuk T, Sherman R: Goal attainment scaling: a general method of evaluating comprehensive mental health programs. Community Ment Health J 4:443, 1968
102. Bailey BD, Simeonsson RJ: Investigation of use of goal attainment scaling to evaluate individual progress of clients with severe and profound mental retardation. Ment Retard 26:289, 1988
103. Stephens TE, Haley SM: Comparison of two methods for determining change in motorically handicapped children. Phys Occup Ther Pediatr 11(1):1, 1991
104. Palisano RJ, Haley SM, Brown DA: Goal attainment scaling as a measure of change in infants with motor delays. Phys Ther 72:432, 1992
105. Clark MS, Caudrey DJ: Evaluation of rehabilitation services: the use of goal attainment scaling. Int Rehabil Med 5:41, 1986
106. Ottenbacher KJ, Cusick A: Goal attainment scaling as a method of clinical service evaluation. Am J Occup Ther 44:519, 1990
107. Heavlin WD, Lee-Merrow SW, Lewis VM: The psychometric foundations of goal attainment scaling. Community Ment Health J 18:230, 1982
108. Palisano RJ: Comparison of goal attainment scaling and behavioral objectives as methods to evaluate change in motor development in infants receiving physical therapy, abstracted. Phys Ther Suppl 71(6):55S, 1991

10 Functional and Naturalistic Frameworks in Assessing Physical and Motor Disablement

Stephen M. Haley
Mary Jo Baryza
Yvette Blanchard

Over the past decade, a major shift to an action-focused conceptualization of infant movement has occurred. In this model, infant movement is driven by the desire to achieve goal-directed activities, move toward new objects, or explore novel physical environments. Movement does not occur for its own sake or in a vacuum void of context, but rather is a product of the infant's responses to the physical and social factors in his or her world. Current developmental literature emphasizes the analysis of motor skills in the practical context of functional behavior and in a broad theoretical context of perceptual, cognitive, and social behavior.[1,2] A comprehensive physical therapy assessment of motor activity must incorporate this environmental and functional orientation to movement activity.

Theories of motor development have traditionally been concerned with the description of the unfolding of motor competencies over time.[3] Although well accepted for decades, this narrow theoretical framework is now recognized as incomplete. Infant mobility is viewed as more than the emergence of isolated

225

movements and the evolution of different sequences of motor behaviors. Instead motor activity represents the goal-directed action of the whole child functioning in a social environment.[4] The emphasis on goal-directed, functionally based behaviors in motor assessment of infants represents a consistent new theme in the pediatric physical therapy literature.[2,5-7] Such a broadened perspective on motor behavior suggests that physical therapists focus attention on the functional nature of motor performance and on the important characteristics of the naturalistic environments in which an infant develops movement and activity.

Functional and naturalistic orientations to motor assessment challenge us to examine alternative assessment approaches. Rather than a sole focus on the infant's isolated motor capabilities, assessment strategies may involve assessing motor patterns in periods of spontaneous activity, obtaining impressions of function from parents and teachers, directly observing the child in a naturalistic setting, or observing how caregivers and the physical and social environments affect motor activity. In this chapter, we provide a theoretical and conceptual basis for functional and naturalistic frameworks for physical therapy assessment in early infancy. Then we review selected infant motor tests and describe to what extent they incorporate orientation toward functional and naturalistic assessment. Finally, we identify potential applications of these concepts in assessment practices for physical therapists who treat infants with physical and motor disabilities.

THEORETICAL AND CONCEPTUAL APPROACHES

The purpose of this section is to present selected theoretical and conceptual approaches that support the utilization of functional and naturalistic frameworks for the assessment of infants with physical and motor disabilities. We discuss how these approaches can guide the physical therapist's strategies for assessing movement dysfunction in early infancy.

Ecologic Framework

The ecologic perspective on motor and perceptual development is based on the work of James and Eleanor Gibson.[4,8,9] In accounting for the emergence of independent mobility, the Gibsons assign primary importance to the infant's perception of the environment in which he or she develops. An important concept of ecology theory is the concept of affordances, that is, what the environment offers or provides as possibilities for action. For example, physical environments "afford" support surfaces, barriers, and passageways. The Gibsons claim that the infant and environment form a whole, as an active, motivated infant meshes with the affordances of the environment. The perception of the environment, including its physical arrangement and perceived challenges, guides action. Two broad functions of mobility are highlighted: (1) getting from place to place and (2) exploration and gathering information. Mobility and exploratory behaviors are not simply described in terms of motor skills but are directly linked to perceptual and cognitive abilities that help the infant to anticipate and predict outcomes.[10] Infants are viewed as inherently motivated to learn about the world and to develop goals and needs that are specific to a given situation. A constant feedback loop is sustained between mobility and perception. Both systems, in effect, jointly support the infant's need for information gathering and exploratory functions. The ecologic framework provides a compelling argument for pediatric physical therapists to assess movement dysfunction within a broad framework that considers the role of perceptual and environmental factors in the emergence of motor abilities.

Skill Theory

Skill theory represents a broad set of principles based on the work of Fischer et al.[11-13] Skill is defined as an ability to carry out a set of actions in a particular type of task; it is characteristic of neither a person nor a context, but of a person in a specific context.[13,14] The organization of skills and abilities is influenced by parameters such as the nature of the task, environmental conditions, degree of environmental support (physical and social), arousal state, and body structure. Skill theory calls attention to a broad set of parameters that may affect the ability of the infant to perform motor skills during a specific assessment session. The infant's skill level on similar tasks may vary depending on slight variations in the tasks, changes in the infant's state, or a modification of the environment. For example, unfamiliarity with the physical surrounding might influence a child to use crawling instead of upright locomotion. Similarly, a tired child at home might be observed to make the same choice even though upright locomotion is the preferred means of mobility in most other situations.

A corollary approach to skill theory, but one that is focused primarily on the development of motor skill, is the skill acquisition taxonomy developed by Gentile.[15] Her taxonomy identifies relevant task and environmental characteristics that influence the performance of motor skills. This approach emphasizes that activities that have intertrial variability (e.g., walking on uneven surfaces, where each step is different) are much more difficult to learn than more predictable tasks (such as walking across a hard floor with a consistent surface). Gentile's work underscores the importance of considering the nature of the specific task during an assessment of motor skill acquisition. Furthermore, this framework argues that a valid assessment of motor skill can only be made when the assessment tasks and conditions are either identical or as close as possible to the natural tasks and environmental conditions.

Social Context and Vygotsky's "Zone of Proximal Development"

Contextual viewpoints of development consider the active participation of parents and caregivers in the organization (social and physical) of the environment as crucial to the emergence of developmental competencies.[16-18] In Vygotsky's theory of development, the origin of knowledge and skill development is fundamentally social.[19,20] A key concept in Vygotsky's theory is the "zone of proximal development,[21] which is defined as the difference between the infant's level of functioning as determined by his or her independent problem solving and the level of potential performance as seen during problem solving under adult guidance. During the development of functional competencies, parents provide the external help necessary for the successful completion of a task and will take away the help as the child's abilities mature and develop. Parents model and structure the expected functional competencies and provide only the assistance necessary for effective completion of the task by the child. As the child masters more of the necessary components of a task or activity, the adult gradually transfers more of the responsibility to the child.[18] The expectations of the adult directly influence the type of demands placed on the child and, to some extent, the child's level of performance.

An appraisal of the quality and appropriateness of this social training process for functional and mobility skills can be an important part of a therapy assessment[22] and can actually provide a model for assessment and intervention approaches.[23] Lyons[23] advocates an assessment format in which independent performance is viewed as a basal level, and then increasing levels of support are given to determine the maximum level of performance. Consistent with this social contextual view of development are two key components that should be included in a physical therapy motor assessment: (1) determination of the level of help given to an infant in order to perform a task and (2) assessment of the parent's strategies for challenging the infant to a higher level of performance. During intervention, therapists often develop home programs aimed at teaching parents how to determine the proper mixture of physical challenge, assistance, and support.

Ecocultural Theory

An interesting perspective for the understanding of the importance of family adaptation and accommodation is the ecocultural theory applied to families of infants and children with disabilities.[24] A main tenet of this theory is that families establish a number of activity settings within their daily routine to provide the opportunity for infants to learn functional and mobility skills through modeling, joint participation, task engagement, and other forms of goal-directed interactions. This approach stresses that children are given the opportunity to become more independent in mobility and other self-care activities not as a deliberate effort on the part of parents, but rather during familiar parts of the family's routine. Assessment of how well parents are able to use these naturally occurring activity settings may help to identify those settings that are efficient and stimulating for motor activity. For example, part of an initial physical therapy assessment may include a parental record of daily activities. This log may help the therapist to identify situations during the day in which the parents could provide their infants with natural opportunities for practicing mobility skills.

Dynamic Systems Theory

Dynamic systems theory regards functional skills as emerging from the dynamic cooperation and interaction of a number of simultaneously developing subsystems.[25,26] Of particular importance to the naturalistic framework noted in this chapter, the dynamic systems approach emphasizes the interlocking roles of the organism's intrinsic neuromotor components in interplay with the specific physical characteristics and social contexts of the motor task.

Thelen and Ulrich[26] have applied this model to the field of motor development in infancy through their work with infant treadmill stepping. They have found that the emergence of infant stepping is not determined solely by isolated neural connections at a certain point in time. Rather, environmental, perceptual, and social support parameters play a significant role in the emergence and specific motor properties of the independent stepping performance.

Disablement Framework

The disablement framework embodies a classification system that describes a hierarchical spectrum of the consequences of pathology or disease. The most widely used framework is one developed by the World Health Organization (WHO)[22] that identifies three levels of disablement. In the WHO classification system as applied to physical and motor function, *impairment* refers to the loss or abnormality of a motor component or process, *disability* is the restriction of a complex functional activity as part of expected social performance (self-care or mobility), and *handicap* is the inability to participate in expected social roles (e.g., attend day care, play with peers). An alternative model of disablement developed by Nagi has recently gained attention in the physical therapy literature.[28] In addition to the level of impairment, Nagi[29] advocates the use of the term *functional limitations,* which can be defined as the inability to perform functional tasks. According to Nagi, *disability* is a term that should be reserved for the performance of less than appropriate age function in important social roles. Campbell[30,31] has applied one or both of these disablement frameworks to the assessment of motor dysfunction in infants and children. Additional work by the Nordic Neuropaediatric Association[32,33] in adapting the disablement framework to the description of motor disability in older children has further highlighted its usefulness for classifying outcomes of childhood illnesses.

The disablement framework supports both functional and naturalistic frameworks for physical therapy assessment of infant mobility in two ways. First, the combined spectrum of outcomes as defined by impairments, functional limitations, disability, and handicap emphasizes the importance of the environment and the social context for the performance of mobility skills. For example, the environment plays a minimal role in the manifestation of a motor impairment; however, it becomes an increasingly important element of assessment when determining the nature of functional limitations, disability, and handicap. Second, the disablement framework provides a basic model from which measurement constructs can be defined and empirically tested. This is particularly important for defining and measuring function, since the word *function* has many different connotations and meanings.

Based on the WHO classification system and Nagi's description of disability, and borrowing from recent work by Guccione[28] in the application of models of disablement to physical therapy practice, we have proposed an elaboration of the disablement framework for the description of disablement in children[34,35] (Fig. 10-1). This working model highlights three measurement constructs within the assessment of disablement in children: (1) capability for discrete functional skills (functional limitations), (2) performance of complex functional activities (disability), and (3) participation in social, family, and personal roles (handicap). Advantages of this adapted model of childhood disablement are that it emphasizes the distinction between capability and performance, recognizes the distinction between discrete functional tasks and integrated functional activities, and incorporates both developmental and contextual frameworks into the description of childhood disability.

This working model of childhood disablement depicted in Figure 10-1 places a strong emphasis on the development of measurement constructs that differentiate between capability and performance. We have chosen to characterize the level of functional limitations as primarily representing capability of functional units of behavior (such as sitting up in bed, using eating utensils, managing clothes before toileting), while we view the level of disability as the actual performance of complex functional activities (such as mobility within the environment, self-feeding, bladder management) that are part of age-expected social roles of the infant. We use the term *handicap* or *social role performance* to apply to the actual level of participation in social, family, and personal roles.

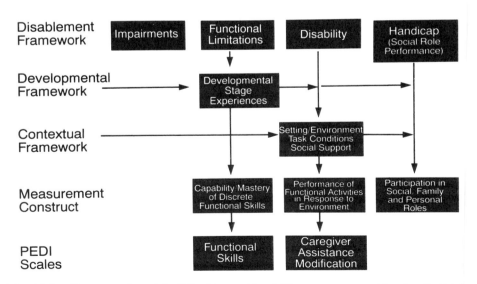

Fig. 10-1. Conceptual model of disablement in children as measured by the Pediatric Evaluation of Disability Inventory. (Adapted from Haley,[34] with permission.)

We believe that continued development and refinement of such models are needed to provide foundations for the accurate measurement and description of physical disablement in infants. These conceptual models become even more important for the measurement of function in preschool children as independent mobility and self-care skills emerge.

In summary, we present a series of conceptual and theoretical approaches that support two important frameworks for the assessment of physical disablement in infants: naturalistic and functional. A consistent theme noted in ecologic theory, skill theory, social context frameworks, ecocultural theory, and dynamic systems theory is the importance of assessing motor activity within the context of the infant's environment. Strategies for more naturalistic assessment are advocated in order to incorporate the broad range of influences that affect the movement performance of the infant. Assessments that incorporate the evaluation of motor performance within naturalistic environments are more likely to identify limitations in motor performance in functional activities that are important to the child and family.

A second major theme noted in many of the conceptual approaches, but particularly emphasized in the disablement framework, is the importance of defining goal-directed functional outcomes as part of a physical therapy assessment. In fact, physical therapy assessments that are focused on motor activities in a naturalistic setting are often, by their very nature, focused on functionally based behaviors. The emphasis of assessing relevant functional behaviors in naturalistic settings should be the cornerstone of the physical therapy motor assessment in young infancy.

In the next section, we use the four levels of disablement that were previously discussed (impairments, functional limitations, disability, and handicap/social role performance) as an organizing structure for the examination of assessment methodologies for the measurement of physical disablement in early infancy. To illustrate applications of assessments using various methodologies, we provide detailed descriptions of our own work in the areas of infant movement assessment and functional assessment.

METHODOLOGIES FOR THE CLINICAL ASSESSMENT OF PHYSICAL DISABLEMENT

A strong correspondence exists between the various levels of physical disablement (impairments, functional limitations, disability, and handicap/social role performance) and the specific methodology employed to measure each outcome level. Five general methodologies are reviewed in order to describe the nature of the linkages between the level of disablement and the assessment methodologies. These proposed linkages are summarized in Table 10-1.

Testing of Neuromotor Behaviors

As noted in Table 10-1, the standardized testing of neuromotor behaviors provides information primarily at the impairment level of the disablement spectrum. Many neuromotor tests are largely based on elicitation of responses or

Table 10-1. Relationship of Assessment Methodology to the Measurement of Physical Disablement

Methodology	Levels of Physical Disablement			
	Impairments	Functional Limitations	Disability	Handicaps
Testing of neuromotor behaviors	Loss or abnormality of a specific motor pattern component or response			
Criterion Testing	Loss or abnormality of a specific prefunctional determinant of movement	Limited capability to accomplish functional/ developmental motor tasks under standardized conditions		
Movement analysis	Loss or abnormality of a specific movement pattern; loss of frequency or quality of movement	Limited capability to move in a specific functional movement pattern or task		
Judgment-based assessment		Limited capability to accomplish functional motor tasks as judged by respondent	Lack of performance of functional motor activities as judged by respondent	Lack of performance of mobility-dependent social roles as judged by respondent
Observation of naturalistic movement			Lack of performance of functional motor activities observed in specific environment	Lack of performance of mobility-dependent social roles observed in specific environment

reflexes and yield no direct information regarding the performance of motor and functional activities. Neuromotor tests may be very dependent on the clinical skills of a trained examiner and are often administered under highly standardized conditions. Neuromotor tests are probably most useful for prediction and diagnosis[36] and are not very useful for treatment planning or treatment monitoring purposes. In a recent review article of neuromotor tests used in pediatric physical therapy, Harris[37] discusses the need to complement the neuromotor test with voluntary movement activities and more naturalistic movement protocols. (see Ch. 9 for a thorough review of neuromotor tests in early infancy.)

Criterion Testing

Criterion testing refers to the administration of a motor test in which voluntary responses to a series of standardized motor items are required. On most criterion tests, the infant does not pass an item unless he or she demonstrates the capability of performing that item during the test administration. Recently some therapist-generated attempts have been made to examine the quality of movements as well as the capability to perform a movement or action using criterion-testing formats.[38,39] Criterion tests require a standardized format and criteria for scoring and primarily assess the motor capability and not necessarily the actual performance of the child in different settings.

The utility of criterion testing for understanding the performance of infants can be further questioned in light of the evidence that many motor skills are highly influenced by task conditions. Gentile[15] has provided a framework with which to classify the different environmental conditions surrounding manipulation and body transport tasks. Haley et al.[40] have used this model to help classify task conditions of motor items from criterion tests when assessing children with brain injury. An appreciation of the different task conditions within motor items may provide additional information regarding the generalizability of the results of criterion tests when estimating actual environmental performance. We must remember, however, that these simulated tasks may not represent the true motor task conditions within the infant's environment.

Movement Analysis

Movement analysis as described here represents a series of methodologies to assess the quality and quantity of movement in structured or semistructured settings. The focus in most of these assessment techniques is the actual movement pattern or the variability of movements and not the successful achievement of goal-directed activities. That is not to say that functionally based movements are never used as the movements of interest; however, the process, sequential pattern, and control of movement, rather than the end result, are typically the major focus of analysis. In most cases, the infant is constrained in some manner by physical boundaries or by task-specific activities in order to facilitate the recording and scoring of the desired movements. This approach differs from strictly naturalistic observations (as described in a section below), which place no constraints on the physical location or the specific activity sequence of the infant.

Movement analysis represents some of the most exciting work in pediatric physical therapy as researchers and clinicians try to blend theoretical and motor control information with clinical practice. Approaches to assessment using movement analysis techniques for very young infants are essentially similar to naturalistic obervations, since the natural environment for very young infants is the crib at the hospital or at home. As the infant becomes older and less confined to one physical space, however, movement analysis techniques are generally administered in standardized conditions that are less similar to the infant's true environment. We first examine studies that focus on the quantity and variability of movement and then discuss selected studies of qualitative aspects of motor control.

Quantity and Variability of Movement

Both real-time[41,42] and interval sampling[43] techniques have been utilized as behavioral methods to measure the quantity and variability of infant movement. Perhaps the most sustained and productive investigation using both interval and real-time analysis to describe postural variety and movement quality in early infancy has been the work of Prechtl and associates.[44-48] Recent work in this area, as discussed by Campbell (see Ch. 12), involves early identification and prediction of cerebral palsy.

With the relative ease of videotape recording in many physical therapy clinics and in homes, the use of real-time movement analysis has become more feasible. Haley et al.[49,50] devised a testing protocol to use real-time videotape analysis techniques to record spontaneous antigravity postures and voluntary movements in infants up to 1 year of age. The protocol, entitled "Assessment of Movement Activity in Infants," involves videotaping spontaneous movements of the infant for 3-minute segments in a 6 ft by 6 ft play enclosure. Spontaneous movements are recorded under two starting conditions: prone and supine. We have noted that in many infants with movement disorders, active attainment of antigravity positions is much more difficult than simply maintaining these positions. This protocol allows us to observe the infant's ability to attain important antigravity positions spontaneously. We have also noted that spontaneous movement activity can vary, especially in infants with low cognitive ability, or with the presence of stimulating objects. Thus spontaneous movements are recorded for conditions in which both toys and no toys are available within the play enclosure. The postures recorded are prone, supine, sitting, four point, kneeling, and standing. Postures that involve more work against gravity are weighted more heavily to reflect greater difficulty. For each posture, behaviors are rated "static," "attempts at transition," "transitions," and "mobility." "Mobility" receives the highest weight, followed by "transitions" from one posture to another. Attempts at transitions that fail are scored lower than transitions that succeed.

Levels of spontaneous movement activity can be quantified, resulting in two summary index scores during each condition, toys and no toys. A frequency score (relative frequency) represents how often the child spontaneously changes positions, with higher scores reflecting more movement variability in developmentally more difficult positions (e.g., kneeling, standing). A duration score (duration probability) represents time spent in various postures, with higher scores reflecting more time spent in developmentally more mature antigravity postures. Data on movement activity have been collected on a small normative sample (n = 40) so that rough age-appropriate comparisons can be made for infants with motor dysfunction.

Figure 10-2 displays the developmental function of duration probability for nondisabled children between the ages of 2 and 12 months in a no toys condition. As noted in Figure 10-2, the slope of the developmental function score dramatically increases between ages 6 and 8 months, reflecting the ability of nondisabled infants to transition spontaneously out of prone and supine positions into sitting and quadruped positions when left on the floor. Rapid changes continue to occur with the attainment and maintenance of developmentally more mature antigravity positions of kneeling and supported standing throughout the period of 8 to 12 months of age.

The underlying objective of this measurement approach is to quantify the spontaneous activity of infants as they explore new movement experiences. Nondisabled infants are highly motivated to practice movements and seem to be interested in new movements only if they are challenging and novel. Learning of new motor skills takes place during intense periods of practice of new movement patterns. Physical therapy intervention is often directed toward stimulating self-practice opportunities in order for the infant to attain new skills actively. The Assessment of Movement Activity in Infants protocol helps to quantify the frequency and duration of spontaneous and active movement exploration.

As expected, children with cerebral palsy routinely fall well below age-expected activity scores.[51] Activity scores can also be used to document change over time if the treatment goals are focused on increasing more spontaneous activity. Data from children who were followed over a 1-year period indicate that scores on the Assessment of Movement Activity are predictive of gains in motor milestone development. Infants who had higher movement activity scores made greater gross motor progress than infants with less spontaneous activity. Children whose movement scores plateaued over time made very little gross motor progress as recorded by standardized motor milestone tests.[51]

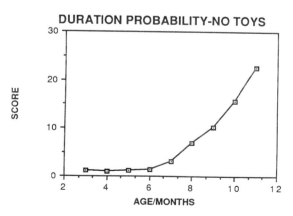

Fig. 10-2. Developmental function of duration probability summary scores for nondisabled children.

Qualitative Aspects of Motor Control

A number of investigators have begun to use computer-based technology to assess kinematic patterns of infant movement in both spontaneous and elicited situations.[25,52] Many movements that are now being examined using quantitative techniques are functionally based behaviors.[2,53,54] This work has been extended to examine postural control of infants and young children in sitting positions and in transitional movements such as sit-to-stand and during ambulation.[55] The use of quantitative methods for the assessment of motor activity is covered extensively by Heriza (see Ch. 11).

Judgment-Based Assessment

Judgment-based assessments collect, structure, and quantify the impressions of professionals and caregivers about a child's performance.[56,57] They can be distinguished from criterion tests since judgment-based assessments do not require observation of the actual performance of the motor task. Instead, the informant or respondent is asked to make a judgment about the ability of the infant to execute the motor task based on prior observation and knowledge of the infant's performance in typical situations. Parents, teachers, and therapists are likely respondents for a judgment-based assessment. This approach to assessment is usually combined with information gathered from neuromotor or developmental tests and can be useful to measure functional performance or behavioral traits that are not easily assessed in clinical settings. In early intervention or rehabilitation settings, judgment-based assessments can not only provide summary profiles of motor performance within and across settings but also help to structure intervention priorities and provider needs.[58]

With information gathered from a variety of people involved in the care of the infant (parents, teacher, therapists, social worker), the child's pattern of functional skill development in different environments can more readily be identified.[57] Judgment-based assessment facilitates the development of a collaborative treatment program and the planning of realistic and functional goals for the child and family.

A number of new assessment approaches in pediatric rehabilitation are adopting a judgment-based format.[59,60] As noted in Table 10-1, judgment-based assessments can be structured to assess the respondent's judgment of the child's capability or performance of functionally based behaviors. Care must be taken to distinguish clearly between capability and actual performance of motor function in this type of assessment.

One example of a new judgment-based assessment for young infants and children is the Pediatric Evaluation of Disability Inventory (PEDI).[60] The PEDI measures both the infant's capability for functional skills and the performance of complex functional activities in the content domains of self-care, mobility, and social function. Measurement dimensions include the capability to perform functional skills (functional units of behavior), the amount of caregiver assistance needed for complex functional activities, and the number and type of modifications needed to complete the activity successfully. Data have been collected on a normative sample to develop a hierarchical model of functional skill attainment and to develop norm-referenced scores for infants and children. In addition to a standardized normative score, the PEDI also provides a scaled performance score within each content domain.

Additional conceptual clarifications are needed to identify the most important measurement dimensions for assessing functional capability and performance in infants and children.[35] For example, in the PEDI we have chosen to measure capability by asking the respondent if the child has any limitations in a functional task. Other possible aspects of limited capability may be the speed or difficulty with which the infant accomplishes the task. In the area of performance, we have chosen to use the amount of caregiver assistance to determine the amount of help a child needs during actual daily routines. Other measurement dimensions may be equally important, such as the frequency with which an infant performs a gross motor activity or the amount of time needed to accomplish the activity.

As an alternative to structured judgment-based assessments, some attempts have been made to record systematically the amount of care given to children during daily routines.[61-63] This type of analysis is most useful when the caregiving burden is extremely demanding. Consistent documentation of parents' care load may provide an important evaluative index for change, and at the very least will enable therapists who are asking parents to change their daily routine to be more sensitive to the high burden of care already experienced by families.[61]

Observation of Naturalistic Movement

Although recognized as an important area of further investigation, few measurement approaches have addressed the naturalistic assessment of infant movement and activity outside of the nursery or a structured environment. This approach differs from standardized movement assessments, since naturalistic observations introduce no constraints on the physical location or the specific activity sequence of the infant. Movement activity in infants must be viewed in a broad context of exploration and development of cognitive and social behaviors. Impaired self-produced locomotion may have a significant impact on the cognitive and psychosocial development of the young infant and child.[64] Many alternative approaches to ambulation are available and are now being advocated for the infant who does not demonstrate the capability for self-locomotion by age 1 year.[64] Naturalistic observation methods are particularly important for tracking the mobility of infants who require alternative systems of mobility, since traditional criterion tests have not developed scoring methods applicable for infants who utilize various means of augmentative mobility.

Several studies have used observation of the child in natural environments with no investigator or environmental influence.[65,66] A recent example of a naturalisitc study of gross motor patterns in children with athetoid cerebral palsy was reported by Yokochi et al.[67] Investigators in other disciplines, primarily speech and language, have pioneered methodologies to operationalize naturalistic behaviors that provide meaningful aggregate scores for performance.[68] Future work in the operationalization of measures of naturalistic movement activity that borrows from methodology developed in other disciplines is needed in pediatric physical therapy.

A number of investigators have employed activity and motion sensors to examine spontaneous movements of infants in naturalistic settings. For example, motion sensors have been used to measure infant activity during sleep[69] and to record extremity motion of infants and young children during 2 days of natural activity at home.[70] A wide variety of technologies are available for accurately recording motor activity with unobtrusive technology so that the effect on the spontaneous movement of the infant is minimal.[71] Pediatric physical therapists, however, are concerned not only with the ability to detect activity but also to be able to discriminate between random and purposeful activity.

In physical therapy practice, naturalistic assessments may be expanded to assess the quality of the physical and social supports for mobility in the infant's environment. Moore[72] found that the configuration of the physical environment in child care settings had a favorable effect on the amount of exploratory behavior and the degree of social interaction in children of preschool age. Although this approach has not yet been applied to infants with movement disorders, it suggests that attention should be given to the physical environments of home, child care center, and physical therapy clinic to develop settings in which independent mobility and functional skill attainment is fostered and encouraged.

Naturalistic observation, as part of the physical therapy assessment, may also include a focus on the parent–child interaction patterns. These patterns can be altered significantly by the presence of a severe motor handicap. Preliminary studies suggest that maternal training can maximize interactional patterns between mothers and infants.[73] A number of research and clinical formats exist that can help structure the observation of parent–infant interactions. An example of a semistructured observational approach to sample the interaction pattern between parent and infant during a developmental teaching situation is the Teaching Scale[74] described by Sparling (see Ch. 4).

SELECTED REVIEW OF INFANT MOTOR ASSESSMENTS

The focus of this section is to review standardized instruments that measure adaptive and mobility content in two primary areas: (1) movement assessment and (2) judgment-based assessment. Some brief comments are made about the functional and naturalistic characteristics of selected criterion-testing scales; however, a more detailed analysis of their technical characteristics will be found in Chapter 9. We are not aware of any published tests that measure purely naturalistic movements in infants. A summary of selected infant motor tests reviewed in this chapter is presented in Table 10-2.

Criterion Testing

A number of criterion tests commonly used by physical therapists in motor assessments incorporate functional content. For example, the Battelle Developmental Inventory (BDI)[75] (which is also normed) samples items such as dressing and toileting within the adaptive content domain. These items can also be scored

Table 10-2. Summary of Selected Infant Motor Tests

Instrument	Mode of Administration	Level(s) of Disablement	Construct	Content Domain
Infant/Toddler Scale for Everybaby (ITSE)[77]	Criterion test/ movement analysis	Functional limitations	Developmental skills	Cognitive, communication, physical, social–emotional, and adaptive
Toddler and Infant Motor Evaluation (TIME)[78]	Movement analysis	Impairments/ functional limitations	Capability to perform typical patterns and sequences of movement	Sequence and quality of movement and motor planning skills
Alberta Infant Motor Scale (AIMS)[79]	Movement analysis	Functional limitations	Capability to perform postural control	Postural alignment and selective control of body parts in supine, prone, sitting, and standing positions
Assessment of Movement Activity in Infants[50]	Movement analysis (videotape format)	Functional limitations	Frequency and duration of spontaneous, antigravity movements	Relative frequency and duration probability of prone, supine, sitting, quadruped, kneeling, and standing positions
Wee-Functional Independence Measure (WeeFIM)[59]	Judgment based	Disability	Caregiver assistance needed in performance of functional activities	Self-care, mobility, sphincter control, communication, social cognitive
Pediatric Evaluation of Disability Inventory (PEDI)[80]	Judgment based	Functional limitations/ disability	Capability of functional skills; caregiver assistance in performance of functional activities	Self-care, mobility, social function

based on parental report, so that actual performance at home and other settings can be more properly assessed. A basic difference, however, between the BDI and more functionally oriented judgment-based assessments is the actual manner in which the items are specified. The BDI structures items within the traditional milestone approach, identifying behaviors representing markers of increasing developmental maturation. Similarly, although the Gross Motor Function Measure[76] samples meaningful gross motor content for many children with cerebral palsy, it does not sample other important functional behaviors such as transfers and alternative means of mobility. In contrast, functionally based tests move from merely specifying items that mark more mature development to including important functional competencies that are meaningful intervention goals for children with motor disabilities (see Ch. 9 for a thorough review of criterion tests).

Movement Analysis

Infant Toddler Scale for Everybaby*

Brief Description of the Test. The Infant Toddler Scale for Everybaby (ITSE)[77] is an individually administered screening test for children aged 3 to 42 months. It covers five developmental domains: cognitive, communication, physical, social–emotional, and adaptive. It is meant to discriminate between normal and abnormal development and has both a screening and an assessment form.

Technical Evaluation. The test was developed with extensive input from panels of experts from many disciplines. It was pilot tested on a sample of 80 normal and 74 children with developmental delays in Colorado. No norms are available yet.

The test demonstrates test–retest reliability coefficients from 0.80 to 0.91. The test is also very good at discriminating between normal and delayed children.

Qualitative Evaluation. The ITSE takes between 30 and 50 minutes to administer and consists of play activities that are administered by the parent with the therapist observing. The play materials are interesting to the child, and the parents seem to understand the instructions well. Only a research edition is available at this time.

Summary Evaluation. The test shows promise as a means to quantify movement capabilities and developmental/functional skills in a semistructured format. It covers all five domains mandated in PL 99-457 using a play format.

---

* The author of this assessment is Lucy Jane Miller. It was published in 1992 (research edition) and is available from the KID Foundation, 8101 E. Prentice Avenue, Suite 518, Engelwood, CO 80111.

Toddler and Infant Motor Evaluation†

Brief Description of the Test. The purpose of the Toddler and Infant Motor Evaluation (TIME)[78] is to measure quality of movement in children with suspected motor dysfunction. It provides information to be used in treatment planning and to measure change over time. The test is applicable for children from birth to age 42 months. Spontaneous movements are recorded for the first 10 seconds that a child spends in each starting position: supine, prone, sit, quadruped, and stand. The sequence of positions assumed is recorded, as are any abnormalities. Some evoked movements are also scored. All positioning and handling of the child is done by the parents, with only verbal cues given by the therapist. Content domains measured include mobility, stability, organization, and dysfunctional positions.

Technical Evaluation. The test was developed with significant input from a panel of experts in pediatric physical and occupational therapy. It has been pilot tested on a sample of over 600 children, including 133 infants and toddlers with motor delays stratified by major demographic variables. Standard scores will be available. Reliability has not yet been reported.

Qualitative Evaluation. The test takes 15 to 30 minutes to administer. It appears easy to administer, and the instructions are clear. Since only the research edition is presently available, it is unclear how much examiner training will be needed for the final form; however, the tester will probably need to have significant experience in developmental testing.

Summary Evaluation. The test appears to be a significant contribution to the area of movement quality evaluation. It incorporates a flexible administrative format in which the examiner observes the child's spontaneous movements, and the parent does any necessary manipulation.

Alberta Infant Motor Scale‡

Brief Description of the Test. The Alberta Infant Motor Scale (AIMS)[79] was designed as a gross motor screening assessment for infants at increased risk for motor disorders from birth through independent walking (0 to 18 months). The AIMS includes 58 items that are divided into four positions: supine, prone, sitting, and standing. The parent should be present during the assessment and should undress the child. Minimal handling is required, and it can be performed by the parent. The infants' postural control in the four posi-

---

† The author of this assessment is Lucy Jane Miller. It is scheduled to be published in 1993 by Therapy Skill Builders, P.O. Box 42050, Tucson, AZ 85733. For the research edition, contact The KID Foundation, 8101 E. Prentice Avenue, Suite 518, Englewood, CO 80111.

‡ The authors of this assessment are Martha Piper, Joanna Darrah, Lynn Pinnell, Thomas Maguire, and Paul Byrne. It is scheduled to be published in 1992 by W.B. Saunders; for more information, contact Martha C. Piper, 3073 UAH Education and Development Center, University of Alberta, Edmonton, Alberta, Canada T6G 2G4.

tions and the actual levels of their performances are scored on a pass–fail scale. The AIMS has few constraints. The infants can be tested at home or in the clinic; use of familiar toys, objects, or pieces of furniture is permitted; and facilitation of motor performance by the examiner is not part of the protocol. The inclusion of the parents, as well as their active participation in the process, provides an optimized context in which the infants' best performance can be elicited.

Technical Evaluation. The work on this assessment is in its final stage of reliability and validity testing, and the construction of norms is in progress.[79] Items were chosen and refined with extensive input from pediatric therapists in Canada. In addition, a panel of experts reviewed the items and established administration and scoring criteria.

Qualitative Evaluation. The assessment takes about 20 minutes to complete. It requires a minimum of equipment (only a mat, appropriate toys, and a stable surface for pull-to-standing activities). The instructions are supplemented with very clear pictures and complete descriptors of scoring criteria.

Summary Evaluation. The major strengths of this test are its ease in administration and clear emphasis on components of motor milestones.

Assessment of Movement Activity in Infants§

Brief Description of the Test. The Assessment of Movement Activity in Infants[50] is an individually administered, videotaped measure of spontaneous antigravity movement and posture. It quantifies information about frequency and duration of movement and is meant to be used as a measure of change in children who are not yet walking. The children are videotaped inside a 6 ft square play enclosure with no examiner influence.

Technical Evaluation. The test was normed on a group of 40 nondisabled infants in the Boston area. Scores represent the proportion of time an infant spends in antigravity positions (duration probability) and how often the child spontaneously changes position (relative frequency). The scores are grouped by age in 2-month intervals, and separate scores are obtained to represent whether or not toys are present in the environment. A small sample of 13 handicapped infants were also administered the test and longitudinal data are available for them.[51]

As expected, both relative frequency and duration probability scores increase with age. Interobserver reliability is high (ICC > 0.90) using trained observers. Based on a small clinical sample, summary scores discriminate between nondisabled infants and infants with disabilities.

§ The authors of this assessment are Stephen M. Haley, Mary Jo Baryza, Jane Coryell, and Carol Zielenski. It consists of an unpublished manual and is available from Stephen M. Haley, Research and Training Center, in Childhood Trauma and Rehabilitation, 750 Washington Street, No. 75K-R, Boston, MA 02111.

Qualitative Evaluation. The test takes about 15 minutes to administer, and the time can be shortened if necessary. Scoring the videotape takes 30 to 45 minutes. The scorers need to be familiar with infant motor development, but need not be experienced pediatric therapists.

Summary Evaluation. This test is a method to quantify observations regarding spontaneous movement. Both the normative and clinical samples are small at this time, but the methodology shows promise in recording spontaneous activities.

Judgment-Based Assessments

Pediatric Evaluation of Disability Inventory ‖

Brief Description of the Test. The Pediatric Evaluation of Disability Inventory (PEDI)[80] is a judgment-based functional assessment that samples content in domains of self-care, mobility, and social function. The test is designed for children between the ages of 6 months and 7.5 years, but it can be used for older children if their functional abilities fall below those expected of nondisabled 7-year-old children. The PEDI measures both capability (197 functional skill items) and performance (20 items that measure caregiver assistance and environmental modifications) of essential functional items. The PEDI is intended to be used as (1) a discriminative device to determine if functional deficits exist, (2) an evaluative instrument to monitor individual or group progress, and (3) an outcome measure for program evaluation or quality assessment programs.

Technical Evaluation. Content validation has been determined by a panel of experts in pediatric rehabilitation.[60] The PEDI has been standardized on a normative sample of 412 nondisabled infants and children between the ages of 6 months and 7.5 years. The PEDI has also been standardized on 102 children with disabilities. A stratified quota sampling technique was utilized to ensure appropriate representation of key demographic and socioeconomic variables in the normative sample. Domain scales have been constructed using the Rasch Rating Scale methodology, yielding a hierarchical model of items within each scale. Two scores are available for each domain: (1) a normative standard score in 6-month increments and (2) a scaled score of performance within each domain. Standard error estimates are available for each individual score. In addition, a goodness-of-fit index can be calculated (with an optional PC-based software program) to determine if an individual profile fits the expected hierarchical model. Inter-interviewer and inter-respondent reliability estimates are reported in the manual and are high (ICC > 0.90). Concurrent and construct validity of

---

‖ The authors of this assessment are Stephen M. Haley, Wendy J. Coster, Larry H. Ludlow, Jane T. Haltiwanger, and Peter J. Andrellos. Version 1.0 was published in August 1992 and is available from PEDI Research Group, Department of Rehabilitation Medicine, New England Medical Center Hospital, No. 75K/R, 750 Washington Street, Boston, MA 02111-1901.

the PEDI on children with moderate[81] and with severe[80] disabilities have also been reported.

Qualitative Evaluation. The PEDI can be scored based on judgment or recall by rehabilitation professionals or educators who are familiar with the child. The items can also be administered to parents through a structured interview that takes approximately 45 minutes. The manual includes specific scoring criteria for each item. Examiners should have a good knowledge of overall child development and be familiar with the functional problems encountered by children with disabilities. Because Version 1.0 has just been published, no critiques from other published sources are available.

Summary Evaluation. The PEDI meets the requirements of a judgment-based performance instrument of function in infants and young children. Summary scores are available and have been derived from the hierarchical model of items developed through the normative sample. An IBM-PC compatible software program is available to assist with data entry, calculation of scores, and storage and retrieval of data.

Functional Independence Measure for Children¶

Brief Description of the Test. The Functional Independence Measure for Children (WeeFIM)[59] is intended to be a minimum data set of functional items to be used as an indicator of severity of disability by measuring "burden of care." It measures what a child actually does in the home or hospital environment, not what he or she is capable of doing. The WeeFIM is designed for children aged 6 months to 7 years. It consists of 18 items across six domains (self-care, sphincter control, mobility, locomotion, communication, and social cognition). Each item is scored on a seven- point scale from "complete independence" to "total assistance." The test is scored by a caretaker to represent the child's usual level of functioning.

Technical Evaluation. The normative sample of 465 children was taken from the Buffalo, NY, area. A national pilot study with a clinical sample is being collected in approximately 25 pediatric hospitals.

Items were selected from the Functional Independence Measure (FIM)[82] and modified as needed for children. Content validity was measured by a panel of eight experts.[83] Summary scores show a good correlation with age for nondisabled children.[84] Reliability data are not yet reported. Summary scores are raw counts, sometimes referred to as *FIM points,* with higher scores reflecting increased independence.

¶ The authors of this assessment are Carl Granger, Susan Braun, Kim Griswood, Nancy Heyer, Margaret McCabe, Michael Msall, and Byron Hamilton. Version 1.5 was published in July 1991 and is available from Uniform Data System for Medical Rehabilitation, State University of New York, Research Foundation, 82 Farber Hall, SUNY South Campus, Buffalo, NY 14214.

Qualitative Evaluation. The test takes about 10 to 20 minutes to administer if the parent is being interviewed. In a clinical setting, various professionals may fill out particular sections. Many clinical sites are already familiar with the FIM and can easily use the pediatric rating scale. A national database is being set up so that clinicians can make comparisons of client progress with other programs.

Summary. The major strengths of this evaluation are the ease of administration and its potential to provide continuity between pediatric and adult functional measures. Because it provides only a minimum database, however, not all clinically significant changes will be reflected in the scores.

EMPIRICAL STUDIES EXAMINING THE CORRESPONDENCE OF ASSESSMENT INFORMATION ACROSS METHODS, RESPONDENTS, SETTINGS, AND LEVELS OF DISABLEMENT

The purpose of this section is to provide a selected review of the literature on the degree of correspondence in the assessment of motor skills across different methods of assessment, by judgments of different respondents, and across different settings. We also examine the issue of a comprehensive approach to assessment using outcome variables from multiple levels of the disablement spectrum.

Criterion Testing Vs. Judgment-Based Assessments

An important concern of pediatric physical therapy programs is the accuracy and efficiency of collecting outcome data in order to monitor progress over the length of the intervention episode. Both criterion testing (observing the infant perform the item) and judgment-based assessment (using parents or therapists as respondents) have been promoted as potential methodologies for routine functional assessment. The accuracy of information of respondents appears to be related to both the characteristics of the test and the respondents.[85] In our own work assessing young infants with the PEDI, we have found that the complexity and contextual specificity of the items are major factors in obtaining accurate information from parent respondents. For example, items such as "mobility outdoors" are difficult for parents of young infants to answer unless the specifics of the items are addressed. Infants as old as 2 years of age might be expected to be independent in locomotion outdoors on some surfaces, but not on others (e.g., ramps, uneven surfaces). Research on parental reports of early childhood measures indicate that parents can best respond to items that incorporate small segments of behavior in specific situations.[86] This may be even more true for parents of children with motor and functional disabilities, whose children often use alternative means for accomplishing mobility functions.

A number of studies have found generally moderate to high correspondence between criterion-testing methods and parental report from judgment-based assessments.[87-92] A consistent finding is the apparent overestimation of parental report in relationship to the results obtained from professionals' administration of a standardized test. The basis of the difference is not straightforward, as parents are often making judgments about the infant at home, while the professionals' judgments are based mainly on performance in a standardized test situation. Bagnato and Neisworth[90] indicate that "large discrepancies between parental and professional judgments can signal the need for parent education or counseling or for professionals to evaluate more closely child functioning *in situ*. When parents are said to *overestimate* child performance, it could also be a case of professional *underestimation*."

Care should be exercised when interpreting the results of studies comparing criterion testing and judgment-based assessments, since the measurement constructs of the testing instruments may be strikingly different. For example, the moderate correlations obtained when comparing the summary scores of the PEDI and BDI Screening Test[81] are largely a function of the difference between developmental milestone content and functional content of the BDI and PEDI, respectively. Sample differences may also affect comparisons. The degree of correspondence between the PEDI mobility scales and the motor scales of the BDI has been reported to be higher for children with severe disabilities[92] than for children with moderate motor impairments or children with no disabilities.[81]

Correspondence Between Different Respondents on Judgment-Based Assessments

Only a few investigators have examined the correspondence between different respondents on judgment-based tests for young infants. As part of a larger study, Bagnato and Neisworth[90] compared the results of the Preschool Attainment Record[94] completed by parents and the Perceptions of Developmental Skills[95] completed by a special educator for 58 children with developmental disabilities between ages 16 and 62 months. Both scales covered traditional domains of development such as motor and self-care and were administered in a structured method in which respondents rated the child's behavior through recall of performance. Correlations were only moderately high for the summary scores ($r = 0.59$); however, differences in the two instruments cause difficulty in determining the relative contributions of content and respondent factors to the discrepancy in scores.

A more direct comparison of the effects of different respondents on judgment-based assessments can be made when studies employ the same assessment across respondents. Gradel et al.[88] reported correlations of 0.42 to 0.87 for content domains on the Developmental Profile[96] administered independently on 30 developmentally delayed infants (aged 2 to 24 months) by parents and teachers. Interestingly, correlations were much higher on a sample of older preschool children (0.95 to 0.98). In a study comparing consensus rehabilitation team (physical therapist, occupational therapist, educator) reports and independent parent reports on the PEDI in children with severe disabilities between the ages of 3 and 10 years, moderately high intraclass correlations (ICC = 0.74 to 0.96) were obtained for summary scores across the three content domains of the PEDI (self-care, mobility, and social function).[97] The relatively high summary score correlations, however, tended to mask the much lower levels of agreement in individual items. We have found that many children with disabilities perform certain functional items (such as mobility and toilet items) differently across settings. These findings highlight the difficulty of interpreting information from only one respondent restricted to one setting. Collectively, these studies point out the importance of adopting a broad framework for the assessment of infants that incorporates information from a variety of respondents across a variety of settings.

Motor Assessment Across Settings

Although home-based assessments and intervention are common in infant early intervention programs, little research has been conducted to compare results of assessments of infants and young children in different settings. Rosenbaum et al.[98] compared the performance results of children who had both an initial assessment performed at home and one performed in a clinical setting. The investigators also examined the parents' perception and satisfaction with the assessments. Although parent reports tended to favor the home assessment, the infants' performance did not differ statistically across settings. Parents of children who were initially assessed at home, however, felt that the play and social behaviors of their child were more typical than did parents whose children were assessed in the clinical setting. The authors suggested that the process of assessment (parental participation, familiar toys, interviews, free play) might be more important in eliciting a broad range of typical infant performance than the actual setting of the assessment.[98]

Assessment of Levels of Disablement

We conclude this section with a discussion of the need for conceptual and empirical work in pediatric physical therapy to address the issue of classifying multiple levels of motor outcomes. Based on an early intervention model of motor training, we developed a hierarchy of motor outcomes for infants and young children, recognizing that different levels of outcomes were important for different purposes[99] (Fig. 10-3). More recently, we have discussed the usefulness of the disablement framework for the classification of motor outcomes in infancy.[34,35] Campbell (see Ch. 12) suggests that the disablement framework provides a uniform approach to the development of a comprehensive assessment strategy for infants and children with motor disorders.

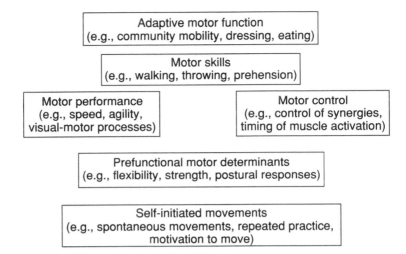

Fig. 10-3. Hierarchy of motor assessment outcomes for infants and young children. (From Haley and Baryza,[99] with permission.)

Clinical research is needed to help delineate the relationships among the levels of disablement (impairments, functional limitations, disability, and handicap/social role performance) in infants with motor disorders. Often the correspondence between physical impairment and motor function is not direct. The extent to which a specific impairment can be related to a functional limitation or disability often depends on the severity of the impairment, the relevance of that deficit to a particular functional skill, the infant's other strengths and weaknesses, and the environmental conditions. One model that may be useful in clinical practice is the comprehensive assessment approach suggested for infants and children with brain injuries that incorporates standardized measures at each level of disablement.[100]

CASE STUDY

To illustrate the use of naturalistic and functional frameworks in the physical therapy assessment of young infants, we present an illustrative case. David is a healthy baby who was born at 31 weeks gestation with no respiratory problems or intracranial bleeding. He was referred for physical therapy because of his premature birth and movement dysfunction related to abnormal postural tone. David exhibited a hypotonic trunk with hypertonic extremities. Shoulder retraction was present in almost all positions, and his postural stiffness increased with movement.

The physical therapy evaluation was carried out at 15 months of age to assess his need for direct therapy and to plan an intervention program. His parents reported a large difference between his performance in the early intervention center and his performance at home. Based on the physical therapy assessment in the clinic, David's motor performance was characterized as strongly influenced by postural tone disorders in which he continually pushed into hyperextension with strongly retracted shoulders. Developmental testing using the BDI Screening Test showed failures in all content domains. He displayed almost no expressive communication, very few cognitive skills, and refused to self-feed. His assessment at home revealed very different mobility skills than those noted in the clinic. At home, his gross motor skills and expressive language were much closer to age-appropriate levels.

The Assessment of Movement Activity in Infants,[50] which measures spontaneous movement, could not be completed in the clinic because David would not separate from his mother in that environment. His activity scores at home were slightly below an 8-month-old level. Scores on the PEDI[80] also showed differences between home and center functioning. In both situations, David scored below his age level, but functioned better at home. His test scores are summarized in Table 10-3.

By having completed assessments at both home and the center, a clearer picture of David's needs for intervention was obtained than by observing him in only one setting. Observations in both settings helped the physical therapist to recognize the influence of the environment on the infant's performance. Although muscle tone problems needed some attention, his higher skill level at home suggested that muscle tone per se was not the major contributor to his level of disability. From the home assessment, we determined that David was capable of moving in and exploring his environment, but he needed strong motivation (i.e., the desire to follow his mother around). Furthermore, the discrepancy between the PEDI and the BDI indicated that motor capabilities were not routinely being translated into performance. For example, David was capable of crawling and exploring his environment, but because he was kept in

Table 10-3. Test Results (David at age 15 months)

Test	Home	Clinic	Comments
	\multicolumn{2}{c}{Months}		
Battelle Screen			
Adaptive	5	3	Dressing and feeding delayed
Gross motor	12	9	Will move around in home but still does not walk or cruise
Fine motor	4.5	4.5	Possibly shows lack of practice and opportunity
Pediatric Evaluation of Disability Inventory			
Functional Skills			Self-care skills (as measured by the PEDI) and
Self-care	9	3	performance are not closely matched.
Mobility	9	4	Mobility skills (as measured by gross motor
Caregiver Assistance			scale on the PEDI) and performance show
Self-care	12	6	wide differences
Mobility	8	4	
Assessment of Movement Activity in Infants	<7	N/A	Score is below age of 8 months showing less than expected spontaneous activity at home

a playpen most of the day at home he did not routinely crawl from place to place. He could put objects to his mouth, but did not finger feed because he was not given the opportunity. Instead of characterizing David as a child with spasticity who lacks movement, the physical therapist could now see David as a child who demonstrated the capability to perform near age-appropriate skills but lacked the opportunity and motivation to use them consistently. In addition to direct motor treatment, an important focus of the intervention program was to change the caretaking environment and expectations so that he would be encouraged to develop self-mobility and self-feeding skills.

IMPLICATIONS FOR ASSESSMENT PRACTICES IN PHYSICAL THERAPY

Because the infant's sensorimotor development cannot realistically be separated from the caretaking environment,[101] the physical therapy evaluation of motor function should be carried out within a naturalistic framework. The caretaking environment includes both the physical environment that the child inhabits and the child's interaction with his or her caretakers. Clearly the motor performance of an infant cannot be separated from the characteristics of the specific motor task.[15] The challenge for pediatric physical therapists is to make the assessment process as naturalistic as possible without sacrificing the traditional assessment components unique to physical therapy (e.g., range of motion, muscle activity patterns).

A number of strategies can be employed to make the physical therapy assessment more naturalistic. Therapists should pay particularly careful attention to the environment, with testing and observation conducted in multiple environments, if possible. If the evaluation is carried out in the clinic, providing an environment that includes appropriate toys will encourage exploration and allow the therapist to observe spontaneous motor activity. Using some of the child's own toys will probably elicit more natural and customary motor responses. Structured parent interviews and standardized judgment-based assessments can often provide valuable information regarding performance in the natural environment.

Newly developed movement activity scales and judgment-based assessments allow for more flexibility in item administration than do more traditional developmental inventories.[77-80] These tests appear to contain items that involve less manipulation of the infant and more emphasis on structuring the environment to encourage active movement. Additionally, parents are more involved in the test administration process and elicit more typical and spontaneous motor responses.

Therapists are encouraged to choose outcome measures that are functionally based. Sampling motor outcomes across the entire disablement framework will allow for a comprehensive assessment approach for multiple assessment purposes. Attention should also be paid to the role of cognition, perception, attention, and motivation to the movement activity of the infant. Bagnato et al.[102]

have developed a model assessment strategy that promotes multidisciplinary, multidimensional, and multienvironmental testing at frequent intervals. Such an approach supports both treatment planning and careful monitoring of functional and adaptive changes within multiple settings.

Strong theoretical bases exist for the incorporation of naturalistic and functional frameworks to the motor assessment of young infants. Increasingly, assessment procedures in pediatric physical therapy are changing to incorporate goal-directed exploration and movement capabilities in the world of the family and other care settings. Our review of a series of assessment methodologies emphasizes the need for continued development and utilization of movement analysis, judgment-based assessments, and naturalistic observation methods in physical therapy.

In conclusion, we agree with Thelen's analysis[103] of the conceptualization of infant movement, as she calls for "no more chapters in introductory texts depicting motor development as a series of milestones." With regard to assessment practices, we would paraphrase her analysis by calling for a broader approach toward motor assessment, with no more assessments by physical therapists depicting the motor dysfunction of infants as merely a problem with the development of motor milestones.

ACKNOWLEDGMENTS

Appreciation is expressed to Wendy J. Coster, PhD, OTR/L, for providing comments on an earlier draft of this manuscript. This chapter was supported in part by grants H133B80009 and H133G80043 from the National Institute on Disability and Rehabilitation Research, U.S. Department of Education, and by Fonds pour la Formation de Chercheurs et l'Avancement de la Recherche (FCAR), Sainte-Foy, Quebec, Canada.

REFERENCES

1. Pick HL: Motor development: the control of action. Dev Psychol 25:867, 1989
2. Fetters L: Measurement and treatment in cerebral palsy: an argument for a new approach. Phys Ther 71:244, 1991
3. McGraw MB: The Neuromuscular Maturation of the Human Infant. Hafner Publishing Company, New York, 1963
4. Gibson EJ, Schmuckler MA: Going somewhere: an ecological and experimental approach to development of mobility. Ecol Psychol 1:3, 1989
5. Campbell SK: Measurement in developmental therapy: past, present and future. Phys Occup Ther Pediatr 9(1):1, 1989
6. Harris SR: Efficacy of physical therapy in promoting family functioning and functional independence for children with cerebral palsy. Pediatr Phys Ther 2:160, 1990
7. Haley SM, Coster WJ, Ludlow LH: Pediatric functional outcome measures. p. 689. In Jaffe KM (ed): Pediatric Rehabilitation (Physical Medicine and Rehabilitation Clinics of North America). WB Saunders, Philadelphia, 1991

8. Gibson JJ: The Ecological Approach to Visual Perception. Houghton-Mifflin, Boston, 1979
9. Gibson EJ: Exploratory behavior in the development of perceiving, acting, and the acquiring of knowledge. Annu Rev Psychol 39:1, 1988
10. Gibson EJ, Riccio G, Schmuckler MA et al: Detection of the traversibility of surfaces by crawling and walking infants. J Exp Psychol [Percept Perform] 13:533, 1987
11. Fischer KW, Pipp SL: Processes of cognitive development: optimal level and skill acquisition. p. 45. In Sternberg RJ (ed): Mechanisms of Cognitive Development. WH Freeman, New York, 1984
12. Fischer KW, Farrar MJ: Generalizations about generalization: how a theory of skill development explains both generality and specificity. Int J Psychol 22:643, 1987
13. Fischer KW, Hogan AE: The big picture for infant development: levels and variations. p. 275. In Lockman JJ, Hazen NL (eds): Action in Social Context. Plenum Press, New York, 1989
14. Fischer KW: A theory of cognitive development: the control and construction of hierarchies of skills. Psychol Rev 87:477, 1980
15. Gentile AM: Skill acquisition: action, movement and neuromotor processes. p. 93. In Carr JH, Shepard RB (eds): Movement Science: Foundations for Physical Therapy in Rehabilitation. Aspen, Rockville, MD, 1987
16. Valsiner J: Parental organization of children's cognitive development within home environment. Psychologia 28:131, 1985
17. Rogoff B: Integrating context and cognitive development. p. 125. In Lamb M, Brown AL (eds): Advances in Developmental Psychology. Vol 2. Lawrence Erlbaum Associates, Hillsdale, NJ 1982
18. Rogoff B: Apprenticeship in Thinking. Oxford University Press, New York, 1990
19. Wertsch JV: Vygotsky and the Social Formation of Mind. Harvard University Press, Cambridge, 1985
20. Hazen NL, Lockman JL: Skill and context. p. 1. In Lockman JL, Hazen NL (eds): Action in Social Context. Plenum Press, New York, 1989
21. Vygotsky LS: Mind in Society: the Development of Higher Psychological Processes. Harvard University Press, Cambridge, 1978
22. Exner CE: The zone of proximal development in hand manipulation skills of non-dysfunctional 3- and 4-year-old children. Am J Occup Ther 44(10):884, 1990
23. Lyons BG: Defining a child's zone of proximal development: evaluation process for treatment planning. Am J Occup Ther 38(7):446, 1984
24. Gallimore R, Weisner TS, Kaufman SZ, Bernheimer LP: The social construction of ecocultural niches: family accommodation of developmentally delayed children. Am J Ment Retard 94:216, 1989
25. Heriza CB: Implications of a dynamical systems approach to understanding infant kicking behavior. Phys Ther 71:222, 1991
26. Thelen E, Ulrich BD: Hidden skills: a dynamic systems analysis of treadmill stepping during the first year. Monogr Soc Res Child Dev 56, 1991
27. World Health Organization: International Classification of Impairments, Disabilities and Handicaps. World Health Organization, Geneva, 1980
28. Guccione AA: Physical therapy diagnosis and the relationship between impairments and function. Phys Ther 71:499, 1991
29. Nagi SZ: Disability concepts revisited: implications for prevention. p. 309. In Pope AM, Tarlov AR (eds): Disability in America. National Academy Press, Washington, DC, 1991

30. Campbell SK: Framework for the measurement of neurologic impairment and disability. p. 143. In Lister MJ (ed): Contemporary Management of Motor Control Problems: Proceedings of the II Step Conference. Foundation for Physical Therapy, Alexandria, VA 1991

31. Campbell SK: Central nervous system dysfunction in children. p. 1. In Campbell SK (ed): Pediatric Neurologic Physical Therapy. 2nd Ed. Churchill Livingstone, New York, 1991

32. Ferngren H, Lagergren J: Usefulness and inter-observer agreement of a child adapted handicap code of WHO's ICIDH. Int Disabil Studies 10:155, 1988

33. Diderichsen J, Ferngren H, Hansen FJ et al: The handicap code of the ICIDH, adapted for children aged 6–7 years. Int Disabil Stud 12:54, 1990

34. Haley SM: Motor assessment tools for infants and young children. In Forrsberg H, Hirschfeld H (eds): Treatment of Children with Movement Disorders: Theory and Practice. Karger, Basel, Switzerland (in press)

35. Coster WJ, Haley SM: Conceptualization and measurement of disablement in infants and young children. Inf Young Child (in press)

36. Harris S: Early neuromotor predictors of cerebral palsy in low birthweight infants. Dev Med Child Neurol 29:508, 1987

37. Harris SR: Movement analysis—an aid to early diagnosis of cerebral palsy. Phys Ther 71:215, 1991

38. Case-Smith J: Reliability and validity of the posture and fine motor assessment of infants. Occup Ther J Res 9:259, 1989

39. Boyce WF, Cowland C, Hardy S et al: Development of a quality-of-movement measure for children with cerebral palsy. Phys Ther 71(11):820, 1991

40. Haley SM, Baryza MJ, Troy M et al: Head trauma in children: application to assessment and treatment of patients with neurological disorders or dysfunction. p. 237. In Lister MJ (ed): Contemporary Management of Motor Control Problems: Proceedings of the II Step Conference. Foundation for Physical Therapy, Alexandria, VA, 1991

41. Horton M, McGuinness J: Movement notations and the recording of normal and abnormal movements. p. 124. In Holt K (ed): Movement in Child Development. (Clinics in Developmental Medicine, No. 55). JB Lippincott, Philadelphia, 1975

42. Downs FS, Fitzpatrick JJ: Preliminary investigation of the reliability and validity of a tool for the assessment of body position and motor activity. Nurs Res 25(6):404, 1976

43. Brand HL, Rosenbaum P: Recording child's movements: the development of an observational method, p. 119. In Holt K (ed): Movement and Child Development. (Clinics in Developmental Medicine, No. 55). JB Lippincott, Philadelphia, 1975

44. Hopkins B, Prechtl HFR: A qualitative approach to the development of movements during early infancy. p. 179. In Prechtl HFR (ed): Continuity of Neural Functions from Prenatal and Postnatal Life. (Clinics in Developmental Medicine, No. 94.) JB Lippincott, Philadelphia, 1984

45. Caesar P: Postural Behavior in Newborn Infants. p. 9. (Clinics in Developmental Medicine, No. 72). JB Lippincott, Philadelphia, 1979

46. Prechtl HFR, Fargel JW, Weinmann HM, Bakker HH: Postures, motility and respiration of low-risk pre-term infants. Dev Med Child Neurol 21:3, 1979

47. Cioni G, Ferrari F, Prechtl HFR: Posture and spontaneous motiliy in fullterm infants. Early Hum Dev 18:247, 1989

48. Prechtl HFR: Qualitative changes of spontaneous movements in fetus and preterm infant are a marker of neurologic dysfunction. Early Hum Dev 23:151, 1990

49. Haley SM: Assessment of motor performance in infants. In Wilhelm IJ (ed): Advances in Neonatal Care. University of North Carolina at Chapel Hill, Chapel Hill, 1985
50. Haley SM, Baryza MJ, Coryell J, Zielinski C: Assessment of Movement Activity in Infants: Videotape Scoring Protocol. Unpublished Test Manual. New England Medical Center, Boston, 1989
51. Baryza MJ: Duration and frequency of spontaneous movement in handicapped infants compared to non-handicapped infants. Unpublished Masters Thesis. Boston University, 1989
52. Gross MT, Cochrane CG: A method for quantifying the activity and rest periods of spontaneous infant kicking. Phys Occup Ther Pediatr 8(2/3):59, 1988
53. Reddihough D, Bach T, Burgess G et al: Objective test of the quality of motor function of children with cerebral palsy: preliminary study. Dev Med Child Neurol 32:902, 1990
54. Reddihough D, Bach T, Burgess G et al: Comparison of subjective and objective measures of movement performance of children with cerebral palsy. Dev Med Child Neurol 33:578, 1990
55. Giuliani CA: Dorsal rhizotomy for children with cerebral palsy: support for concepts of motor control. Phys Ther 71:248, 1991
56. Neisworth JT, Bagnato SJ: Assessment in early childhood special education. p. 23. In Odom SL, Karnes MB (eds): Early Intervention for Infants and Children with Handicaps. Paul H. Brookes, Baltimore, 1988
57. Fleischer KH, Belgredan JH, Bagnato SJ, Ogonosky AB: An overview of judgment-based assessment. Top Early Child Spec Ed 10:13, 1990
58. Bagnato SJ, Neisworth JT: System to Plan Early Childhood Services (SPECS). Administration Manual. American Guidance Service, Circle Pines, MN, 1990
59. Uniform Data System, State University of New York: Guide for the Functional Independence Measure for Children (WeeFIM). Version 1.5. Center for Functional Assessment Research, SUNY, Buffalo, 1991
60. Haley SM, Coster WJ, Faas RM: A content validity study of the Pediatric Evaluation of Disability Inventory. Pediatr Phys Ther 3:177, 1991
61. Johnson CB, Deitz JC: Time use of mothers with preschool children: a pilot study. Am J Occup Ther 39:578, 1985
62. Hagberg B, Edebol-Tysk K, Edstrom B: The basic care needs of profoundly mentally retarded children with multiple handicaps. Dev Med Child Neurol 30:287, 1988
63. Edebol-Tysk K: Evaluation of care-load for individuals with spastic tetraplegia. Dev Med Child Neurol 31:737, 1989
64. Butler C: Augmentative mobility: why do it? In Jaffe KJ (ed): Pediatric Rehabilitation. (Phys Med Rehabil Clin North Am) 2:801, 1991
65. Pickler E: Learning of motor skills on the basis of self-induced movement. p. 5. In Hellmuth JH (ed): Exceptional Infant: Studies in Abnormalities. Vol. 2. Brunner Mazel, New York, 1971
66. Carter RE, Campbell SK: Early neuromuscular development of the premature infant. Phys Ther 55:1332, 1975
67. Yokochi K, Hosoe A, Shimabukuro S, Kodama K: Motoscopic analysis of gross motor patterns in athetotic cerebral palsied children. Brain Dev 11:317, 1989
68. Stone WL, Caro-Martinez LM: Naturalistic observations of spontaneous communication in autistic children. J Autism Dev Disorders 20:437, 1990
69. Erkinjuntti M: Body movements during sleep in healthy and neurologically damaged infants. Early Hum Dev 16:283, 1988

70. Eaton WO, McKeen NA, Lam CS: Instrumented motor activity measurement of the young infant in the home: validity and reliability. Inf Behav Dev 11:375, 1988

71. Tryon W: Principles and methods of mechanically measuring motor activity. Behav Assess 6:129, 1984

72. Moore GT: Effects of the spatial definition of behavior settings on children's behavior: a quasi-experimental field study. J Env Psychol 6:205, 1986

73. Hanzlik JR: The effect of intervention on the free-play experience for mothers and their infants with developmental delay and cerebral palsy. Phys Occup Ther Pediatr 9(2):33, 1989

74. Barnard KE, Eyres SJ: Child Health Assessment, Part 2: First Year of Life. U.S. Department of Health, Education and Welfare, Public Health Service, HRA, Bureau of Health Manpower, Division of Nursing, KHEW Publ. No. HRA 79-25, Hyattsville, MD, 1979

75. Newborg J, Stock JR, Wnek L: Battelle Developmental Inventory. DLM Teaching Resources, Allen, TX, 1984

76. Russell D, Rosenbaum P, Gowland C et al: Gross Motor Function Measure. Chedoke-McMaster Hospitals, McMaster University, Hamilton, Ontario, Canada, 1990

77. Miller LJ: Infant Toddler Scale for Everybaby (ITSE). 2nd Research Edition. KID Foundation, Englewood, CO, 1992

78. Miller LJ: Miller Motor Assessment. Research edition. KID Foundation, Englewood, CO, 1992

79. Pinnell L, Piper MC, Darrah J et al: Reliability and validity of the Alberta Infant Motor Scale (AIMS). Paper presented at the meeting of the Canadian Physiotherapy Association, Montreal, Quebec, Canada, 1991

80. Haley SM, Coster WJ, Ludlow LH, Haltiwanger JT et al: Pediatric Evaluation of Disability Inventory (PEDI): Development, Standardization and Administration Manual. New England Medical Center Hospitals, Boston, 1992

81. Feldman AB, Haley SM, Coryell J: Concurrent and construct validity of the Pediatric Evaluation of Disability Inventory. Phys Ther 70:602, 1990

82. Granger CV, Hamilton BB, Keith RA et al: Advances in functional assessment for medical rehabilitation. Top Geriatr Rehabil 1:59, 1986

83. McCabe MA, Granger CV: Content validity of a pediatric functional independence measure. Appl Nurs Res 3:120, 1990

84. Braun SL: Granger CV: A practical approach to functional assessment in pediatrics. Occup Ther Pract 2(2):46, 1991

85. Klein-Parris C, Clermont-Michel T, O'Neill J: Effectiveness and efficiency of criterion testing versus interviewing for collecting functional assessment information. Am J Occup Ther 40:486, 1986

86. Holden GW, Edwards LA: Parental attitudes toward child rearing: instruments, issues and implications. Psychol Bull 106:29, 1989

87. Knobloch H, Stevens F, Malone A et al: The validity of parental reporting of infant development. Pediatrics 63(6):872, 1979

88. Gradel K, Thompson MS, Sheehan R: Parental and professional agreement in early childhood assessment. Top Early Child Spec Ed 1:31, 1981

89. Goldstein DJ: Accuracy of parental report of infants' motor development. Percept Motor Skills 61:378, 1985

90. Bagnato SJ, Neisworth JT: Assessing young handicapped children: clinical judgment versus developmental performance scales. Int J Partial Hosp 3:13, 1985

91. Kenny TJ, Hebel JR, Sexton MJ, Fox ML: Developmental screening using parent report. Dev Behav Pediatr 8:8, 1987

92. Sexton D, Thompson B, Perez J, Rheams T: Maternal versus professional estimates of developmental status for young children with handicaps: an ecological approach. Top Early Child Spec Ed 10(3):80, 1990

93. Schultz CI: Concurrent Validity of the Pediatric Evaluation of Disability Inventory. Unpublished Masters Thesis, Tufts University, Boston, 1992

94. Doll EA: PreSchool Attainment Record. American Guidance Service, Circle Pines, MN, 1966

95. Bagnato SJ, Neisworth JT: Perceptions of Developmental Skills (PODS). HICOMP, University Park, PA, 1977

96. Alpem GD, Boll TJ: Developmental Profile. Psychological Development Publications, Indianapolis, IN, 1972

97. Sundberg KB: Inter-Rater Reliability of the Pediatric Evaluation of Disability Inventory; Parental and Professional Agreement. Unpublished Masters Thesis. Boston University, Boston, 1992

98. Rosenbaum P, King S, Toal C et al: Home or children's treatment centre: where should initial therapy assessments of children with disabilities be done? Dev Med Child Neurol 32:888, 1990

99. Haley SM, Baryza MJ: A hierarchy of motor outcome assessment: self-initiated movements through adaptive motor function. Inf Young Child 3(2):1, 1990

100. Haley SM, Baryza MJ, Lewin JE, Cioffi MI: Sensorimotor dysfunction in children with brain injury: development of a data base for evaluation research. Phys Occup Ther Pediatr 11(3):1, 1991

101. Horowitz FD: Targeting infant stimulation efforts. Clin Perinatol 17(1):185, 1990

102. Bagnato SJ, Mayes SD, Nichter C et al: An inter-disciplinary neurodevelopmental assessment model for brain-injured infants and preschool children. J Head Trauma Rehabil 3:75, 1988

103. Thelen E: The (re)discovery of motor development: learning new things from an old field. Dev Psychol 25(6):946, 1989

11 | Kinematic Motion Analysis

Carolyn B. Heriza

HISTORICAL REVIEW

Interest in the movement patterns of humans and animals dates back to prehistoric times, as depicted in cave drawings, statues, and paintings.[1] Not until the last century, however, were the first motion picture cameras used to record locomotion patterns of humans and animals. In 1885, a French physiologist, Marey, used a photographic gun to record human gait and chronophotographic equipment to provide stick diagrams of the movement. During the same period, Muybridge, in the United States, sequentially triggered 24 cameras to record the patterns of a man running.

In this century, over a period of approximately 30 years, Nicolai Bernstein, a Soviet physiologist, developed the techniques of recording movement in real time.[2] Progress has been rapid since Bernstein's work in view of advances in both measurement and experimental procedures. These advances have taken place as the result of the development of automatic data acquisition and processing technology, including computer mathematical and statistical software packages. Currently we can record and analyze everything from the gait of children with cerebral palsy to the motoric performance of a trained athlete. Recently, these procedures have been used to study movement in infants. The term used for these descriptions of human movement is *kinematics*.

KINEMATICS AS A MEASUREMENT TOOL

Kinematics is that branch of biomechanics that is concerned with the detailed descriptive analysis of a movement pattern. It is not concerned with the forces involved in the production of the movement pattern. This latter aspect of movement is the preserve of kinetics.

Traditional measures of motor milestones, reflexes and reactions, muscle "tone," as well as other parameters have not been adequate for determining the effectiveness of therapeutic programs for infants with movement dysfunction. While these tools may be quantitative in nature, they are subjective and yet are addressing a qualitative issue of movement change. Qualitative aspects of movement may be the most amenable to change through intervention.[3]

Kinematic analysis reveals how the segments of the body are coordinated with one another and with the structure of the movement. It describes and analyzes movement according to the objective kinematic variables of joint or segment position, joint angles, time, linear and angular displacements, velocities, and accelerations. By tracking the position of a body part during a movement, sampling many times per second, we can determine which segment initiates the movement, the sequence in which the segments become involved, the joint angles, and the accuracy of the movement. The velocity and acceleration of movements can also be mathematically derived from the position-time data. Thus kinematics allows us to transform a visually observed movement into quantifiable measurements.

In addition to use in infant evaluation and treatment, kinematics is capable of transforming ideas about movement dysfunction into testable clinical hypotheses.[4] These hypotheses allow researchers to develop and test others about motor control, motor learning, and motor development at the behavioral level.

Infant kinematics, using imaging techniques, provides a permanent record of the movement from which the therapist objectively can (1) describe the movement pattern, (2) identify infants early who may have movement dysfunction, (3) classify movement dysfunction, and (4) determine the effectiveness of treatment. In addition, kinematic analysis can provide data that may help to answer the following questions: How do motor coordination and control develop? What fundamental processes drive developmental change? What mechanisms are responsible for producing abnormal movement? What precisely happens when an infant practices a movement?[5] Such analysis will contribute to a basic understanding of the neuromotor system and the effects of various debilitating conditions on movement. It will provide techniques for diagnosis and for assessing the effects of therapeutic interventions and will help clinicians to develop theory-based regimens of treatment.

MEASUREMENT TECHNIQUES

Imaging Techniques

Technology is playing an increasingly important role in the management of infants with movement dysfunction. As most movements are complex, the only system that can possibly capture all the data is an imaging system.[1] Imaging techniques have traditionally been used in research settings to provide objective kinematic analysis of movement. Recent advances in technology have seen these systems being transferred to clinical settings. Since the impact of technology is wide ranging, that is, it affects both the diagnostic and therapeutic capabilities as well as research protocols, we must stay abreast of new and different applications of such technology. The imaging techniques vary in cost and sophistication. This discussion is limited to three major types: cinematography, videography, and optoelectric systems.

Cinematography

Cinematography (high-speed photography) allows for frame-by-frame analysis of movement. Many different-sized motion picture cameras are available, but the most commonly used is the high-speed 16 mm camera. Cameras with high speed rates are necessary for high velocity movements such as athletic events, but for clinical purposes frame rates greater than 64 frames per second (fps) are seldom required. Several types of 16 mm cameras are available: spring driven or motor driven by either batteries or power supplies. An advantage of the battery driven camera is that it is portable and can be used where power is unavailable. Disadvantages involve the cost of the camera, the necessity for additional lighting, and the time to reduce the data.

Videography

A major difference between videography and cinematography is that videography is a fixed frame rate. The name given to each television image is a *frame*. A frame consists of two visual fields. In North America, there are 60 fields/s; in Europe the standard is 50 fields/s. Thus videography has a high enough field rate for most movements, but probably too low for a quantitative analysis of rapid movements such as athletic events or tremors. A major advantage of television is the capability for instant replay, which serves both as a quality control check and as an initial qualitative assessment.[1] Since the television camera can be battery driven, it can be transported and used in naturalistic settings such as the home or hospital. The light required with videography is not as extensive as that needed with cinematography; thus videography can be used where the lighting cannot be increased, such an in neonatal intensive care nurseries.

Optoelectric Systems

Computer-based, optical tracking systems have recently been developed. In these imaging systems, the infants wear special lights, minature infrared emitting diodes (IREDs), on desired body points. The systems track the IREDs at high sample rates, so are suited for fast movements. A primary advantage of optoelectric systems over conventional cinematography is in the speed of data reduction. These systems necessitate a designated room for filming infants and are not portable. They are costly and technically sophisticated. Typically, optical tracking systems are coupled with videotape recordings.

In all systems, with the exception of the optoelectric systems, markers are easily placed and do not interfere with movement. Markers are placed on particular points of the body, and these points are tracked in space over some period of time. Points can be the extremes of limb segments or key anatomic prominences, depending on the goals of the assessment. Markers can be pieces of tape of contrasting color, high contrast reflective tape or balls, IREDs, or marks made with hypoallergenic pencils. Time to attach or draw the markers is minimal with the exception of the IREDs, which require more careful attention for placement.

The spatial reference system can be either relative or absolute.[1] A relative spatial reference describes the position of one limb to that of another limb and does not provide information about where the infant is in space. An absolute spatial reference analyzes movement of the infant in relation to the ground or the direction of center of gravity.

Event markers or other indicators of temporal events are required for analysis of infant movement. Many of the kinematic systems have the timing units on the film. Others need to incorporate a timer into the field of view, or a time code needs to be superimposed on the image for frame-by-frame analysis.

Two-dimensional (2D) coordinates of the position of selected body points can be determined from a single camera or from two synchronized cameras. Calculation of three-dimensional (3D) positions is possible if two cameras are used and if a view of a standard calibration grid is available for each camera. Some kinematic systems have the option of both 2D and 3D coordinates. A disadvantage of a 2D system is that movement frequently occurs outside the sagittal plane because of segment rotation. A 3D system more accurately assesses rotation.

Table 11-1 provides a summary of the advantages and disadvantages of each of the imaging techniques. The particular system chosen should yield reliable and valid measurements and answer the particular question under study.

Data Conversion Techniques

The points of interest (the markers on the joints or limb segments) may be digitized in real time, that is, at the time of filming, or identified and digitized after data collection. Digitization can be done by hand or automatically. Digitizing by hand is labor intensive. In the automated systems, digitization is rapid but the cost of automated imaging measurement techniques is high. Digitized data can be stored in a computer for later reduction and analysis. The coordinates of each marker are determined and yield the time and spatial course of each body marker, which in turn form the basis of all successive kinematic analysis. Raw kinematic data, the coordinates of each marker, must be smoothed to eliminate error and noise in the process of collecting and converting the raw data. The smoothed data can be transformed to yield a variety of kinematic variables.

Table 11-1. Summary of Advantages and Disadvantages of Kinematic Systems

Consideration	Cinematography	Videography	Optoelectric
Sophistication (ease of use)	Somewhat sophisticated	Sophisticated	Very sophisticated
Cost (capital and running)	Moderate to high, except cost of conversion equipment	Moderate, except cost of conversion equipment	Expensive
Frequency	≥64 Hz	60 Hz (U.S.A.) 50 Hz (Europe)	≥64 Hz
Encumbrance to movement	Minimal	Minimal	Some
Time to attach	Minimal	Minimal	Moderate
Availability of data for analysis	Film processing and conversion of data high	Instant replay; has capability for instant conversion	Instant conversion
Lighting	Extra lighting required indoors	No extra lighting required for 2D, but may be useful; required for 3D	Extra lighting required
Visual record	Available	Available	Not available unless coupled with video
Laboratory vs. naturalistic setting	Both	Both	Laboratory

Visual Display

Kinematic data conventionally have been displayed graphically, resulting in a visual permanent record of movement.[5-7] Such graphic display provides useful interpretative data about the movement path of a body segment with respect to time or the movement path of one body segment versus another, as well as the movement path's velocity, acceleration, direction, and magnitude. Plotting formats used in the presentation of normal and pathologic kinematic data can be either time-dependent representations or time-independent representations.

Time-Dependent Graphics

In time-dependent graphics, the patterns of joint or segment displacements are plotted as a function of time and are referred to as *angle-time diagrams* (Fig. 11-1). Typically, displacement of the joint or segment is plotted on the vertical axis and time on the horizontal. The shape of the displacement, the complexity of the movement path in relation to the task,

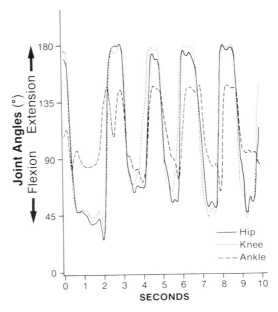

Fig. 11-1. Typical angle–time diagram of joint angles of spontaneous kicking movements of a 34-week gestational age infant. Decreasing angles indicate flexion. (From Harris and Heriza,[5] with permission.)

and directional changes, such as the curvature, jerkiness, or straightness of the path, can be studied. Patterns of joint velocity or acceleration have been plotted as a function of time (Fig. 11-2). In these graphics, the number of peaks and valleys have been utilized as variables to address changes in movement with age and the efficacy of treatment. These have been referred

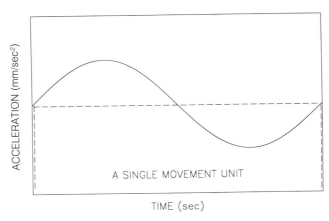

Fig. 11-2. A single movement unit including one acceleration and one deceleration. (From Kluzik et al.,[8] with permission.)

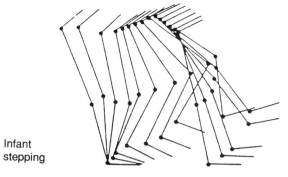

Infant
stepping

Fig. 11-3. Stick diagram of infant stepping from a 6-week-old infant. (Modified from Forssberg,[23] with permission.)

to as *movement units* (MU),[8] *functional units,*[9] and *curvature-speed relationships.*[10] Stick figure tracings, in which each body segment is represented by a straight line or a stick, may also be generated for visual representation of the movement (Fig. 11-3). By joining the sticks together, the spatial orientation of all segments is displayed at any point in time.

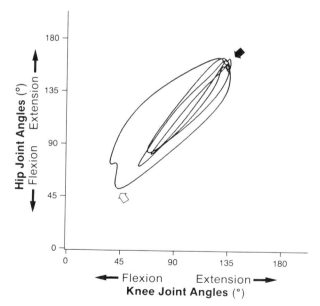

Fig. 11-4. Typical angle–angle diagram of hip joint amplitude versus knee joint amplitude during spontaneous kicking of a 35-week gestational age infant. Note that, as the hip flexes, the knee flexes, and as the hip extends, the knee extends. The filled arrow indicates the beginning of a kick flexion movement; the open arrow indicates peak flexion. (From Harris and Heriza,[5] with permission.)

Time-Independent Graphics

Time-independent graphics are used for inferring causal patterns (i.e., revealing underlying motor control mechanisms) from dynamic data.[7,11] The plots have characteristic shapes that can be used to differentiate disordered movement from normal limb kinematics.[7] A disadvantage of time-independent plots is that time is omitted from the graphic representation. This problem can be remedied by incorporating tick marks on the path trajectory of the movement at constant time intervals.[7]

The two types of time-independent graphics are angle–angle diagrams and phase plane trajectories. In angle–angle plots (Fig. 11-4), the joint angle of a moving limb is plotted against another joint angle of the same limb. Such representation of kinematic data provides insights into intersegmental coordination which are difficult, if not impossible, to see in other geometric plots.[7] Typical shapes of trajectory segments in angle–angle space with dynamic interpretations are described in Figure 11-5.

In phase plane plots, the kinematic variables are plotted against their time derivatives.[11] A common example is a plot of the joint velocity of a moving limb plotted against the joint angle of the same limb at every instance in time (Fig. 11-6). This graphic representation is referred to as an *amplitude–velocity phase plane plot* and demonstrates the relationship be-

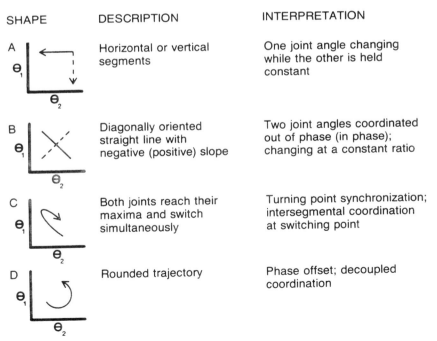

SHAPE	DESCRIPTION	INTERPRETATION
A	Horizontal or vertical segments	One joint angle changing while the other is held constant
B	Diagonally oriented straight line with negative (positive) slope	Two joint angles coordinated out of phase (in phase); changing at a constant ratio
C	Both joints reach their maxima and switch simultaneously	Turning point synchronization; intersegmental coordination at switching point
D	Rounded trajectory	Phase offset; decoupled coordination

Fig. 11-5. Selected shapes of trajectory segments in angle–angle space with dynamic interpretations. (From Winstein and Garfinkle,[7] with permission.)

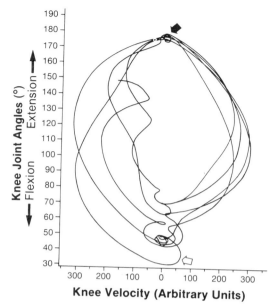

Fig. 11-6. Typical phase plane trajectory of the amplitude of movement and peak velocity of the knee joint during spontaneous kicking of a 34-week gestational age infant. The filled arrow indicates the beginning of a kick flexion movement; the open arrow indicates peak flexion. Phase plane trajectories progress clockwise. (From Harris and Heriza,[5] with permission.)

tween velocity, its changes, and position. The position is typically plotted on the x-axis and its velocity on the y-axis, although the orientation of the phase plane plot can be reversed. Phase plane diagrams progress clockwise. To assist in visual analysis of the movement, a line is often drawn through zero velocity to determine whether the path trajectory demonstrates self-intersections (i.e., crossings or reversals of the movement path at zero velocity). The kinematic data presented graphically represent the resultant action of motor control mechanisms. If the movement pattern has a recognizable shape, it can be compared with the shapes seen in dynamic systems for which the underlying control processes are known. Particular styles of causal action can be associated with particular segment shapes and vice versa. The typical shapes of trajectory segments in phase plane space with dynamic interpretations are displayed in Figure 11-7.

Phase plane plots have also been referred to as phase portraits[12-14] or phase diagrams.[15] These are dynamic terms used to describe motion using both position and velocity. Recently, a phase angle, the angle describing the relationship between two segments in the same limb or the relationship between two limbs, has been mathematically calculated from the phase portraits. This phase angle is considered a measure of coordination. The phase angle may not quantitatively describe the coordination of all types of

SHAPE	DESCRIPTION	INTERPRETATION

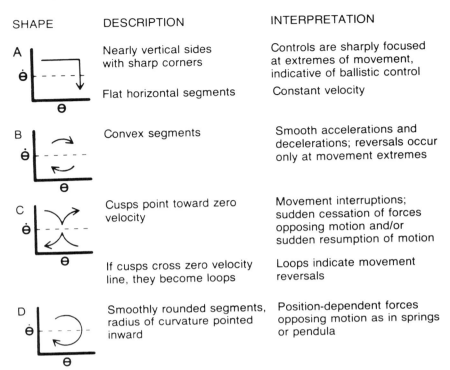

	Nearly vertical sides with sharp corners	Controls are sharply focused at extremes of movement, indicative of ballistic control
A	Flat horizontal segments	Constant velocity
B	Convex segments	Smooth accelerations and decelerations; reversals occur only at movement extremes
C	Cusps point toward zero velocity	Movement interruptions; sudden cessation of forces opposing motion and/or sudden resumption of motion
	If cusps cross zero velocity line, they become loops	Loops indicate movement reversals
D	Smoothly rounded segments, radius of curvature pointed inward	Position-dependent forces opposing motion as in springs or pendula

Fig. 11-7. Selected shapes of trajectory segments in phase plane space with dynamic interpretations. The dotted line indicates zero velocity. (From Winstein and Garfinkle,[7] with permission.)

movement. It has been suggested for use for independent walking in infants but may not be a useful measure for reaching in infants. The phase portrait is a visual qualitative picture of the movement pattern while a phase angle, if calculated, is a quantitative measure of the coordination of the same movement pattern.[12-15]

CLINICAL APPLICATIONS

Numerous investigators have used kinematics analysis to analyze infant movement. Kicking and stepping movements have been described in normal and in low- and high-risk preterm infants.[16-19] Changes in motor coordination during the transition from prelocomotion to crawling have been documented.[20] Others have delineated the time and spatial characteristics of first independent walking, walking over the second year, and walking in infants with Down syndrome.[21-25] The kinematics characteristics of reaching movements have been described in full-term infants and infants ranging in age from 3 to 9 months.[9,10,26-28] The relationship between speech events and arm movements also has been studied.[29] The development of sitting behavior has been described for full-term and preterm infants as well as infants with cerebral palsy.[30-32]

Following are reviews of selected studies that have used kinematics to describe the development of movement in normal and at-risk infants and to determine the effectiveness of therapeutic intervention. When appropriate, graphic representations of various infant movements are presented. As the technology for assessing infant movement using imaging is now being transferred to the clinic from the research area, clinicians must feel comfortable interpreting the graphic information produced by kinematics analysis.

Kicking and Walking

Normal Infants

Thelen and her colleagues[33-37] have used kinematics coupled with electromyography (EMG) and behavioral analysis to analyze infant leg movements. Supine kicking and upright stepping in eight 2-week-old infants were recorded with two videocameras, one in the sagittal plane and one in the frontal plane.[16] Kinematics data (joint angles, amplitude, duration of the four phases of the kick or step cycle) were obtained by analyzing the videotapes in the sagittal plane frame-by-frame at a speed of 60 fields/s. Concurrent EMG was collected. Kicking and stepping movements were displayed visually using stick figures (Fig. 11-8). Kinematic analysis of kicking and newborn stepping demonstrated that these two movements were similar on a number of measures. Both behaviors were initiated with simultaneous flexion of the hip, knee, and ankle, followed by extension of the three joints in unison. Both behaviors had similar temporal organization with similar flexion phase mean durations, with slightly longer extension phase mean durations. Nonmovement phase durations for both behaviors were more variable than movement phase durations. The major difference between kicking and stepping was that spontaneous kicking was observed in the supine position while stepping was demonstrated in the supported upright position. This similarity suggests that the two apparently different behaviors are one behavioral pattern with different developmental profiles (i.e., spontaneous kicking does not disappear with age in contrast to the disappearance of newborn stepping). The disappearance of newborn stepping was attributed to the biodynamic consequences of the upright posture due to asynchronous development of muscle mass and concomitant strength. By manipulating the environmental context, that is, from the upright position to supine, Thelen and Fisher[16] demonstrated that newborn stepping does not disappear with age, as infants continued to kick throughout the first year. In other kinematics studies, investigators have manipulated the environmental context by placing infants in water,[37] placing small weights on their legs,[37] or supporting them over a mobilized treadmill[36,38] and have also elicited more mature leg coordinations in infants. Some of these behaviors were believed to have disappeared while others were elicited months earlier than they were normally expected. These studies bring into question the

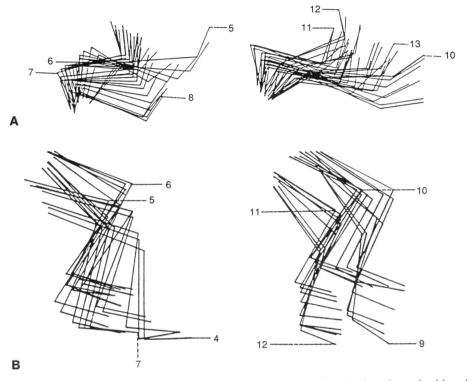

Fig. 11-8.   Stick figure diagrams of kicking (**A**) and stepping (**B**) in a 2-week-old male infant. (From Thelen and Fisher,[16] with permission.)

theory that motor development is the result of developmental changes of the central nervous system (CNS). They emphasize the importance of a systems perspective for understanding development and the importance of the environmental context in eliciting functional movement.

Forssberg[23] also used kinematics to study the development of walking in normal infants. Locomotor patterns of infants during stepping in the newborn period (first 2 months of life), during supported locomotion (ages 6 to 12 months), and during independent locomotion in children who were just able to walk by themselves without external support (ages 10 to 18 months) were recorded by an automated kinematics system in the sagittal plane. Reaction forces and EMG recordings were also collected. Kinematics data consisted of segment position, joint angles, velocity, duration, and step length. Kinematics plots consisted of time-dependent plots (angle–time plots, stick figures) and time-independent plots (angle–angle plots, position plots). In contrast to Thelen and colleagues' proposition that mature walking emerges from the interaction of subsystems around the task of walking, Forssberg argued that his results indicated that early infant stepping is controlled by motor programs in the CNS and that the development from the early pattern to mature walking is reflected by changes within the nervous system as well as learning.

The coordination between two limbs, interlimb coordination, has been described in infants during the first 6 months of walking.[21] Infants were filmed using a 16 mm camera according to the speed of the movement and therefore differed with walking age. New, 0.5- and 1-month walkers were sampled at 32 fps and 3- to 6-month walkers were sampled at 50 fps. Time–space kinematics data were obtained by digitizing the heel at heelstrike. The phasing relationship between the two limbs served as the variable of study. Phasing was calculated as the proportion of the ipsilateral limb cycle when footstrike occurred in the contralateral limb. In mature stepping, the step cycle of one leg is initiated at 50 percent of the cycle of the opposite leg (the limbs are precisely 180 degrees out of phase). Graphics were not utilized. At the onset of independent walking, infants were quite variable in their interlimb phase relationship. After walking 3 months, however, their variability was similar to that of an adult.

Thelen and Ulrich[36] have also used interlimb phasing as a variable to capture the patterned leg action of infants on a treadmill. Nine infants were tested twice each month throughout the age range of 1 to 7 months. Leg excursions on the treadmill were tracked by means of an optoelectric system through a series of trials beginning with the treadmill belt turned off and continuing through seven more in which the speed of the belt was gradually increased. As an additional condition, each leg was driven by the treadmill at a different speed. Results indicated that, as infants aged, they more closely approximated the mature interlimb phase relationship (180 degrees out of phase). The studies by Clark and colleagues and by Thelen and collaborators indicate that changes in stepping and walking with age can be studied by using interlimb phasing as a variable.

Atypical Infants

Kinematics analysis has also been used to address movement change in kicking and stepping in atypical infants.[17–19,22] Forty-nine infants participated in the kicking studies.[17–19] Fifteen were term infants, 10 were low-risk preterm infants, and 24 were high-risk preterm infants with documented intraventricular hemorrhages. Videography was used in these studies with one camera positioned in the sagittal plane of the kicking limb. Ten seconds of kicking were digitized at a sampling rate of 60 fields/s. Kinematics data consisted of joint position of the hip, knee, and ankle; amplitude; peak velocity; and duration of four phases of the kick cycle (flexion, intrakick pause, extension, and interkick pause). In addition to these variables, the relationship of individual joints to each other and the phase lags between joints were calculated. A phase lag was defined as the elapsed time between the onset or termination of the movement of one joint and that of another joint divided by the duration of the kick cycle. Graphic displays of the kinematics data included time-dependent representations (angle–time) and time-independent representations (amplitude–velocity phase plane trajectories) of the knee.

Results indicated that intralimb kicking was similar in all infants regardless of age, environment, or risk factors. The top panel of Figure 11-9 displays the angle–time displacement of the joint angles of the hip, knee, and ankle plotted as a function of time for four infants at different gestational or postgestational ages. The patterns of intralimb kicking among the infants are similar. The relationships between the joints demonstrated that the joints moved in unison. The hip–knee relationship was especially strong. When the hip flexed, the knee flexed, and when the hip extended, the knee extended. The durations of the movement phases (flexion and extension) were constrained, and the nonmovement phases (intra- and interkick pauses) demonstrated variability.

Although intralimb kicking of the high-risk preterm infants, as a group, was similar to that of term and low-risk preterm infants, some infants showed individual profiles in which kicking appeared disorganized. The time-dependent diagrams (Fig. 11-10, top panel) show that the ankle is out of phase with the knee and hip in infant A, a preterm infant with a grade IV intraventricular hemorrhage, and that the knee is out of phase with the hip and ankle in infant B, a preterm infant with a grade IV intraventricular hemorrhage and hip dysplasia. Although the timings of the movement phases of flexion and extension were similar to those of the other infants, the correlations between the joints were weak and phase lags were long.

Time-independent graphics (amplitude–velocity phase plane trajectories) of the knees of all infants demonstrated that the path trajectories were confined to particular regions of the plot and showed particular ordered patterns. Figure 11-9 (bottom panel) shows that the amplitude and peak velocities of the kicking movements of each infant are similar with the exception of those of the high-risk infant, which show variability of amplitude and peak velocity for the four kicks. No self-intersections occurred (i.e., no crossings or reversals of movement at zero velocity) during the flexion and extension movements. Although the 40-week-postgestational age high-risk preterm infants, as a group, demonstrated preferred behavioral patterns, some infants showed individual profiles. Phase plane diagrams of two of these infants (Fig. 11-10, bottom panel) demonstrated differences in their kick patterns. The kicks show simple closed curves with oscillations at the extremes of the movement, variability in the amplitude and velocity, and self-intersecting loops (i.e., self-crossing or reversals of movement at zero velocity), which primarily occur during the extension phase. The author concluded that the use of graphics visually demonstrated differences between organized and disorganized intralimb kicks and that these visual representations were supported quantitatively by joint correlations and phase lags. As such, these kinematics variables and graphic representations could be used clinically to evaluate intralimb kicking behavior.

Although the patterns of kicking were stable among low-risk preterm and full-term infants, differences were found in the amplitude and velocity of movement, the pauses during the kick cycle, and the joint angles at the initiation of flexion and at peak flexion. With age, low-risk preterm infants showed decreased movement amplitude and peak velocity (Fig. 11-9A,B, bottom panel). At 40 weeks postgestation, all low-risk preterm infants were more extended at all

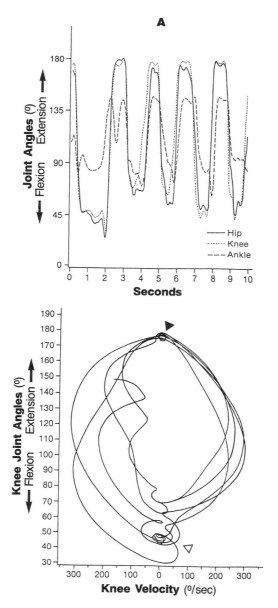

Fig. 11-9. Kicking movements of representative infants. Top panel shows angle–time diagrams of the displacement of hip, knee, and ankle joints. Bottom panel illustrates corresponding phase plane trajectories of the knee joint amplitude of movement and peak velocity. The filled triangle in the bottom panel indicates the beginning of kick flexion movement; the open triangle represents peak flexion. Phase plane trajectories progress clockwise. **(A)** Low-risk infant at 34-weeks gestational age. (*Figure continues.*)

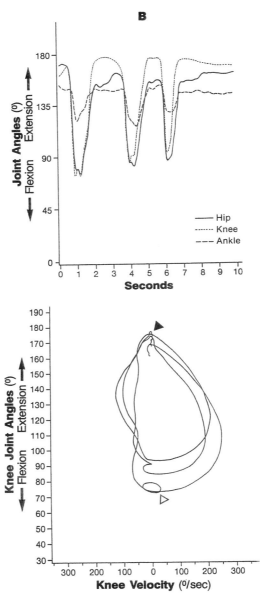

Fig. 11-9. (*Continued*).   (**B**) Same low-risk infant at 40-weeks postgestational age. (*Figure continues.*)

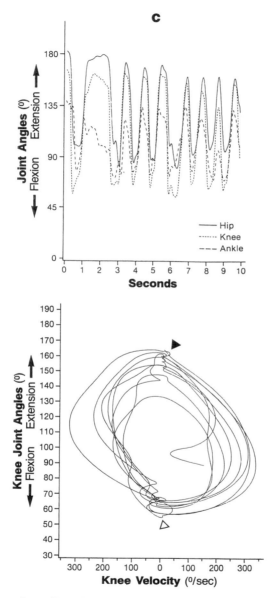

Fig. 11-9. (*Continued*).   (**C**) Full-term infant at 40-weeks gestational age. (*Figure continues.*)

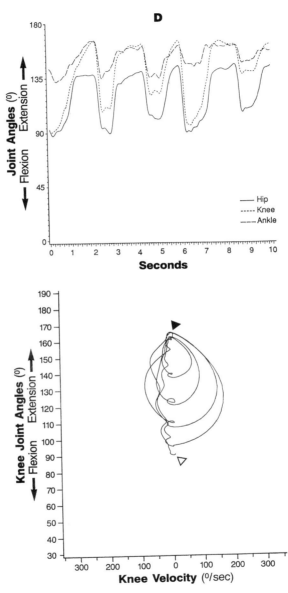

Fig. 11-9. (*Continued*).   **(D)** High-risk infant at 40-weeks postgestational age. (From Heriza,[19] with permission.)

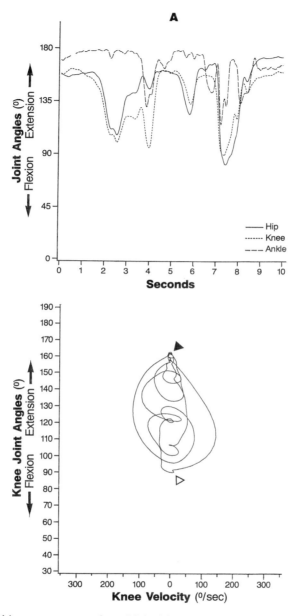

Fig. 11-10. Kicking movements of two high-risk preterm infants at 40-weeks postgestational age. Top panel shows angle–time diagrams of the displacement of hip, knee, and ankle joints. Bottom panel illustrates corresponding phase plane trajectories of knee joint amplitude and peak velocity. The filled triangle in the bottom panel indicates the beginning of kick flexion movement; the open triangle represents peak flexion. Phase plane trajectories progress clockwise. **(A)** High-risk infant with grade IV intraventricular hemorrhage. (*Figure continues.*)

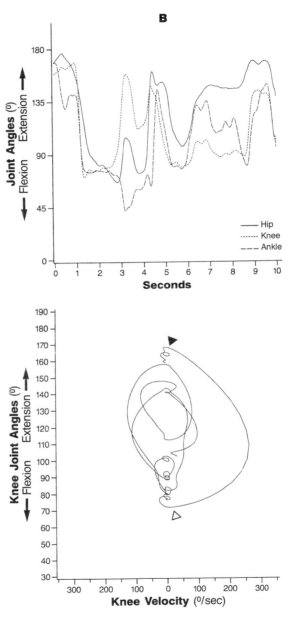

Fig. 11-10. (*Continued*).   **(B)** High-risk infant with grade IV intraventricular hemorrhage and hip dysplasia. (From Heriza,[19] with permission.)

joints, especially the ankle, than full-term infants (Fig. 11-9B,C, top panel). The same infants also paused more during kicking than did full-term infants, resulting in longer kick periods and in a trend toward less frequent kicking. The author hypothesized that differences in kicking outcome may be that (1) larger masses of the limbs in a gravity environment contribute to decreased movement amplitude and velocity and inhibit the extreme flexion of the youngest preterm infant; (2) the long confinement in the intrauterine space for full-term infants may bias muscle and joints toward flexion, contributing to the flexor dominance of the full-term infant; and (3) increases in arousal level may contribute to small angles at peak flexion and short pauses in the kick cycle, resulting in increased frequency of kicking.

Figure 11-11A is an amplitude–velocity phase plane graphic of the thigh of two infants (one normal, one with Down syndrome) who have been walking for 3 months.[22] Although both infants have been walking the same amount of time, the infants are about 1 year apart chronologically. The swing phase of the gait cycle (the large circular portion on the top of the plot) is similar for both infants. Differences, however, are evident in the stance phase of the gait cycle (bottom of the plot). These differences are primarily related to the displacement of the movement rather than to the shape of the plot. The phase portrait of the lower leg segment of the same step cycle of these two infants shows more similarity (Fig. 11-11B). Although the infant with Down syndrome did not walk for almost 1 year after the normal infant, walking behavior seems to be similar for infants who have had 3 months experience walking.

Reaching, Grasping, and Catching

Normal Infants

The emergence of manual skills has been documented through a series of studies by von Hofsten.[9,26–28] In one study, five infants aged 12 to 36 weeks reached toward a suspended stationary object and a suspended object moving at three velocities (3.4, 15, and 30 cm/s) placed 11 or 16 cm from the infant's nose.[9] The infants sat in a semireclining seat on a table. Movements were recorded with two videocameras, one above and one in front of the infant, enabling the investigators to reconstruct three-dimensional trajectories of the hand movements, preserving the time–space properties of the reaching task. The reach was digitized at a sampling rate of 10 Hz.

To allow for the calculation of reaching, the movements were subdivided into functional units. A *functional unit* was defined as one acceleration and one deceleration. Kinematics data calculated to analyze manual movements consisted of distance (relative length of the movement path defined as the actual distance traveled by the hand divided by the shortest distance between the hand and the object); velocity; acceleration; duration of the reaches; and the number, duration, and direction of functional units. Time-dependent plots were utilized to display movement paths (angle–time graphics), velocity plots (velocity–time

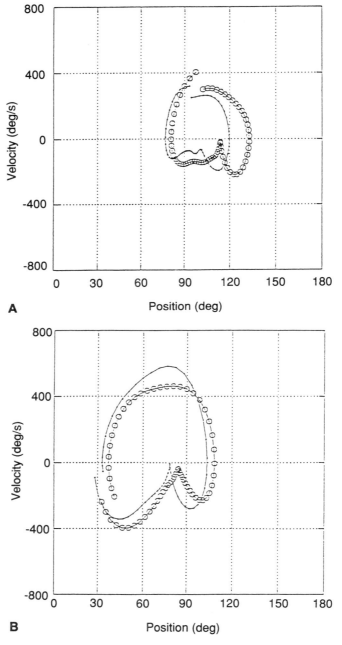

Fig. 11-11. Phase plane trajectories of the thigh **(A)** and lower leg **(B)** of two 3-month-old walkers. Trajectory marked 0–0 indicates a normal infant; the other trajectory indicates an infant with Down syndrome. (From Clark,[22] with permission.)

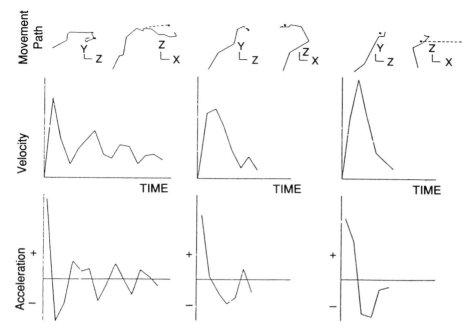

Fig. 11-12. Movement path trajectories, velocity and acceleration profiles of three reaches. Profiles to the left consist of four functional units (age of infant, 30 weeks; object velocity, 3.4 cm/s; duration of reach, 1.4 s). Middle profiles consist of two functional units (age of infant, 27 weeks; object stationary; duration of reach, 0.7 s), and the one to the right consists of one functional unit (age of infant, 36 weeks; object velocity, 15 cm/s; duration of reach, 0.6 s). (From von Hofsten,[9] with permission.)

graphics), and acceleration plots (acceleration–time graphics). Figure 11-12 shows three examples of movement paths, velocity and acceleration profiles during reaching for a suspended moving object (left and right panels) and a suspended stationary object (middle panel). Note that the number of functional units depicted in the acceleration profiles decreases in this representative infant from four functional units at age 30 weeks (left panel) to one at 36 weeks (right panel). In addition, jerky movements are present in the movement path at 30 weeks, whereas smooth movements are predominant at 36 weeks.

The use of kinematic data indicated that reaching skill improved with age. The number of functional units decreased with age. The relative length of the movement path decreased with age, becoming straighter. For the two slowest conditions (object velocity 3.4 cm/s or stationary), duration of approach time decreased with age whereas for the two fastest conditions (object velocity 15 or 30 cm/s) no changes in approach time were evident. Functional unit duration changed with age depending on the position of the functional unit in the reach. Duration of the first functional unit increased with age, while subsequent units decreased with age.

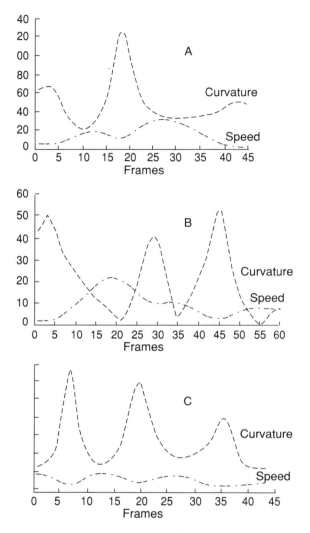

Fig. 11-13. Curvature graphed against speed. Peaks in curvature are associated with speed valleys (slowing). A, B, and C are reaches from a 5-, 7-, and 9-month-old infant, respectively. (From Fetters and Todd,[10] with permission.)

Fetters and Todd[10] filmed 10 infants at ages 21, 33, and 41 weeks reaching for far and near stationary objects placed in front of them on a table. Infants were seated in an infant seat with the back reclined 70 degrees from the horizontal. Three high-speed cameras captured the movement; one overhead and one each to the left and right of the infant. The reach was digitized frame by frame at a sampling rate of 100 Hz.

To allow for calculation of reaching, the speed-curve relationship was subdivided into units of action (Fig. 11-13). The unit was defined by inflection

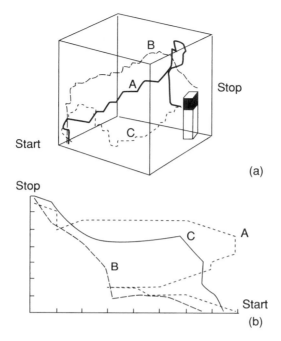

Fig. 11-14. Trajectory path of three reaches from the same 9-month-old infant. Shape of each path is unique. **(a)** side view. **(b)** overhead view. (From Fetters and Todd,[10] with permission.)

points in the reach when a speed valley (slowing) occurred at a curvature peak. A MU was defined as that portion of the reach occurring from one curvature peak to the next. Time-dependent graphics were used to denote curvature-speed plots (Fig. 11-13) and position-time plots (Fig. 11-14).

Kinematics data showed no developmental trends with age. MUs remained consistent, being comprised of 2 to 4. MU durations remained the same regardless of age, whether the MU was the first unit or subsequent units, and whether the object was placed near or far. The path of the reach was jerky (Fig. 11-14) and did not become straighter with age. The duration of the reach showed no obvious developmental pattern and was variable within and between infants.

Although these two studies present different results, they demonstrate that kinematics analysis has the ability qualitatively and quantitatively to describe reaching movements in infants. The discrepancies in findings between the studies are important, as these results demonstrate that a minimal change in the reaching context, reaching for a suspended moving object in the von Hofsten[9] study and for a stationary object on a table top in the Fetters and Todd[10] study may change the kinematics behavior of the reach.

The clinical assumption that proximal trunk support improves distal function was studied by Clary-Trimm.[39] Five term infants aged 4 to 5 months were tested in two supported sitting conditions, minimal and maximal trunk support, with the infant sitting on a floor mat. Reaching for a suspended toy was recorded with two videocameras, one positioned anterior to the infant and one lateral. The mid-dorsal wrists of the three best reaching trials in each condition were digitized in two dimensions at 15 or 30 Hz.

Kinematics data included average wrist velocity, average wrist trajectory movement ratio (defined as the shortest distance between the hand and the object divided by the actual distance traveled by the hand [note that this is the reverse ratio from Fetters and Todd[10] and von Hofsten[9] in their definition of straightness]), and the average number of peaks in the wrist velocity plot. A peak was defined as one acceleration and one deceleration of 2.5 cm/s. Time-dependent plots were used to display wrist velocity visually (Fig. 11-15C,D); time-independent plots were used to display the wrist trajectory patterns (Fig. 11-15A,B).

Although results did not support the assumption that proximal support improves reaching, a trend was evident for the average velocity to increase and the number of velocity peaks to decrease, indicating an improvement in the control of velocity in the maximal support condition. A trend for the average movement ratio to decrease, indicating decreased control of the reaching trajectory and an increase in the average movement time, was also observed when maximal support was given. Figure 11-15 shows three reaching trials for a

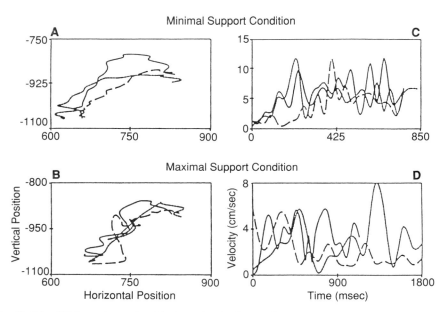

Fig. 11-15. Wrist trajectories **(A,B)** and velocity profiles **(C,D)** for representative infant for three trials of reaching in the minimal **(A,C)** and maximal **(B,D)** support condition. The wrist trajectories during the maximal condition exhibit less linearity compared with the minimal support condition. The velocity profile is multipeaked across trials in both support conditions. (From Clary-Trimm,[39] with permission.)

representative infant. Note that fewer directional changes occur in the movement path during the minimal support condition (A) than the maximal support condition (B). The velocity profile is multipeaked across trials in both support conditions (C,D).

Atypical Infants

Reaching for a stationary object was assessed in 8 term and 11 low-risk preterm infants at ages 7, 9, and 12 months.[40] The experimental design and procedures were similar to those of Fetters and Todd.[10] Kinematics data were analyzed for straightness, duration, number of start–stop phases (MUs), and relative duration of the first MU of the reach. The MU was defined as that portion of the reach between one accelaration and one deceleration and thus is analogous to the functional unit as defined by von Hofsten.[9] Results indicated that developmental changes occurred with age, and, although changes in preterm reach often paralleled those of term reach, subtle group differences were present. With age, term and preterm reaches became straighter and had fewer MUs. The relative duration of the first MU became greater but not faster for term infants. In contrast, the relative duration and speed of the first MU did not change with age in preterm infants.

Movement units have also been used to assess the effectiveness of neurodevelopmental treatment on reaching for a stationary object in preadolescent children with spastic quadriplegia cerebral palsy.[8] Prior to intervention, the children demonstrated multiple MUs or jerky stop–start movements during reaching. After the treatment, the number of MUs significantly decreased in the immediate posttreatment period (Fig. 11-16). Although this study did not involve infants, it demonstrates the use of kinematics to ascertain the efficacy of intervention strategies.

Sitting

The development of postural control in sitting in response to a natural perturbation has been described in 10 normal infants, 7 preterm infants, and 8 infants with cerebral palsy.[30–32] Two stages of sitting were analyzed: stage 1, defined as sitting with support with head erect and steady and only slightly bobbing; and stage 2, defined as sitting alone momentarily with the head well controlled and using the arms to control the sitting position momentarily. Trunk support was removed from the infants while they were sitting erect on a mat table or bench. Postural responses were recorded with one videocamera at a rate of 30 fields/s. The kinematics variables of angular displacement and angular velocity were used to determine kinematics differences between stages 1 and 2 sitting in the three infant samples. Graphics were not used to display the kinematics data. EMG data were also collected. Results indicated a significant decrease in angular displacement and angular velocity from stage 1 to stage 2

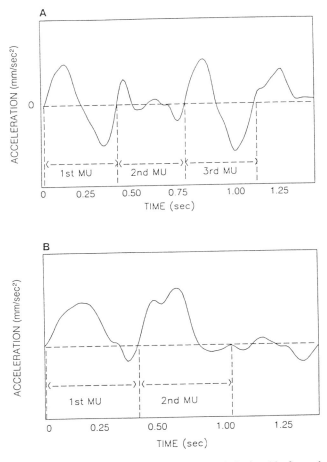

Fig. 11-16. **(A)** Graph of three movement units (MUs) derived before physical therapy from the acceleration profile of a single reach by a preadolescent with CP (cerebral palsy). **(B)** Graph of 2 MUs derived after physical therapy from the same subject. The reduction in the number of MUs suggests a smoother reach. (From Kluzick et al.,[8] with permission.)

in normal and preterm infants. Although infants with cerebral palsy demonstrated a decrease in these kinematic parameters, the decrease was not significant. In addition, no significant differences in angular displacement and velocity were observed between normal infants and infants with cerebral palsy at either stage 1 or stage 2. The authors concluded that the measurement of angular displacement and angular velocity of trunk movement during the acquisition of sitting provided valid measures of the development of independent sitting and that these variables could be used clinically to evaluate and measure improvement in sitting control of infants with sitting dysfunction.

IMPLICATIONS FOR CLINICAL PRACTICE

The uses of kinematic analysis with infants, including atypical or handi-capped infants, are just now being explored. Preliminary data indicate that kinematics provides alternative measuring tools to (1) describe the develop-ment of movement, (2) differentiate between normal and atypical movement, (3) determine the efficacy of therapeutic intervention, (4) test clinical assump-tions of treatment intervention, and (5) test hypotheses about motor control, motor learning, and motor development. Kinematics allows us to look at the process of how new movement is generated and thus holds the potential to identify how abnormal movement is produced. This will lead to alternatives in treatment. Kinematics focuses on functional movements and age appropriate tasks in specified environmental contexts, in contrast to evaluating the product or outcome of the movement. It is a sensitive measurement tool, being respon-sive to changes in the environment even though the task remains the same. Such analysis therefore holds promise for evaluating a variety of therapeutic interventions for the same functional task and identifying the best intervention for the specific infant.

Traditionally, efficacy studies on the effectiveness of physical therapy interventions have used changes in gross motor milestone attainments as the outcome variable. This measure is a product measure and does not address how the infant is progressing toward accomplishing a motor activity. Kinematics offers the use of alternative variables that might be expected to change during an intervention program of physical therapy. These include joint correlations, phase lags, and movement durations in the lower extremities; and the concept of movement units, functional units, or speed curvature relationships in reaching and grasping tasks. The use of visual graphics assists in measuring infant move-ment and provides information concerning the causes of movement. The shape of the graphics provides valuable information concerning path trajectories and has the ability to differentiate between the movement patterns of nonhandi-capped infants and those with possible neurologic dysfunction.

Kinematic analysis is used often in conjunction with videography. By viewing videotapes, movement can be evaluated by the use of behavioral analy-sis. Variables that have been used in videotape analysis include the frequency and types of kicks and steps. Kicks have been defined as single, bilateral, alternating, and simultaneous[41]; steps have been defined as single, alternating, parallel, and double.[36] Duration of the step cycle and phase lags have also been computed using behavioral analysis for kicks and steps.

Data presented here have led us to question our theoretical assumptions regarding the development of movement and have provided alternative develop-mental theories. Kinematic analysis has also provided a means for testing current assumptions about the treatment of infants with movement dysfunction.

Major disadvantages of kinematic analysis include the cost and sophistica-tion of the equipment. In addition, data reduction is labor intensive even in the automated systems. With advances in technology, however, the sophistication, cost, and time to reduce data will decrease. As this occurs, the systems will become a preferred method of describing, analyzing, and evaluating movement. In the future, we may be able to use motion analysis to simulate our treatments on a computer before we apply them to the patient.[42]

Kinematics is a sensitive measurement system that quantifies the quality of movement, describes the movement according to objective kinematic variables, and provides a permanent graphic record of the movement that can be reviewed for evaluation purposes, compared with other movement sequences of the same infant, or compared with movement patterns of other infants. A challenge for physical therapists is to determine the efficacy of treatment, intervention, and prevention programs. Kinematics analysis coupled with videography provides alternative measurement tools to assist us in this challenge.

KINEMATICS COUPLED WITH EMG AND KINETICS

Electromyography

Electromyography provides useful information about the neural control of movement.[5,6] It describes the fundamental patterns of neural output to muscles during on-going behavior and analyzes the relationship of muscle activity to movement. We must remember, however, that a pattern of muscle activity does not always have a one-to-one relationship with the kinematics. Behaviorally, identical movement patterns may result from dissimilar patterns of muscle contractions; thus identifying consistent patterns of individual muscles within an infant or across an infant population may be impossible. We should be alerted in advance not to expect predictable muscle patterns even in the presence of highly consistent kinematics. At the same time, EMG recordings are nearly impossible to interpret without corresponding movement analysis, especially in infants who cannot voluntarily contract muscles on command.[16,43,44]

Kinetics

Kinematics is essential for conducting advanced motion analysis of the underlying kinetics of the movement. Kinetics represents the distribution of forces that provide information on the underlying cause of movement. As with EMG, the pattern of forces that produce the movement may be produced by substantially different patterns of forces and their associated torques.

In a coordinated research effort a team of scientists has recently studied the question: How does an infant move in a world of forces?[45,46] To begin to address this question, the forces involved in kicking in the supine and vertical postures by 3-month-old infants were delineated. Using inverse dynamics, the contributions of active (muscular) and passive (motion-dependent and gravitational) torque components at the hip, knee, and ankle joints from three-dimensional limb kinematics were calculated. In kicking, active muscle contractions (which include passive deformations of muscles, tendons, ligaments, and other periatricular tissues) flex the leg, gravity extends the leg, and the inertial forces generated by other moving segments of the body operate in complex ways. Of the three forces that tend to rotate the limbs around the center of mass, active muscle contraction, gravity, and inertial properties, only one, muscle, is an active force, while the other two are passive.

Figure 11-17 shows the kinematics of the joint angle excursions of two kicks in the vertical posture by the same infant, one of low intensity (A), as demonstrated by the relatively small amplitude and velocity, and the second of high intensity (B), as demonstrated by the relatively large amplitude and velocity. In these kicks, simultaneous flexion and extension of the hip and knee occurred while the ankle remained relatively stable throughout the kick. A more complex picture emerges if we look at the underlying hip joint torque profiles for the two kicks. Figure 11-17 shows the partitioning of the torques acting around the hip joint (C,D). In the small amplitude kick (C), we can see that throughout the kick gravity acts to extend the leg and the muscle torque acts primarily to counteract gravity. Note that the muscle torques in this kick are flexor throughout the kick, even though the leg actually flexes and then extends. Figure 11-17D shows the passive or motion-dependent torques, the torques acting on the hip from the actions of the other segments. Here we see the large dynamic effect of the vigor of the kick. The vast, vigorous kick generates much larger muscular torques. Note again that the muscle torques are precisely modulated to counteract the gravity and the inertial torques.

Although infant vertical kicks appear stereotyped and have no apparent goal, and their kinematics profiles are similar, no single pattern of interactive torques characterize the two kicks. The infant uses two different strategies to manage the torques. In the slow kick, the infant's muscular torque counteracts the force of gravity, whereas in the fast kick the muscular torque counteracts the torques of the inertial forces of the other segments of the kicking limb. The intrinsic dynamics of the leg appear to be assembled with respect to the context or task goal to produce smooth kicking patterns. By measuring the forces underlying spontaneous movement, we can begin to describe how the infant adapts these movements for intentional and goal-directed movements.

A full understanding of movement production comes only with coupling descriptive kinematics with EMG and kinetics analysis that identify the forces acting on the body.[4,46,47] Although the analysis of intersegmental dynamics is in its infancy and cannot be accomplished in a clinical setting at this time, it provides researchers with a potent method for gaining greater insight into the control of natural movements. The real power of this analytical technique is to understand the processes by which movements change, either in the immediate task context or over ontogenetic time.[46] In addition, questions concerning how infants adapt inherent movements to the demands of functional tasks in which limbs must bear weight and move forward or how they reach for objects in an accurate manner can begin to be elucidated. The use of descriptive kinematics with EMG and kinetics analysis has the potential to identify how the process becomes changed in infants with movement dysfunction and to provide information for therapeutic intervention.

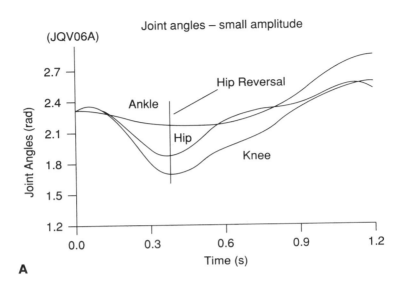

A

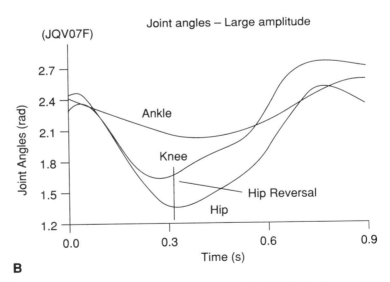

B

Fig. 11-17. Joint angle changes associated with a single kick in the vertical posture. **(A)** Small amplitude kick. **(B)** Large amplitude kick. (*Figure continues.*)

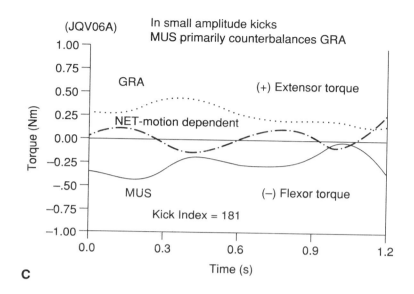

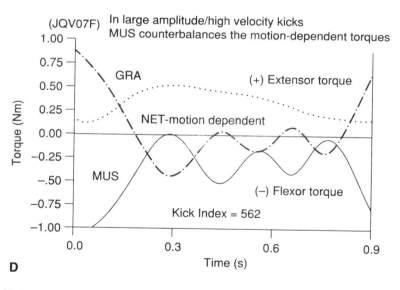

Fig. 11-17. (*Continued*). **(C)** Hip joint torque profiles accompanying the small amplitude kick shown above. **(D)** Hip joint torque profiles accompanying the large amplitude kick shown above. (From Jensen et al.,[45] with permission.)

REFERENCES

1. Winter DA: Biomechanics and Motor Control of Human Movement. 2nd Ed. John Wiley & Sons, New York, 1990
2. Whiting HTA: Human Motor Action: Bernstein Reassessed. Elsevier Science Publishing, New York, 1984
3. Fetters L: Measurement and treatment in cerebral palsy: an argument for a new approach. Phys Ther 71:246, 1991
4. Kamm K, Thelen E, Jensen JL: A dynamical systems approach to motor development. Phys Ther 70:763, 1990
5. Harris SR, Heriza CB: Measuring infant movement: clinical and technological assessment techniques. Phys Ther 67:1877, 1987
6. Heriza CB: Motor development: traditional and contemporary theories. p. 99. In Lister M (ed): Contemporary Management of Motor Control Problems. Proceedings of the II Step Conference. Foundation for Physical Therapy, Alexandria, VA, 1991
7. Winstein CJ, Garfinkel A: Qualitative dynamics of disordered human locomotion: a preliminary investigation. J Motor Behav 21:373, 1989
8. Kluzik J, Fetters L, Coryell J: Quantification of control: a preliminary study of effects of neurodevelopmental treatment on reaching in children with spastic cerebral palsy. Phys Ther 70:65, 1990
9. von Hofsten C: Development of visually directed reaching: the approach phase. J Hum Movement Stud 5:160, 1979
10. Fetters L, Todd J: Quantitative assessment of infant reaching movements. J Motor Behav 19:147, 1987
11. Beuter A, Garfinkel A: Phase plane analysis of limb trajectories in nonhandicapped and cerebral palsied subjects. Adapt Phys Activity Q 2:214, 1985
12. Clark JE, Truly TL, Phillips SJ: A dynamical systems approach to understanding the development of lower limb coordination in locomotion. p. 363. In Bloch H, Bertenthal B (eds): Sensory-Motor Organization and Development in Infancy and Early Childhood. Kluwer Academic, Hingham, MA, 1990
13. Kelso JAS, Saltzman EL, Tuller B: The dynamical perspective on speech production: data and theory. J Phonetics 14:29, 1986
14. Schoner G, Kelso JAS: Dynamic pattern generation in behavioral and neural systems. Science 239:1513, 1988
15. Scholz JP: Dynamic pattern theory—some implications for therapeutics. Phys Ther 70:827, 1990
16. Thelen E, Fisher DM: Newborn stepping: an explanation for a "disappearing" reflex. Dev Psychol 18:760, 1982
17. Heriza CB: Organization of leg movements in preterm infants. Phys Ther 68:1340, 1988
18. Heriza CB: Comparison of leg movements in preterm infants at term with healthy full-term infants. Phys Ther 68:1687, 1988
19. Heriza CB: Implications of a dynamical systems approach to understanding infant kicking behavior. Phys Ther 71:222, 1991
20. Benson JB, Welch L, Campos JJ et al: The Development of Crawling in Infancy. Presented at the Eighth Biennial Meeting of the International Society for the Study of Behavioral Development, July 6–10. Tours, France, 1985
21. Clark JE, Whitall J, Phillips SJ: Human interlimb coordination: the first 6 months of independent walking. Dev Psychobiol 21:445, 1988

22. Clark JE: On viewing atypical and normal development as dynamical systems. Presented at the International Conference on Infant Studies, April 21. Montreal, Canada, 1990

23. Forssberg H: Ontogeny of human locomotor control, I. Infant stepping, supported locomotion, and transition to independent locomotion. Exp Brain Res 57:480, 1985

24. Thelen E, Cooke DW: The relationship between newborn stepping and later locomotion: a new interpretation. Dev Med Child Neurol 29:380, 1987

25. Sutherland DH, Olshen R, Cooper L et al: The development of mature gait. J Bone Joint Surg 62:336, 1980

26. von Hofsten C: Predictive reaching for moving objects by human infants. J Exp Child Psychol 30:369, 1980

27. von Hofsten C: Eye-hand coordination in newborns. Dev Psychol 18:450, 1982

28. von Hofsten C: Catching skills in infancy. J Exp Psychol [Hum Percept] 9:75, 1983

29. Dowd JM, Tronick EZ: Temporal coordination of arm movements in early infancy: do infants move in synchrony with adult speech? Child Dev 57:762, 1986

30. Harbourne RT: A Kinematic and Electromyographic Analysis of the Development of Sitting Posture in Infants. Master's Thesis. University of North Carolina at Chapel Hill, Chapel Hill, NC, 1988

31. Scalise-Smith D: The Response to Postural Pertubation in Premature Infants in Two Stages of Sitting: a Kinematic and Electromyographic Analysis. Master's Thesis. University of North Carolina at Chapel Hill, Chapel Hill, NC, 1989

32. Owen PL: Postural Responses of Children With Cerebral Palsy at Two Stages of Sitting Development. Master's Thesis. University of North Carolina at Chapel Hill, Chapel Hill, NC, 1989

33. Fogel A, Thelen E: Development of early expressive and communicative action: reinterpreting the evidence from a dynamic systems perspective. Dev Psychol 23:747, 1987

34. Thelen E: Self-organization in developmental processes: can systems approaches work? p. 747. In Gunnar M, Thelen E (eds): Systems and Development: The Minnesota Symposium on Child Psychology. Vol. 22. Lawrence Erlbaum Associates, Inc., Hillsdale, NJ, 1989

35. Thelen E, Kelso JS, Fogel A: Self-organizing systems and infant motor development. Dev Rev 7:39, 1987

36. Thelen E, Ulrich BD: Hidden skills: a dynamic systems analysis of treadmill stepping during the first year. Monogr Soc Res Child Dev 56(1):1, 1991

37. Thelen E, Fisher DM, Ridley-Johnson R: The relationship between physical growth and a newborn reflex. Inf Behav Dev 7:479, 1984

38. Thelen E: Treadmill-elicited stepping in seven-month-old infants. Child Dev 57:1498, 1986

39. Clary-Trimm BL: The Effect of Proximal Support on Upper Extremity Reaching. Master's Thesis. The University of North Carolina at Chapel Hill, Chapel Hill, NC, 1990

40. Rose-Jacobs R, Fetters L: Kinematic assessment of reach in term and preterm infants. Inf Behav Dev 13:596, 1990

41. Thelen E, Ridley-Johnson R, Fisher DM: Shifting patterns of bilateral coordination and lateral dominance in the leg movements of young infants. Dev Psychobiol 16:29, 1983

42. Gage JR: President's message. Am Acad Cerebral Palsy Dev Med News 42:1, 1991

43. Beckoff A: A neuroethological approach to the study of the ontogeny of coordinated behavior. p. 19. In Burghardt GM, Bekoff M (eds): The Development of Behavior: Comparative and Evolutionary Aspects. Garland, New York, 1978
44. Winter DA: Biomechanical motor patterns in normal walking. J Motor Behav 15:302, 1983
45. Jensen JL, Ulrich BD, Thelen E: Limb dynamics of infant kicking in supine and vertical postures. Presented at the Society for Research in Child Development, April. Kansas City, MO, 1989
46. Schneider K, Zernicke RF, Ulrich BD et al: Understanding movement control in infants through the analysis of limb intersegmental dynamics. J Motor Behav 22:493, 1990
47. Bradley NS: Animal models offer the opportunity to acquire a new perspective on motor development. Phys Ther 70:776, 1990

12 Future Directions for Physical Therapy Assessment in Early Infancy

Suzann K. Campbell

The currently available assessment methods, while excellent in many respects, do not collectively represent a systematic protocol for comprehensive assessment of development in infancy. Rather, they are a set of individual tests of different constructs and, sometimes, of multiple constructs. Furthermore, they have weak diagnostic capabilities and limited predictability of long-term outcome. Few assessment tools are available that are adequately prescriptive (i.e., that assist physical therapists in designing intervention programs and evaluating their outcomes). The sum of these problems results in a weak linkage among problem identification, treatment, and expected outcomes. The purposes of this chapter are (1) to review what is known about the predictability of outcomes based on assessments in infancy, (2) to review various theoretical and decision-making approaches to incorporating what we know into systematic assessment protocols, and (3) to review tests under development for consistency with such a conceptual framework. Consideration of these topics suggests the work of the future.

THE PROBLEM OF PREDICTABIITY

What do we know about prediction of outcomes from early assessment? The bulk of the literature on assessment in infancy suggests that very little regarding outcome in later years can be successfully predicted for individual

293

children and certainly not from typical developmental assessment scales.[1-3] For example, poor motor performance scores early in life have some capacity for identifying children at risk for developmental problems, but in a nonspecific way. Poor motor scores may later be associated with cerebral palsy, mental retardation, or even blindness and behavioral problems.[4-6] The process of recovery from early nonoptimal medical conditions also complicates the situation as Piper and others (this volume) have pointed out. For example, the presence of early brain insult may reveal itself in transient dystonia that simulates cerebral palsy but later subsides to result in normal development or, alternatively, reappears as subtle problems in learning, perceptual skills, or behavior.[4]

The Importance of Process-Oriented Research

A major problem in predicting motor and other outcomes is the failure to concentrate on *process* rather than product when assessing children. Two important papers have brought this issue into clear focus. The first is a review of the history of research on cognition by Kopp,[1] and the second is a monograph by Thelen and Ulrich[7] on dynamic systems analysis of the process of motor development in infancy.

Kopp[1] reviews the history of attempts to define and identify developmental risk. Key findings have included the following:

1. The earlier the appearance of a biologic risk factor, the greater the risk of long-term adverse developmental outcome.
2. Little continuity of risk across ages has been found. Some risk factors disappear unpredictably over time, some are non-specific predictors of later dysfunction, and some children show no early signs of risk but nevertheless develop severely disabling conditions. Although the tests used as predictors may be one source of the problem, until the time at which a specific brain area usually begins to mature, dysfunction related to earlier damage of that area is not likely to be identified accurately.
3. Environmental factors strongly influence the outcome of biologic risk. Social factors can play a strong ameliorating role or, conversely, can magnify the likelihood of adverse outcome, at least for cognitive development. Environmental effects on motor development are not well defined.

What these findings suggest is that multifactor assessment of the individual and his or her environment across time is essential to improving predictability. Kopp's review[1] elegantly demonstrates that recent studies on the *processes* of cognitive development have finally yielded important predictive information that could not be obtained by the study of products, or milestones. For example, her data, based on an information processing model, have revealed the importance, in the development of cognition, of sustained attention, of response to novelty, and of exploration in the first 1 to 1.5 years. The continuum progresses from selective attention to visual stimuli in early infancy to sustained attention to seen and held objects. Along the way, visual attention to the hands at 3 to 4 months, heralding the switch to sustained attention to what the hands can do with objects (e.g., shaking, banging, crumpling),[8] is followed by a focus of attention on the objects themselves. Focus on and continued engagement with objects is essential for cognitive growth; however, work with children with cerebral palsy has indicated that actual physical manipulation is not required.[9] Qualitative differences arise in children with developmental disabilities, however, because they often have difficulty sustaining performance of the mature behaviors of which they are capable and thus tend to use cues, attention, and other cognitive processes inefficiently for successful learning.[1]

These concepts fit well with recent emphasis in the physical therapy literature on motor learning models for use in intervention. These models stress the importance for therapists of helping children to recognize the salient features of a motor task that are regulatory in achieving successful task performance.[10] For the present purpose, however, the crucial lesson for therapists to derive from this work is the importance of identifying and studying not only the cognitive processes important in motor learning but also the underlying motor control processes themselves. Here the work of Thelen and colleagues is instructive.[7,11,12]

Thelen and her colleagues are engaged in identifying the processes involved in the development of walking. They have found that use of a dynamic systems model for designing studies and interpreting their results has lead to rich new information on motor development. Their approach has involved rejecting the idea that development is guided only by maturation of the nervous system and instead recognizing that concurrent development in multiple interacting systems leads to the overt behaviors we recognize as the products of motor development. Some of these systems include the postural control system, strength, and the anthropometric characteristics of the performer (including weight and the location of the center of mass of the body (see Ch. 5). The information already obtained clearly shows that one of the slowest developing (and potentially rate-limiting) systems is that of postural control (see Ch. 8). Therapists have long understood that postural control develops only after the ability to assume a position in space has been attained (i.e., postural control develops through experience), but we have not been able to define it operationally in a way that has led to useful clinical assessment tools.

Although the creative experiments of Thelen and colleagues do not yet lend themselves to use for assessment in clinical situations, they have already led the way to a fresh look at how we assess motor performance in children. The drive to look, to move, and to obtain the upright position in space appears to be innate. Developmental processes that develop over time and with experience, in addition to those involved in controlling the center of mass, such as anticipatory postural control, appear to include (1) selective control of individual segments, particularly distal segments (hands in the first year, feet in the second); (2) the ability to change positions at will; (3) orientation to stimuli, both attentionally and physically; (4) evaluation and use of sensory inputs to enhance motor control; and (5) the ability to control and modulate the force and speed of movement. Other control parameters are discussed by Shumway-Cook and Woollacott (Ch. 8). Clearly, independent assessment of multiple characteristics of the performer, the task, and the environment will be necessary in order to understand motor development and developmental risk.

Two additional types of currently available information are likely to be useful as we consider what new tests we need and how they should be developed: (1) information regarding early diagnostic indicators of cerebral palsy or delayed development and (2) information regarding the value of early therapy in reduction of disability at later ages as it relates to the natural history of abnormal developmental functions. Information from these two types of inquiry should be helpful in deciding what new assessments of motor processes might be helpful in both identifying children who will have problems and in planning and assessing intervention.

Prediction of Cerebral Palsy

Although early neurologic tests and therapist-designed tests such as the Movement Assessment of Infants have been successful in identifying *groups* of children at risk for cerebral palsy, no currently available test has been successful in identifying *individual* children who have sustained permanent brain damage.[2] Recently, however, Prechtl[13] in the Netherlands has reported successful differentiation, before the age of 5 months, of prematurely born children who will or will not develop spastic cerebral palsy after the recognition of a brain pathology via ultrasound examination. The diagnostic indicator that proved predictive was the presence of "cramped synchronized" movement quality during spontaneous motor behavior. The suggestion that children with spastic cerebral palsy begin life with hypotonia, stereotyped patterns, and poverty of movement and gradually become spastic and lack isolated movement has long been espoused, but this work is the first to use *Gestalt* assessment of the presence of synchronized movement as a successful predictor.

Cioni and Prechtl[14] have also identified a sequence of movement patterns that characterize normal development in the first 3 to 5 months. This sequence involves a qualitative change from movement that is writhing, yet complex and elegant in form, to successively looser and wider ranging writhing, then fidgety, oscillating and ballistic movements before the development of more obviously goal-directed and controlled motor behaviors. Exactly what the processes might be that lie behind this normal sequence of development of general movements and the abnormal distortion represented by cramped synchrony remains to be ascertained. One point their work makes clear, however, is that new types of general movements develop in concert with development of head centering, upright head control, extension of the legs, and trunk stability in prone and supine.

Clinical work by Amiel-Tison and Grenier[15] in France suggests that postural control mechanisms that anticipate the development of postural control in spontaneous motor behavior can be elicited in the first weeks after birth.[15] They use examination maneuvers that are similar to neurodevelopmental treatment (NDT) handling techniques to elicit head, limb, and trunk postural control strategies that are normally demonstrated only later during children's spontaneous activity. Failure to elicit these precursors of normal development is correlated with the presence of cerebral palsy. These clinical maneuvers have not, however, been documented with formal research and do not appear to be reliably elicited in all children. They seem to be useful primarily in documenting normality when present, rather than abnormality when absent. They once again suggest, however, the importance of developing methods for measuring postural control strategies as an important process in motor skill development.

These newly successful approaches to diagnosing spastic cerebral palsy fit extremely well with the clinical data on the primary impairments in this condition. The hallmarks of cerebral palsy of the spastic type include impaired force production, muscle coactivation in abnormal synergies during movement with inability to perform isolated joint and limb movement, and poor postural control mechanisms both for self-initiated movements involving anticipatory postural set and for reacting to postural perturbations from the environment.[16] Because these types of abilities have been demonstrated to be important roles of the cerebral motor–sensory systems, especially the corticospinal tracts and supplementary motor areas, not surprisingly such dysfunction in movement is associated with damaged periventricular white matter in premature infants.[17]

Another approach to identifying important predictors involves review of the clinical literature on primary impairments that ultimately affect later-developing functions, especially those that can be reduced or prevented by early intervention. Very little research exists on this point. One of the few studies that suggests such a result is a comparison of NDT and Vojta therapy, which produced the result that children treated with Vojta walked earlier, on average, and with better postural alignment than those treated with NDT.[18] The significant factor was believed to be the prevention of postural abnormalities in creeping that later impaired functioning in walking. Other possible examples of natural history factors in the development of abnormal movement include early hypoextensibility in hip adductors and hamstrings and in shoulder extensors that are likely early warning signs of cerebral palsy long before the more typical hallmark of shortening in the ankle plantar flexors. Lack of selective activation of individual body parts is another primary impairment that would appear to be a key parameter in early identification of cerebral palsy.

Formal diagnostic tools that incorporate these types of clinically based knowledge need to be developed and studied in the primary care pediatric setting so that they can be extended to high-risk children born at term and to children in whom no history of risk for cerebral palsy is known to exist, that is, to large-scale populations of a diverse nature. Research elucidating the processes involved in accomplishing motor tasks is also needed. One of these processes is clearly anticipatory postural control. Others may include the ability to activate prime movers selectively, to control force production appropriately for given tasks, and to recognize regulatory parameters of the task and the environment.

Prediction of Motor Delay

Much less information is available about populations of children who will have motor dysfunction that is primarily delayed (i.e., children with overall developmental retardation). Most of what has been reported has involved the study of predictors of deviant *cognitive* development; motor performance delay (without deviance in postural control) has not been the subject of much recent study (however, see Molnar[19]). Retained primitive reflexes and even an early diagnosis of cerebral palsy can indicate risk for developmental retardation rather than a cerebral motor disorder.[4] Most of the outcome studies of children at risk for developmental delay because of premature birth have used the Bayley Scales of Infant Development for prediction, which is problematic because of the outmoded norms on this test.[20] Until the revised scales are available, new knowledge regarding prediction of motor delay is unlikely to be attained; however, tests of milestones have not previously proven to be predictors with high specificity.[1] Whether studying the underlying processes of motor development will also aid in better predictability of motor delay remains to be discovered. Here, a primary process problem may be in the cognitive area (such as failure to recognize the affordances or regulatory parameters of the environment) or in the behavioral area (such as lack of motivation or attentional capacity).

How can we translate new findings on the importance of assessing process into clinically useful tools for problem identification, treatment planning, and outcome evaluation? I have argued previously that clinical measurement suffers from lack of a conceptual framework for organizing information and defining constructs of importance.[21] The next section presents several theoretical frameworks that might prove useful.

THE STRUCTURE OF A SYSTEMATIC ASSESSMENT PROTOCOL

Three conceptual frames of reference can contribute to a theoretical, structural base for establishing a systematic assessment protocol for diagnosis, treatment planning, and outcome assessment for infants at risk for developmental disability. These frameworks include (1) the transactional analysis approach to understanding and interpreting developmental functions,[22] (2) the decision theory model for making clinical decisions,[23] and (3) a system for classifying levels of dysfunction and disability.[21,24,25] The first—the transactional sytems approach—takes into account the effects of environmental and social forces on child development and recovery from potentially adverse medical and other events. These forces evolve from family and community level reciprocal interactions between children and the significant people in their lives within a total environmental context. Second, the decision theory model takes the results of research and clinical expert judgment to develop mathematical models for making diagnostic and treatment decisions. In general, the results exceed the ability of even the best clinicians to make complicated conceptual syntheses of signs, symptoms, and prognostic indicators.[26] Finally, the process of disablement framework is a hierarchical conceptual model for understanding the multiple physiologic and functional levels of the disabling process. This approach emphasizes the need for longitudinal information on the course of disabling conditions during the life span and the importance of linking underlying impairment to functional performance in ecologically valid settings. Development of a measurement protocol based on these three types of conceptual frameworks would combine knowledge from multiple disciplinary perspectives at multiple time-points to guide clinical decision making and outcome evaluation.

The Transactional Model

The transactional model of development postulates that children develop in interaction with their environment and in turn produce effects on their environment.[22] A comprehensive assessment protocol, then, would also assess the characteristics of the child's environment and the child's interaction with significant persons in his or her life. The processes of importance include the ability to help a child establish a sense of trust, gain inputs needed for learning, explore novelty, and experience the affordances offered by the environment. Parents best able to do this are those with responsive children and those who (1) have knowledge about developmental processes, (2) are psychologically attached to their children, (3) possess their own personal support network and interests, and (4) have their own physical and emotional needs met.

Tests based on some of these concepts include the Brazelton Neonatal Behavioral Assessment Scales,[27] Barnard's Nursing Child Assessment Scales,[28] and the Assessment of Premature Infant Behavior.[29] The Home Observation for Measurement of the Environment[30] assesses the stimulating characteristics of the home environment while the Parenting Stress Index[31] assesses parental perceptions of stressful characteristics related to the child and other environmental variables. Sparling (Ch. 4) describes others as well. Although such tests exist, they are seldom used by therapists. Such data are often considered in predictive models of risk for aberrant outcome as well as for planning and assessing outcomes of intervention. They will be absolutely essential for use by therapists working in family-focused early intervention under the new provisions of PL 99-457.

Clinical Decision Theory

For years, developmental specialists have been conceptualizing models for tracking risk for developmental deviance in infants, but none have yet been demonstrated to have sufficient predictive validity to be useful at the level of the individual infant. Some systems have high sensitivity for detecting deviance but low specificity for predicting normality and vice versa. Either problem creates unacceptable conditions for practical use in clinical practice. Gordon and

Jens[32] recently reviewed the history of attempts to construct clinical decision-making models for tracking children at risk for developmental disability and clearly described their problems. Based on new knowledge and the previous experience gained with assessing older models, several new models have been proposed. Gordon and Jens, for example, propose a Moving Risk Model for implementation in clinical settings that may overcome some of the previously existing problems; however, their model has not yet been scientifically tested.

The model Gordon and Jens suggest is contrasted with the Risk Routes Model of Aylward and Kenny.[33] The Risk Routes Model assesses risk in three areas: medical/biologic, environmental/psychosocial, and behavioral/developmental. Degree of risk is additive across areas at each time of testing and cumulative across time. Additivity of domains at any one point in time ignores the fact that not all aspects of development proceed at the same rate. The second feature of cumulativity across time means that once assessed as at risk for developmental deviance, a child is never removed from the risk register.

The Moving Risk Model, in contrast, conceptualizes risk as synergistic across areas of development at any one point in time and noncumulative across time.[32] Thus children can move in and out of at-risk status. The model also provides for weighting of individual domains of development based on research-based knowledge indicating that certain areas of development are in especially sensitive stages at particular points in time. For example, they suggest that visual memory is a particularly important developmental process during the period from 3 to 7 months and that mental development is undergoing a sensitive period during the ages of 9 to 24 months.

From the viewpoint of physical therapy, a problem with the Moving Risk Model is that the list of tests suggested for use within this conceptual framework does not include any motor assessment until 9 months of age. At 9 months, the Bayley Scales of Infant Development are suggested as useful. I cannot recommend use of these scales for clinical decision making until the revision and renorming project currently underway has been completed. The fact that the model does not require the use of any particular test, however, means that assessment teams are free to test the model using their own preferred assessments.

From my point of view, however, neither the Moving Risk Model nor the Risk Routes Model is entirely satisfactory. The argument of Gordon and Jens that children must be allowed to move out of the at-risk category at points when development is proceeding normally, even though previous risk might have been very high, is not entirely compelling. The danger of releasing children from careful follow-up too soon is too great when we know that some risk factors are covertly expressed for many months, especially in the case of mild disabilities. Nevertheless, their point that risk should not continue to be completely cumulative across time is well taken.

Clinical decision theory presents an alternative approach that allows a mathematical calculation of the probability of risk at any point in time based on prior degree of risk *and* present degree of risk.[34] In such a model, when contemporary risk is low (because all developmental assessments are well within normal limits), the probability of deviant development *given* previously existing risk can be calculated. The probability outcome that results from that assessment then becomes the prior risk probability at the next assessment point. Risk can move up or down from one point to another, decrease at subsequent points in time when previous developmental tests provide normal results, and increase over time when development falls progressively further behind normative performance levels for age.

The conceptual framework for clinical decision theory[35] assumes that clinical judgment encompasses such a complex set of tasks that mathematical algorithms and decision models incorporating the results of research on important clinical problems are likely to be more successful than clinical judgment for making diagnostic and treatment decisions. In decision theory, probabilities of various outcomes are assessed based on variables such as previous historic events or assessments, potential negative results of various decisions, and patient or family judgments regarding the value of various potential positive and negative results.

In the diagnostic area, for example, risk for cerebral palsy or motor developmental delay could be estimated based on ultrasound results at birth, general movement assessment findings, and tests of postural control and motor milestone achievement at successive ages. Bayesian statistical models allow the degree of risk calculated at earlier points in time to be incorporated as factors in an equation using current test results, thus establishing a risk probability that takes into account prior history as well as current functioning. Studies of decision equations based on variables such as these have almost universally found that diagnostic decisions made with such algorithms are much more reliable than clinicians' judgments.[26] In the area of treatment planning decisions, models could be developed that allow parents to choose frequency or type of treatment based on their judgment of the value and probability of various types of outcomes and risks.

Classification of Impairment and Its Consequences

Two similar but complementary approaches exist for classifying levels of function from the cellular to the societal in the presence of potentially disabling conditions. One is the World Health Organization (WHO) International Classification of Impairments, Disabilities, and Handicaps[24]; the other is the classification of pathology, impairment, functional limitations, and disability developed by Nagi and elaborated by others.[21,25,36,37] Haley (Ch. 10) has described the key concepts of these models; thus the definitions will not be repeated here.

The National Center for Medical Rehabilitation Research (NCMRR) has adopted a slight variation of the Nagi model and added a fifth domain, that of Societal Limitations.[38] The disabling process in the latter domain, which has some similarities to the concept of Handicap in the WHO model, involves societally imposed barriers that prevent individuals with disabilities from functioning at the highest level at which they are capable. Examples include architectural barriers, denial of insurance coverage for necessary services, the shortage of therapists, and societal attitudes toward the disabled that limit employment or opportunities to be educated in the least restrictive environment.

The classification of disability within such a framework could be used to develop a comprehensive assessment protocol. Within the usual purview of rehabilitation professionals are the levels of impairment, functional limitations, and disability. A comprehensive protocol would consist of tests at each level that avoid the serious confounding of variables now found in most frequently used tests. Tests at the level of impairment are likely to be the most discipline specific, whereas tests at the level of disability will be the most interdisciplinary.

The example I will use to illustrate categorization of the disabling process using the NCMRR model is the infant with spastic diplegia,[21] emphasizing the motoric dysfunction characteristic of this condition; the framework for classifying the disabling process, however, can be broadened to include all aspects of disability. In the child with spastic diplegia, *pathophysiology,* the underlying medical or injury processes at the cellular and tissue level, typically involves a white matter infarct in the periventricular areas of the brain caused by hypoxia. Primary prevention strategies at this level are aimed at prevention of hypoxic–ischemic events that lead to brain damage.

In the domain of *impairment,* we classify the cell, tissue, and organ system disorders that are present and will potentially impair functioning. These are not necessarily located in the area of the lesion (in cerebral palsy, the brain) but result from it. In spastic diplegia, sensorimotor impairments include decreased force and power output by the neuromuscular system, poor selective control of the movements of joints and body segments, and poor anticipatory regulation of postural set for movement.[16] These impairments are all well known abnormalities resulting from damage to the corticospinal tracts that descend in the periventricular area of the brain or to the supplementary motor areas involved in motor planning and coordination. Impaired balance, efficiency, endurance, and coordination of movement result.

The combination of impairments in one or more systems leads to *functional limitations* involving whole body function, for example, slow and inefficient gait, tendency to lose one's sitting balance while using the arms for dressing, and so on. Functional limitations result from impairments and are typically assessed in a clinical setting, but may or may not be remediable. On the other hand, not all impairments need result in limitations of function. For example, a slight contracture of the hamstrings will not cause obvious functional limitation; at some level, however, tight hamstrings begin to impair gait and other activities.

If primary impairments can be limited by early therapy, some functional limitations that otherwise result as a part of the natural history of a condition may be avoided. Thus prevention at this level of the disabling process involves attempts to limit impairment resulting from the lesion. For example, most therapists believe that early intervention for children with spastic diplegia produces a more efficient gait; however, very little research exists to document such effects.[18] Theoretically, early treatment should also result in prevention or reduction of secondary impairments, such as contractures and deformities, which are generally not present as primary impairments in children. Rather, they develop later as a result of habitual movement using abnormal compensatory patterns or overactive muslces with paretic antagonists, or from overall poverty of movement.

On the other hand, the research of Palmer et al.[39] suggests that a full year of physical therapy for children with spastic diplegia (which presumably concentrated on treating impairment and functional limitations) is less success-ful than parent programming for facilitation of overall developmental progress *followed* by physical therapy in accelerating the rate of motor and cognitive development. Because the course of developing impairments in areas such as strength, range of motion, postural control, and endurance were not adequately assessed, we do not know whether they suffered even as developmental mile-stone progress was facilitated. Treatment was also infrequent and initiated after 1 year of age, which may have been a factor in the results.

Until we develop tests that clearly separate the elements of underlying impairment from functional limitations that may be primary or may result from use of compensatory strategies to enhance function, we will be unable to docu-ment the value of early or preventive intervention for cerebral palsy or interpret results like those of Palmer and colleagues. As mentioned previously, diagnostic tests that incorporate natural history data (e.g., identifying hamstring tightness that will impair sitting or postural patterns in creeping that predict later problems in walking) also are needed for commonly treated disabling conditions.

When functional limitations persist over long periods of time and are not remediable or cannot be compensated for through use of assistive devices or orthotics, *disabilities* result. Children fail to accomplish normal life roles, such as participation in school, play, or family activities. Therapy planning should start with interdisciplinary assessment at this level. This involves asking which roles and skills are needed and appropriate for a specific child. When disabilities are present or need to be prevented, each discipline considers what contribu-tions it has to make and plans intervention accordingly, in concert with other team members. The process involved may be finding the compensatory strategy that will allow successful functional performance despite functional limitations. In the case of our example of the child with spastic diplegia, a therapist may decide that independent locomotion is a future goal but that the child needs an assistive device at the moment to allow him to keep up with his ambulatory peers. Using the NCMRR model allows one to identify clearly the treatment emphasis—whether it is aimed at reducing impairment (emphasizing strength, endurance, tone, or other factors), at overcoming functional limitations through practice of compensatory strategies, or at preventing disability through provi-sion of an assistive device.

Societal limitations for the child with spastic diplegia might include a physician unwilling to refer a child to physical therapy, architectural barriers to mobility, or inability to attend a day care center because of the presence of cognitive or motor delay or the need for special equipment or transportation. Most problems like these are not within the usual purview of rehabilitation, but must be attacked through problem identification and action at the community and societal level.

Classification of Tests

Most currently available tests for infants would be classified as assessing functional limitation, especially delay in attainment of motor and cognitive developmental milestones (Ch. 9). The Revised Gesell Developmental Schedules might be considered to provide the greatest separation of constructs across developmental domains, as they provide separate subscales for gross and fine motor behavior as well as cognitive and adaptive behavior.[40] Kopp[1] found that Gesell scores were most highly correlated with her measures of sustained attention, while the Bayley Mental Scale scores correlated with measures of exploration. Gesell scores do not by themselves, however, possess discrimination capability for use with very young infants.

Few tests for infants successfully capture aspects of impairment, and those that do test elements of impairment have conceptual bases that have not tended to be predictive. For example, most infant tests include assessment of postural tone and primary reflexes, and none of these tests have diagnostic validity sufficient for use in decision making at the level of the individual baby. The most promising test at the level of impairment is currently the general movement assessment of Prechtl[13] and colleagues. This test appears to tap aspects of coordination and modulation of movement, such as speed, smoothness, variability, amplitude, and selective control, expressed as a *Gestalt* perception. The diagnostically specific pattern for identifying spastic types of cerebral palsy, that of cramped, synchronized movement, implies impairment of selective control and ability to grade the force of movement to perform large amplitude displacements. Predictive validity for use in large populations with varying risk characteristics, however, remains to be demonstrated.

Other aspects of impairment for which tests are under development include the coordination of movement sequences and postural control and alignment. Shumway-Cook and Woolacott (Ch. 8) describe the assessment of postural control that they are developing. Other examples include Levine's test of postural alignment,[41] which is based on the assumption that normal movement begins from an anatomically appropriate alignment of body parts. The Miller Toddler and Infant Motor Evaluation contains a motor test developed under the assumption, supported by Prechtl's recent work, that the variety of motor sequences engaged in from the supine or prone position is an expression of nervous system competence.[42] Because this test has subscales for each of the five required assessment areas under PL99-457, it may come closest to the ideal of a truly comprehensive measurement protocol; it is not yet clear, however, whether its underlying constructs cross the levels of the disabling process model. The Alberta Infant Motor Test, although intended as a normative test of motor development in the first 18 months, defines each milestone in terms of the appropriate postural alignment and selective control of body parts in a developmental continuum that leads to the child's mastery over the force of gravity.[43] Thus it may be a test of functional capacity or limitation based on specific impairment in the area of postural control. These two tests are reviewed by Haley (Ch. 10).

The Test of Infant Motor Performance (TIMP) that I and my colleagues are developing has a similar emphasis on the development of postural control and selective movement. The TIMP was developed to capture aspects of movement that infants from the age of 3.5 months (adjusted age) down to 8 weeks prior to expected date of delivery (32 weeks conceptional age) use for functional purposes in daily life, such as changing positions, looking, self-comforting, and interaction with caregivers. The items include some of Amiel-Tison and Grenier's techniques[15] for eliciting precocious evidence of developing postural control strategies, a strong emphasis on head control, and observation of spontaneous behavior, including instances of isolated movements, especially those of the hands and feet.

The overall construct guiding development of the TIMP was postural control and alignment needed for age-appropriate functional activities involving movement. According to our conceptual model for test development, the processes tested by the items on the TIMP include (1) the ability to orient and stabilize the head in space and in response to auditory and visual stimulation in supine, in prone, while sidelying, while upright, and during transitions from one position to another (facilitated rolling, supine to sit, sit to supine, tilting in upright suspension, and prone suspension; (2) body alignment when the head is manipulated; (3) distal selective control of the fingers, wrists, hands, and ankles; and (4) antigravity control of arm and leg movements.

When the items comprising the TIMP have been sufficiently developed to conform to a Rasch measurement model,[44] future research will be aimed at assessing whether infants actually *do* use the behaviors they performed during TIMP testing when performing normal functions in their natural environment of the home or nursery. Tests at the level of impairments or functional capacity must be studied for correlation with performance of daily tasks (disability level), because we know that functional limitations and the presence or absence of disabilities are not necessarily perfectly correlated.

These promising new tests may overlap with each other, may cross levels of analysis in the model of the disabling process, or they may provide tests of single or multiple constructs of unique importance in defining the processes of motor development. Each has a process, rather than a product, orientation that derives from clinician's concerns for assessing and defining "quality" of movement. Although quality of movement has never been operationally defined in a scientific manner, it certainly includes the use of efficient postural control strategies; other important processes underlying motor development, motor control, and motor learning remain to be clearly identified.

No satisfactory test at the level of disability exists for use with infants, because most of the tests in use or under development primarily assess the need for assistance in older children and rarely are intended for use in the child's natural environment (see Ch. 10 for discussion of those available). A satisfactory test in the domain of disability would assess the infant's ability to master appropriate life roles within the context of the family. Examples of these roles include play, exploration as a basis for learning, and mobility. Within the larger context of a transactional model, one could also include developing the ability to interact with people in the environment. Such tests need to be designed for use by multiple disciplines; indeed, they should *not* be disciplinary specific but should cover the areas of disablement affecting daily life that are of interest to all rehabilitation disciplines.

At present only tests of play, adaptive behavior, and activities of daily living come close to providing an assessment at this level. For example, the Pediatric Evaluation of Disability Inventory is being developed on the basis of a conceptualization of disability as encompassing mobility, personal care, communication and social skills.[45] Some of its items are appropriate for assessment of infants over age 6 months; however, most of the test will be useful primarily for children of an age at which independence in daily skills is expected. This area represents a continuing challenge for development of assessment tools for both infants and older children and for families that are ecologically relevant. Conceptualizing measurement on the basis of the theoretical frameworks that have been described has a number of potential benefits, including

1.   Better delineation of the goals of treatment, for example, clarifying whether treatment is aimed at remediation of primary impairment, prevention of secondary impairment, or compensation for functional limitations in order to prevent disability
2.   Improved predictive validity for developmental outcome
3.   Decision making based on research, family values and needs, and multidisciplinary teamwork
4.   Clarification of the constructs and processes underlying development, disability, and treatment effectiveness
5.   Improved intervention outcomes for infants and their families.

REFERENCES

1. Kopp CB: Developmental risk: historical reflections. p. 881. In Osofsky JD (ed): Handbook of Infant Development. John Wiley & Sons, New York, 1987
2. Piper MC, Darrah J, Pinnell L et al: The consistency of sequential examinations in the early detection of neurological dysfunction. Phys Occup Ther Pediatr 11(3):27, 1991
3. Harbst KB: Indicators of cerebral palsy 1985–1988. Phys Occup Ther Pediatr 10(3):85, 1990
4. Nelson KB, Ellenberg JH: Children who "outgrew" cerebral palsy. Pediatrics 69:529, 1982

5. Ferrari F, Cioni G, Prechtl HFR: Qualitative changes of general movements in preterm infants with brain lesions. Early Hum Dev 23:193, 1990
6. Campbell SK, Wilhelm IJ: Development from birth to three years of fifteen children at high risk for central nervous system dysfunction. Phys Ther 65:463, 1985
7. Thelen E, Ulrich BD: Hidden Skills: A Dynamic Systems Analysis of Treadmill Stepping During the First Year. Monogr Soc Res Child Dev, Serial No. 223, Vol. 56, No. 1. University of Chicago Press, Chicago, 1991
8. Karniol R: The role of manual manipulative stages in the infant's acquisition of perceived control over objects. Dev Rev 9:205, 1989
9. Fetters L: Object permanence development in children with cerebral palsy. Phys Ther 61:327, 1981
10. Keshner EA: How theoretical framework biases evaluation and treatment. p. 37. In Lister M (ed): Contemporary Management of Motor Control Problems. Foundation for Physical Therapy, Alexandria, VA, 1991
11. Heriza C: Motor development: traditional and contemporary theories. p. 99. In Lister M (ed): Contemporary Management of Motor Control Problems. Foundation for Physical Therapy, Alexandria, VA, 1991
12. Thelen E, Kelso JAS, Fogel A: Self-organizing systems and infant motor development. Dev Rev 7:39, 1987
13. Prechtl HFR (ed): New studies in movement assessment in fetuses and preterm infants. Early Hum Dev 23:151, 1990
14. Cioni G, Prechtl HFR: Preterm and early postterm motor behaviour in low-risk premature infants. Early Hum Dev 23:159, 1990
15. Amiel-Tison C, Grenier A: Neurological Assessment During the First Year of Life. Oxford University Press, New York, 1986
16. Campbell SK: Central nervous system dysfunction in children p. 1. In Campbell SK (ed): Pediatric Neurologic Physical Therapy. 2nd Ed. Churchill Livingstone, New York, 1991
17. Graham M, Levene MI, Trounce JQ et al: Prediction of cerebral palsy in very low birthweight infants: prospective ultrasound study. Lancet 2:593, 1987
18. D'Avignon M, Noren L, Arman T: Early physiotherapy ad modum Vojta or Bobath in infants with suspected neuromotor disturbance. Neuropediatrics 12:232, 1981
19. Molnar G: Motor deficit of retarded infants and young children. Arch Phys Med Rehabil 55:393, 1974
20. Campbell SK, Siegel E, Parr CA et al: Evidence for the need to renorm the Bayley Scales of Infant Development based on the performance of a population-based sample of twelve-month-old infants. Top Early Child Spec Educ 6(2):83, 1986
21. Campbell SK: Measuring motor performance in cerebral palsy. Med Sport Sci 36; 1992 (in press)
22. Kolobe HTA: Family-focused early intervention. p. 397. In Campbell SK (ed): Pediatric Neurologic Physical Therapy. 2nd Ed. Churchill Livingstone, New York, 1991
23. Watts NT: Clinical decision analysis. Phys Ther 69:569, 1989
24. World Health Organization: International Classification of Impairments, Disabilities, and Handicaps. World Health Organization, Geneva, 1980
25. Nagi SZ: Disability concepts revisited: implications for prevention. p. 309. In Pope AM, Tarlov AR (eds): Disability in America: Toward a National Agenda for Prevention. National Academy Press, Washington, DC, 1991
26. Dawes RM, Faust D, Meehl PE: Clinical versus actuarial judgment. Science 243:1668, 1989

27. Brazelton TB: Neonatal Behavioral Assessment Scale. 2nd Ed. Clinics in Developmental Medicine No. 88. JB Lippincott, Philadelphia, 1984
28. Barnard K: Nursing Child Assessment Learning Resource, Manual Feeding and Manual Teaching. NCAST Publications, Seattle, WA, 1979
29. Als H, Lester BM, Tronick EZ, Brazelton TB: Toward a research instrument for the Assessment of Preterm Infants' Behavior (APIB). p. 65. In Fitzgerald HE, Lester, BM, Yogman MW (eds): Theory and Research in Behavioral Pediatrics. Vol. 1. Plenum Press, New York, 1982
30. Caldwell B, Bradley RH: Home Observation for Measurement of the Environment (birth to three years). University of Arkansas, Little Rock, 1984
31. Abiden RR: Parenting Stress Index. 2nd Ed. Pediatric Psychology Press, Charlottesville, VA, 1986
32. Gordon BN, Jens KG: A conceptual model for tracking high-risk infants and making early service decisions. J Dev Behav Pediatr 9(5):279, 1988
33. Aylward GP, Kenny TJ: Developmental follow-up: inherent problems and a conceptual model. J Pediatr Psychol 4:331, 1979
34. Slovic P, Lichtenstein S: Comparison of Bayesian and regression approaches to the study of information processing in judgment. Org Behav Hum Perform 6:649, 1971
35. Dowie J, Elstein A (eds): Professional Judgment: a Reader in Clinical Decision Making. Cambridge University Press, New York, 1988
36. Guccione AA: Physical therapy diagnosis and the relationship between impairments and function. Phys Ther 71:499, 1991
37. Schenkman M, Butler RB: A model for multisystem evaluation, interpretation, and treatment of individuals with neurologic dysfunction. Phys Ther 69:538, 1989
38. National Advisory Board on Medical Rehabilitation Research: Report and Research Plan for the National Center for Medical Rehabilitation Research. National Institutes of Health, Bethesda, MD, 1992
39. Palmer FB, Shapiro BK, Wachtel RC et al: The effects of physical therapy on cerebral palsy: a controlled trial in infants with spastic diplegia. N Engl J Med 318:803, 1988
40. Knobloch H, Stevens F, Malone AF: Manual of Developmental Diagnosis. Harper & Row, New York, 1980
41. Levine S: Development of a posture scale for children: preliminary analysis of concurrent validity of the Posture Scale for Children, abstracted. Pediatr Phys Ther 3(4):212, 1991
42. Miller LJ: Miller Toddler and Infant Movement Evaluation. Foundation for Knowledge in Development, Englewood, CO (in press)
43. Piper MC, Darrah J, Pinnell L et al: Alberta Infant Motor Scale (Preliminary Manual). University of Alberta Faculty of Rehabilitation Medicine, Edmonton, 1989
44. Wright BD, Masters GN: Rating Scale Analysis: Rasch Measurement. Mesa Press, Chicago, 1982
45. Haley SM, Faas RM, Coster WJ et al: Pediatric Evaluation of Disability Inventory. New England Medical Center, Boston, 1989

Index

Note: Page numbers followed by f indicate figures, and those followed by t indicate tables.

Physical therapy assessment
in early infancy